Hidden Suicides and Fatal Overdoses

Hidden Suicides and Fatal Overdoses

A Forward Path

Ian Rockett

foreword by Hilary S. Connery

JOHNS HOPKINS UNIVERSITY PRESS BALTIMORE

Printed in the United States of America on acid-free paper
9 8 7 6 5 4 3 2 1

Johns Hopkins University Press
2715 North Charles Street
Baltimore, Maryland 21218
www.press.jhu.edu

Library of Congress Cataloging-in-Publication Data is available.
A catalog record for this book is available from the British Library.
ISBN 978-1-4214-5364-4 (hardcover)
ISBN 978-1-4214-5365-1 (ebook)

EU GPSR Authorized Representative
LOGOS EUROPE, 9 rue Nicolas Poussin, 17000, La Rochelle, France
E-mail: Contact@logoseurope.eu

To the memory of my parents,
other dearly departed,
and the principal affiliates of
the Los Angeles Suicide Prevention Center

Contents

Foreword

Ian Rockett's latest contribution to the field, *Hidden Suicides and Fatal Overdoses: A Forward Path*, draws from and integrates multidisciplinary perspectives on the modern opioid and suicide crises. His work is composed of medical and forensic history, epidemiology, clinical psychiatry and behavioral health research, public health systems and data registries, and colorful personal witness and professional encounters. As such, this book has an immediate appeal to a broad collaborative of specialists involved in finding improved solutions for the nation's relentless problem of premature deaths due to drug use and suicide. Dr. Rockett's expertise and holistic dedication offer value to anyone seeking a more unified perspective and hoping for a more effectively coordinated response to the modern opioid and suicide crises.

As an addiction psychiatrist, I had been treating patients with opioid use disorder (OUD) for more than a decade during the initial two waves of increased opioid overdose deaths due to prescription opioid poisoning, and later heroin poisoning. As this national tragedy mushroomed, and with drug trafficking supplies progressing in 2013 to include highly lethal versions of illicitly manufactured fentanyl analogs (the third wave), I also observed an increasing frequency of OUD patients presenting to treatment with severe despair, hopelessness, and a spectrum of suicidal cognitions, ranging from thoughts that it could be a relief to get high and "just not wake up," to those who episodically considered suicide but didn't consider themselves at risk for suicide, to those who articulated their own risk for suicide because life was intolerable, pointless, hopeless. It surprised me how few colleagues providing OUD care believed that suicide risk assessment was an important preventive intervention. It seemed that nearly everyone assumed that drug poisoning deaths were "accidental," unplanned. In different clinical discussion forums this belief was so prevalent that I began to think I was missing some critical piece of evidence apparent to all other clinicians—but I knew this would be inconsistent with earlier research. This research had demonstrated that OUD populations have significantly higher risk for suicide (up to 14 times that of the general population).

In 2016, I finally discovered Dr. Rockett's seminal 2014 perspective in the *American Journal of Public Health*, "Confronting Death from Drug Self-Intoxication (DDSI): Prevention Through a Better Definition." I emailed him immediately because I needed to understand why nobody else was talking about this or seemed very interested when I raised the subject. I had no idea whether he would reply, but he did. In his reliably generous style, Dr. Rockett spent an hour on the phone with me explaining how the separation between "addiction treatment" and "mental health care" I observed in the clinical world was mirrored by a separation in research. It was exemplified in funding streams and database registries for those investigating death by "overdose" versus those investigating death by suicide. The critical information I lacked was the structural separation of systems addressing drug poisoning deaths and suicide deaths. He then connected me with Eric Caine, MD—also very generous with his time—who discussed this nexus in clinical care. Dr. Caine offered the rare perspective of a leader in psychiatric research of suicide prevention who had also worked in methadone opioid treatment programs and other substance treatment settings.

Since then, I have had the great privilege to work with Dr. Rockett and Dr. Caine. I have also worked alongside many other prestigious experts and community advocates addressing the care and prevention gaps that remain in the field as the American opioid and suicide crises persist. We are collectively making progress in bringing suicide risk assessment and prevention into addiction care, where the need continues to be high.

There is now a vast accumulation of evidence that medications for OUD also achieve suicide prevention. Such medications need to be administered in all health care settings—particularly those focused on mental health. Multidisciplinary collaborations can bend the curve on these treatable conditions and markedly reduce the unacceptable number of premature injury deaths, which leave too many children, families, and communities bereft. Highlighted in this book, these efforts must include attention to mismeasurement and modification of the upstream factors that fuel the suicide and drug overdose epidemics.

HILARY S. CONNERY, MD, PHD
McLean Hospital and the Department of Psychiatry, Harvard University

Preface

This book recounts my long-term but sometimes intermittent efforts to evaluate the medicolegal detection or determination of suicide—a process highly susceptible to undercounting. Suicide undercounting and differential misclassification are problematic for clinical medicine, public health, and the forensic sciences—for research, treatment, and prevention.

Peter Cowan introduced me to the poetry of Robert Frost during my final year of secondary education at Scotch College in my hometown of Perth, Western Australia. At the time, it was considered to be an Antipodean outpost as the most geographically isolated city in the world. Cowan was a superb high school English teacher and a nationally recognized short story writer and novelist. Frost's masterpiece, "The Road Not Taken," captured my imagination. While I have resisted taking the easier pathway as a scholar and researcher, I have frequently felt like an academic fringe dweller. A prominent injury epidemiologist reinforced this feeling when she said that I was a data nerd. I interpreted her comment to mean that I had a penchant for studying the esoteric and cryptic. This perhaps acted as a spur. My research on suicide data quality has since edged closer to the mainstream.

As a history major from the University of Western Australia with a Canadian master's degree in sociology from Western University, I pursued doctoral training in demography and medical sociology at Brown University. This training included a pivotal course in mortality and morbidity with Gerry Hendershot and a comprehensive course in demographic techniques with Sidney Goldstein. I had entered these courses harboring a personal prejudice against the topic as an aspirational researcher, engendered in part by another esteemed professor's question: "Who would want to study mortality? It is such a morbid topic."

During a three-year return to Australia from Canada in the early 1980s, I became acquainted with the discipline of epidemiology as a senior research fellow in community medicine at the University of Melbourne. Fortuitous exposure to injury epidemiology, first at the Rhode Island Department of Health and then at Harvard University during my master of public health degree program, paved the way for suicide data quality to become my premier research interest. In summary: I am a population scientist whose research target is population health. I specialize in injury epidemiology, with a subspecialization in the mismeasurement of suicide and the mischaracterization of most drug overdose deaths as "accidents."

Arcane but inspirational influences on my evolution as a critical thinker and data skeptic include the Australian historian Frank Crowley, novelist and satirist George Orwell (aka Eric Blair), the Vienna Circle, psychiatrist-provocateur Thomas Szasz, Nobel laureate physicist Richard Feynman, and the doyen of data visualization, Edward Tufte. Another key source of inspiration was David Fraser's highly innovative essay "Epidemiology as a Liberal Art," which was published in the *New England Journal of Medicine* in 1987. I got to know David as a fellow judge of the Young Epidemiology Scholars (YES) Competition. He told me that the essay was his job talk in a successful application for the presidency of Swarthmore College.

From a 5-mile-high vantage point, I can detect data anomalies and discrepancies, as well as patterns and trends in suicide rates. However, borrowing from the Renaissance English poet John Donne, no man is an island, and adapting an African proverb, it now takes a cyber village to raise a book. I have progressively enlisted the expertise of distinguished colleagues for reality checks and help in interpreting research findings and translating them for wider audiences. This village represented a myriad of disciplines, from the social sciences and humanities, to psychiatry and emergency medicine, to forensic pathology and medical toxicology.

I conducted most of my research on suicide data quality at West Virginia University's health sciences center. There, books were not the currency of the realm in determining promotion, tenure, and job security—peer-reviewed articles (especially grant-funded ones) were. Written within the cloistered confines of retirement (with an assist from isolation precipitated by the COVID-19 pandemic), this book afforded me the latitude I have been denied in preparing and writing scientific articles.

Despite the privileges in my career, I am very familiar with fear, frustration, and setbacks. I have integrated lived experiences, both positive and negative, into many parts of the book to further comprehension and readability. To ground my research and seek wide application, I have devoted increasing time and energy to translating and disseminating it to audiences that transcend the academic readership of my articles. Injury epidemiology attracted me because it offered obvious opportunities to conduct research that can make a difference. From attending national and regional injury-related conferences during the 1980s, I learned and embraced an important lesson: that people can conduct dispassionate, high-quality research and yet also advocate for public health. The eloquence of Leon Robertson, Julian Waller, Susan Baker, Jerome Barancik, Stephen Teret, and Garen Wintemute in presenting and discussing their injury research in public arenas exemplified this marriage for me. In the spirit of detached concern, and supplanting a prior belief, I recognized and accepted that separation of advocacy from research is not a sine qua non for a dedicated scientist.

I hope the book will serve as a cautionary tale for active and aspirational researchers; spark awareness and heighten understanding among readers of the importance of the economic, sociocultural, and political context in which suicide accounting transpires; and sensitize them to the societal imperative to confront drug addiction and other mental health problems in a unified rather than a piecemeal or siloed fashion. A lofty aim is to elevate the prominence of suicide and other fatal self-injury as a clinical and public health problem in the United States and elsewhere. My motivation is to attract more societal resources to improve their characterization, detection, and certification in order to enhance their scientific understanding and, most importantly, save lives.

Executive Summary

A heavily stigmatized and socially condemned phenomenon, suicide is perennially prone to undercounting. Suicide is difficult to characterize and prevent since susceptibility to undercounting varies across demographic groups and methods. Focusing on the United States, this book tells the story of suicide undercounting for research, prevention, and treatment from the viewpoint of one who has been studying suicide data quality for over 30 years.

The introduction delineates the scope and outlines the approach of the book. Chapters 1 and 2 document the contributions of important domestic and foreign suicide research pioneers, predominantly from the twentieth century, who have enlightened the quest to understand and improve suicide accounting and reporting. Chapter 3 compares suicide data quality for the United States in the later twentieth and early twenty-first centuries with that of other democratic, high-income countries, highlighting the importance of indirect methods when direct ones are infeasible.

Chapter 4 addresses the racial paradox that registered suicide rates for Blacks—a politically and socioeconomically vulnerable minority with a shorter life expectancy—are far lower than those for Whites. Might these discrepant rates in whole or part be an artifact of differential detection of suicide between the two groups by medical examiners and coroners? Health data disparities are distinguished from health disparities in documenting deficits in evidence that would help corroborate suicide among Blacks relative to Whites. This chapter also speaks to the importance of translating and disseminating research findings and advocating for change beyond the narrow scope of academic audiences.

Chapter 5 examines differential detection of suicide by methods used—especially drug poisoning versus shooting and hanging—within the confluence and overlap of twin opioid mortality and suicide epidemics. Under the shadow of overstressed and underresourced medicolegal death investigation systems, American suicide data quality has likely deteriorated substantially in the twenty-first century.

Chapter 6 reports on two multilevel (individual/county), multivariable studies that used the enriched database of the US Centers for Disease Control and Prevention's National Violent Death Reporting System. This database provides individual-level information on demographics, risk factors, death circumstances, and details of the death investigations conducted by medical examiners and coroners. Most notable is the performance of an autopsy and toxicologic testing. The two studies jointly show that the most formidable problem for medical examiners, coroners, and government agencies in accurately accounting for suicide by drug poisoning is the absence or deficiency of corroborative evidence. Such evidence includes an authenticated suicide note, record of any prior suicide attempt, and psychiatric history.

Chapter 7 introduces "death from drug self-intoxication" (DDSI) as a novel concept that emphasizes premortem decedent behavior rather than postmortem inference of decedent intent. DDSI is the building block for another novel concept, self-injury mortality (SIM), which transcends registered suicides in expanding the domain of fatal self-injury. Operationalized and applied in chapter 8, SIM comprises all registered suicides plus estimated "nonsuicide" drug fatalities that implicate patterns of repeated self-injurious behaviors, irrespective of whether the decedents intended to die on their day of death. By mitigating racial/ethnic health data disparities and related bias in suicide detection, the concept of SIM challenges the separation and siloing of suicides and fatal drug overdoses in research and prevention.

Chapter 9 presents the findings from a trio of interstate studies that map, characterize, and estimate the economic costs of suicide and SIM. The first study portrays a geographic regional bias in suicide measurement. Application of SIM reveals that the United States now has a mental health crisis that is national in scope, rather than being confined to the Western and Mountain regions—particularly when registered suicides serve as the sole representative of mortal self-injury and imminent personal and societal distress. The second study characterizes suicide and SIM at the state level. Suicide is associated with "downstream" individual-level characteristics, namely, being male, being a military veteran, owning a firearm, living in a rural area, and misusing a pain reliever. In contrast, SIM primarily connects to macro/ecological factors such as labor underutilization, low prevalence of manufacturing employment, and chronic prescription opioid use. The third and final study presents economic estimates of SIM and suicide costs to society by state from medical expenditures, lost work productivity, and the pain, suffering, and lost enjoyment of life of the people who died and their immediate families. Annual-averaged national costs of SIM in 2019 US dollars increased 143% from $0.46 trillion in 1999/2000 to $1.12 trillion in 2018/19, while the crude SIM rate rose by 112%—from 14.6 to 30.9 deaths per 100,000 population. Corresponding costs for suicide, while high, were appreciably lower than those for SIM. This gap widened over the observation period. Peer-reviewed literature and mass media stories disseminated the findings from the three studies. The chapter also questions the reported decline in the American suicide rate during the onset of the COVID-19 pandemic.

Chapter 10 summarizes the status of the author's research agenda and offers recommendations for future research to improve SIM and suicide accounting and reporting using mixed qualitative and quantitative research methods. Insertion of a self-injury checkbox on the death certificate would enable direct measurement of SIM—supplanting indirect estimation—across three manners of death: suicide, accident, and undetermined (injury intent). Ensuing studies would benefit through medicolegal (medical examiner/coroner) and researcher application of digital technologies and information from social media that centered on the decedents, improving the validity of SIM.

The conclusion ties together the main ideas motivating and driving the book and addresses suicide underreporting quantitatively and the need for death scene investigations to be standardized and aided by mobile technology. It closes with a plea for public and private research agencies to stop viewing suicides and fatal drug overdoses as distinct phenomena in funding research and prevention initiatives. It also stresses the importance of multidisciplinary research in enhancing mental health, and hence population health.

Hidden Suicides and Fatal Overdoses

Introduction

Suicide undercounting

Suicide is a highly emotional and socially stigmatized phenomenon that often goes unreported. Undercounting and differential misclassification of suicide under other mortality categories, such as accident or undetermined intent (Rockett et al., 2011; Snowdon, 2023), distort observed suicide trends, patterns, and their interpretation (Rockett, 2017; Rockett et al., 2020b, 2021). These distortions are dysfunctional for clinical medicine, public health, public safety, and the forensic sciences because they inhibit suicide-related research, treatment policy, and planning and the financing, designing, targeting, implementing, and evaluating of interventions and prevention programs.

In sharing this cautionary story of suicide undercounting and differential misclassification, I admit that there are formidable impediments to remediation. That said, the quest for perfection should not shackle us. To lessen the challenges of suicide accounting, I will propose broadening the fatal self-injury domain by deploying a concept that is a more appropriate representative than registered suicides alone.

Losing a loved one through suicide is excruciating for families and other intimates of the deceased. The impact of such losses often reverberates through neighborhoods and communities. According to the bereavement literature, close relatives of the deceased often experience a wide range of emotions, such as sadness, fear, guilt, shame, blame, embarrassment, confusion, second-guessing, helplessness, rejection, and anger (Hanschmidt et al., 2016; Evans & Abrahamson, 2020).

Most people affected by suicide, and seemingly many suicide researchers as well, are oblivious to the problems inherent in suicide undercounting. Forces depressing suicide counts include social stigma, religious prohibitions, punitive provisions in life insurance policies, training deficits among first responders and death investigators, scarce resources, and inadequate infrastructures for conducting comprehensive medicolegal death investigations. Forces enabling differential suicide nonrecognition and misclassification include oppression—graphically exemplified by political gerrymandering, intimidation, nullification, and kindred forms of voter suppression—discrimination, segregation, poverty, and separation or distance from the health care system.

Although some individuals may protest to medical examiners, coroners, or other medicolegal officials in multiple ways, from outrage to simple denial, survivors generally suffer in silence when a loved one's manner of death is to be recorded on the death certificate as suicide rather than "accident" or natural causes; such is the potency of the social stigma that envelops this manner of death. Consequently, I am not surprised that societal investment in the medicolegal investigation of suicides is inadequate.

If the popular adage "we get what we pay for" is true, then suicide accounting in the United States is in a dubious and fragile state, posing a threat to clinical medicine and public and population health. This situation constitutes my central hypothesis and the motivation for this problematic story of suicide records. The train of scientific evidence that I will present for affirming the hypothesis stems from research on discrepancies and disparities in suicide records conducted by me and my colleagues, as well as that of others, over the past 30 years. Remarkable predecessors have informed this research dating back to the turn of the twentieth century and earlier.

Twin epidemics and a pandemic

The suicide rate in the United States has risen progressively in the twenty-first century, following a prolonged decline. It was 44% higher in 2022 than in 2000, at 15.0 versus 10.4 suicides per 100,000 population, respectively (Centers for Disease Control and Prevention, n.d.-d). Besides this suicide epidemic, an epidemic of opioid and other drug poisoning mortality and the SARS-CoV-2 (hereafter labeled COVID-19) pandemic have complicated matters for suicide accounting. All three phenomena stress scarce medicolegal resources and strain infrastructures. Society is much more informed about factors that cause or enable suicide than those ensuring that medical examiners and coroners can distinguish suicides from deaths attributable to homicide, accident, undetermined (injury intent), and natural causes or disease. Collectively, these five categories represent manner of death. In injury cases, manner of death reflects the circumstances under which someone died versus the underlying cause of death, which specifies the injury that initiated the sequence of events culminating in death (e.g., blunt force trauma, asphyxiation).

As a researcher who studies the determinants of suicide detection or ascertainment, rather than the determinants of suicide, I became interested in the factors contributing to suicide misclassification and, more particularly, suicide undercounting. I accept that economic constraints, together with political and sociocultural ones, impede a full accounting of suicide. I sought to circumvent their deleterious impact on public health by provoking a shift in the research paradigm—aided and reinforced by a cadre of gifted and dedicated multidisciplinary researchers and practitioners. Chapter 8 describes a shift motivated by the goal of preventing suicide and other self-injury mortality. While the bulk of the book speaks to my evolving research agenda on suicide, chapters 1 and 2 offer background that provides a historical, philosophical, and intellectual context for this work.

Defining suicide and delineating the domain

A product of the US Centers for Disease Control and Prevention (CDC), the *Medical Examiners' and Coroners' Handbook on Death Registration and Fetal Death Reporting* defines suicide as "result[ing] from an injury or poisoning as a result of an intentional, self-inflicted act committed to do self-harm or cause the death of one's self" (Department of Health and Human Services et al., 2003, 21). The World Health Organization (WHO) defines suicide as "the act of intentionally carrying out an action to kill oneself" (World Health Organization, 2019, 1). Interpretation of alternative definitions for case ascertainment or detection by medicolegal authorities can be highly variable and problematic, as likely with the accumulation of potential corroborative evidence, such as from the sealing and protection of the integrity of the death scene, performance of an autopsy and toxicologic testing, search for a suicide note, existence and access to psychiatric and other medical records, and interviews with witnesses and survivors by qualified death investigators. Some of the common causes of suicide deaths are asphyxiation, gunshot wound, sharp force injuries, poisoning, and blunt force injuries incurred by jumping from a height. There are also many rarer causes. Diseases such as anorexia nervosa and alcohol-related liver disease and risky behaviors like chronic tobacco smoking could be considered slow suicide. However, the term "suicide" typically refers to acute, intentional, fatal self-inflicted injuries caused by methods such as the use of a firearm, knife, or toxin.

There are two notable exclusions from my research domain. The first is euthanasia (physician-assisted deaths or medical aid in dying). In principle, my general perspective on euthanasia is that it aligns with the concept of "dying with dignity" in response to a terminal illness and related hopelessness. However, some grave ethical problems, needing more attention from clinicians and preventionists, arise when individuals are making this choice because of inadequate pain management, cost, and/or lack of access to medical, nursing home, or hospice care, or when the precipitating condition is severe mental illness.

The second exclusion is martyrdom-associated deaths. U03 is a code in the WHO's *International Classification of Diseases, Tenth Revision* that is reserved for fatal terrorism-related self-harm (World Health Organization, 2004). To date, these deaths have primarily occurred in the throes of war in such countries as Afghanistan and Iraq. They qualify as manifest suicides, but many may truly qualify as homicides, where the contingencies are intimidation and coercion, false promises of heavenly glory, and other gross deceit.

In my preliminary research, I relied on official government suicide rates, which were derived from death certificates and population census data, as the foundation for my investigation into the accuracy of suicide data. Informing my skepticism was seemingly discrepant reporting in some, if not many, of the large differentials I observed in rates by age and sex across nations.

Suicide measurement inhibitors

A systematic review summarizes the findings from scientific studies on a common research question or set of questions according to a predetermined set of criteria in searching the relevant literature and is typically reliant on accessing online databases (Egger et al., 2001; Khan et al., 2003; Petticrew & Roberts, 2006). Such studies suggest that up to 90% of people dying by suicide in high-income European / European-descent countries have a diagnosable mental illness at their time of death (Cavanagh et al., 2003; Arsenault-Lapierre et al., 2004), although this upper limit may be an artifact of methodological flaws in diagnostic assessments (Hjelmeland et al., 2012). Other systematic reviews show that people with depression, affective disorders, and alcohol and other substance use disorders exhibit increased risk of suicide (Harris & Barraclough, 1997; Cherpitel et al., 2004; Wilcox et al., 2004; Too et al., 2019); a host of physical diseases similarly exhibit excess suicide risks (Berman & Pompili, 2011). Less well studied and understood is the association between a documented mental disorder or psychiatric illness, as stigmatized conditions, and ascertainment of suicide cases by medical examiners, coroners, and other officials. In contrast to dire poverty, mental illness is likely much less prevalent among people dying by suicide in poorer countries than in wealthier counterparts (Rane & Nadkarni, 2014). However, less access to psychiatric care means that diagnosis of mental illness is far less likely.

Religious proscriptions and legal penalties against suicide grossly inhibit its reporting in some countries, such as Egypt, Turkey, Iran, Malaysia, Qatar (Pritchard & Amanullah, 2007), Kenya, and the Bahamas (Hasnain, 2022; Mishara & Weisstub, 2016). At the time of writing, a minimum of 17 countries still criminalize suicide, although recently some countries, including Pakistan, Ghana, and Malaysia, have reversed course, and others are poised to follow suit (Johnson, 2023). Nonetheless, most societies socially condemn and highly stigmatize both mental illness and suicide. Expounding a truism, Ken Obenson, a forensic pathologist in Canada, stated that "no other manner of death classification carries the same stigma, or is likely to provoke as much protest from relatives, as a classification of suicide" (2013, 576). In sum, stigma and other forces, such as legal, cultural, and religious prohibitions (Mishara & Weisstub, 2016), together with punitive life insurance policies (Yip et al., 2010) and underresourcing of medicolegal death investigation systems (Kapusta et al., 2011), plausibly depress suicide counts and rates worldwide—an inconvenient truth. An important distinction is between stigma against a suicidal person, which is a barrier to help seeking and mental health treatment, and stigma against the act of suicide—a force that may inhibit acts of suicide and their normalization (Cato & Canetto, 2003; Eskin et al., 2016; Canetto et al., 2021).

Heterogeneity and suicide determination

Complicating comparisons, within and across geographic and other demographic entities, is heterogeneity or variation in the influence and relevance of definitions and inhibitors of reporting suicide. I will expand on artifactuality in suicide accounting throughout this book, as I trace my incremental and circuitous route in investigating suicide determination—most recently using a rich and unique database on suicide and other selected injury deaths, CDC's National Violent Death Reporting System. In so doing, I will endeavor to present empirical evidence for unsubstantiated statements I make in the introduction and first two chapters. Motivating my research on suicide data quality was a recognition that misclassification and undercounting of suicide were most problematic among certain geopolitical entities, suicide methods, and subpopulations. My eventual analytic interest in the role of psychological and psychiatric variables in suicide case ascertainment coincided with an awareness that in the early twenty-first century the United States was undergoing a latent epidemic of suicide and a manifest epidemic of opioid and other drug poisoning mortality.

To reiterate, the principal measure I used in my early research was the rate, a suicide or other specified manner- or cause-of-death count related to a population at risk (e.g., 12 suicides per 100,000 population in a given year). The rate is essential in profiling countries and subnational groups for a comparative assessment of their suicide burdens, as well as for targeting and evaluating the effectiveness of suicide prevention programs and other suicide interventions. At first, my geographic focus was cross-national, as I examined suicide undercounting and associated questions about data quality and data disparities. My attention subsequently shifted primarily to the United States. However, I have assumed a secondary role in suicide or suicide-related research and scholarship conducted in Australia, Austria, Canada, and China. Additionally, my Chinese collaborations have variously involved research on tobacco-related addiction and on migration, the topic of my doctoral dissertation.

Western centricity and hypothetico-deductive reasoning

I acknowledge the Western centricity of the research and scholarship that have influenced or aligned with my investigations into medicolegal determination of suicide. The great preponderance originated in the United

States, the United Kingdom, and Australia. In pursuing my research agenda, I have implicitly or explicitly employed hypothetico-deductive reasoning to address a series of questions in a stepwise process. More recently, I have learned that most of my studies conducted during this century basically conform to what the eminent Cambridge University statistician David Spiegelhalter describes as a PPDAC problem-solving cycle: problem, plan, and data analysis to conclusion (and I add communication or dissemination; Spiegelhalter, 2019). From a hypothetico-deductive perspective, evaluation of a hypothesis to affirmation or falsification induces new hypotheses, which likewise need to be evaluated. This process gives rise to continuing cycles of new questions, hypotheses, and evaluations. Subscribing to the perspective of Karl Popper, a renowned philosopher of science, I consciously use the word "affirmation" not "confirmation." He convincingly reasoned and deduced that a hypothesis could be falsified but never proven (Popper, 2002).

A personal story on suicide

This book blends science with my lived experience, primarily academic. Indeed, it possesses many elements of a research autobiography. My initial awareness of suicide and its personal impact came in my childhood years, through my general (medical) practitioner father, (Richard) Hildreth Rockett, who shared sketchy details about the suicide of a long-time family friend, Hugo Throssell. In 1933, Throssell shot himself in the head with a revolver in the hillside community of Greenmount, which lay in the Darling Range just east of my hometown of Perth, Western Australia. My father had been called to the death (dying) scene. Keeping Throssell's name confidential, he told me that the experience was shocking, bloody, and deeply distressing.

Courtesy of a snippet sent to me in 2023 by a close friend, Perth barrister Bruce Duckham, I surprisingly learned not only Throssell's name but also his celebrity status as a war hero. Later, I extracted details on his life and exploits in World War I from his biography, *The Price of Valour*, written by the English-born and Australian-raised journalist John Hamilton. Hamilton states that Throssell's brother-in-law, George Withers, was the first person to see him after the shooting. Withers called my father and asked him to render medical care—a hapless task. My father objectively described the scene as follows: "[Hugo] was still alive on my arrival. There were three or four pints of blood on the veranda and deck chair. With Mr. Withers' aid, I removed him to a couch where he expired about ten minutes later. I then found the bullet lying on the veranda behind the chair [and a] note in the bookcase, which was located next to Katharine's books and read 'I can't sleep. I feel my old war head. It's going phut, and that's no good for anyone concerned'" (Hamilton, 2012, 344).

One of 14 children of a former state premier (equivalent to an American governor), Throssell was the first West Australian recipient of the Victoria Cross, the highest military honor a soldier from the British Commonwealth can earn in battle. He achieved his medal for valor in 1915 at Gallipoli, Turkey, during the First World War, a conflict where historians say Australia and New Zealand came of age as nations. Throssell received his medal at Buckingham Palace from the reigning British king, George V, Charles III's great-grandfather.

Captain (later General) Horace Robertson reported Throssell's heroics at Gallipoli in glowing terms, having served with him there in the Tenth Light Horse Regiment as an officer in the Australian Imperial Force:

> Hugo was to prove himself with a vengeance. [Major Thomas] Kidd's cool brain directed the fight, but Hugo's reckless active bravery met force with force and gave more than it received.
>
> There is little room in this machine fighting of today for the personal abandon and courage leader . . . [he] carried sandbags and inspired by example rather than words. When bombs ran out he it was who first started catching Turkish bombs and throwing them back before they exploded. . . . In spite of his recklessness, he seemed to bear a charmed life. Bombs exploded all round him, and many fragments [shrapnel] struck him, but he ignored these minor wounds and stuck to his post. And he succeeded. (Hamilton, 2012, 186)[1]

Throssell's actions at Gallipoli were in part his reaction to the deaths in minutes of 9 officers and 71 regular soldiers from his regiment. After a lengthy recuperation from his war wounds in England, he returned to a front line in 1917, at the Second Battle of Gaza—an active war zone as I write—where he sustained minor wounds to the thigh and foot. He then endured severe intestinal damage because of an infestation of tapeworm (9 feet long upon extraction) from eating undercooked pork or drinking contaminated water. Barely recovered from that illness, his suffering multiplied when he contracted malaria following relocation to the mosquito-ravaged Jordan Valley. Ensuing fevers resulted in six months of intermittent therapy in various Middle Eastern military hospitals, clinics, and rehabilitation facilities. Throssell had recurrent bouts of the disease in the 1920s.

One can easily infer from Throssell's war experience that he sustained post-traumatic stress disorder. He later developed dementia because of bacterial meningitis,[2] likely associated with nasal surgery unrelated to his wounds from the Gallipoli campaign. At first a hero upon repatriation to Australia, Throssell fell into public disfavor and endured economic hardship in his home state. The initial stimulus for these adversities was his conversion to socialism and adoption of a passionate antiwar stance, in part emanating from his revulsion to the massive profiteering of the munitions industry during a conflict raining down unprecedented waves of death, disability, and material destruction. These positions were shared by his wife, Katharine Susannah Prichard (her professional name), a cofounder of the Australian Communist Party. Katharine was a staunch and outspoken advocate for the party, with its working-class ties and opposition to fascism. Hugo himself did not embrace communism. While his socialism was inimical to the ambitions of the colonial and postcolonial establishment for political domination and sociocultural assimilation and conformity, it mirrored a long-standing Australian egalitarian and working-class value from the early 1890s—the notion of a "fair go," which as an expression originated in Australian mid-nineteenth-century sports like track, horse racing, and boxing.

Prichard was a highly acclaimed novelist, poet, and journalist, which enhanced her reputation more positively in Australia. In 1951, she received a nomination for the Nobel Prize in Literature. Prichard learned of her husband's death while in London, shortly after touring Joseph Stalin's Soviet Union. The news of Throssell's suicide spread rapidly across Australia and around the world. Without the stigma of the socialist/communist label, the Throssells would certainly have constituted a power couple, using contemporary parlance. Katharine had emerged in Melbourne as a budding intellectual, feminist, and political activist by age 20. However, a combination of genteel poverty and a father who believed that a woman's place was in the home denied her the university education she craved.

Additional information on Hugo Throssell's suicide and its aftermath surfaced in *The Red Witch*, a biography of Prichard written by Nathan Hobby (2022), a self-described biographer and librarian. Afflicted with both physical and mental illness, Throssell died at age 49 during the height of the worldwide Great Depression in Australia; he had been reeling under the crippling weight of unemployment, more than 20 heavily mortgaged properties (including his house, and all of which became markedly undervalued), and indebtedness from running rodeos. Besides the absence of his wife, guilt over marital infidelity, lack of cooking skills, and home degradation compounded his related imminent distress.

None of the accounts I have read of Throssell's life and death intimate an alcohol or other substance use disorder, and there is evidence that his wife Katharine abhorred drunkenness. However, as someone who grew up in Australia during the 1950s and 1960s, I can attest that heavy consumption of alcohol was a hallmark of the culture. Enactment of stringent drunk driving laws and subsequent strong enforcement may have tempered this behavior to a certain extent. Alcohol is a major depressant. Use, especially excessive use, retards brain functioning, reduces inhibitions, and depresses the central nervous system.

Officials questioned the role of Throssell's war service in his suicide, which could have meant that his widow would not receive a war pension from the federal government. A coronial (coroner) inquest determined that he was "mentally deranged" when he shot himself. In the penultimate chapter, I will discuss possible incompatibility between his pronounced mental instability and capacity to form suicidal intent. This issue has implications for suicide undercounting. Prichard did secure a pension, likely expedited by a note from Hugo, written on the back of his final will. It read, "I have never recovered from my 1914–18 [World War I] experiences, and, with this in view, I appeal to the State to see that my wife and child get the usual war pension. No man could have a truer mate" (Hamilton, 2012, 341). My father received three mentions in Hobby's biography as the on-scene "doctor," but never by name, despite Hobby having cited Hamilton's biography of Throssell, which had identified him.

Other familial suicides

Suicide was a shadowy presence in Katharine Susannah Prichard's story and fiction. Besides her husband, her father, Thomas Prichard, died by suicide in his early sixties—burdened by sometimes thwarted ambitions as a newspaper editor, as well as economic insecurity, insomnia, depression, psychosis, and temporary institutionalization in an "asylum"—as did her son Ric Throssell, at age 76, three decades after her death in 1969.

The suicide of Ric Throssell, a diplomat and part-time playwright and writer, immediately followed the death of his second wife from cancer. His first wife had died early in their marriage in a Russian hospital in Moscow—where the Australian government had posted Ric—from an unknown illness that induced rapid paralysis and a coma. Thinking of contemporary Russia, I do wonder whether she was poisoned, either deliberately or inadvertently. Ric's autobiography, *My Father's Son*, displayed literary talent reminiscent of his mother's (Throssell, 1989). Unproven allegations during the 1950s that he was a Russian spy—fueled by intelligence gleaned from American intercepts of Soviet diplomatic cable messages—intensified his emotional baggage. Making Ric an easy target for authorities, of course, was an invidious Cold War legacy—his mother's long-documented and unabashed loyalty to communism (Comrade Katya) and her misguided besottedness with Joseph Stalin (Joseph Dzhugashvili),[3] one of history's most notorious tyrants. Stalin directly or indirectly caused the deaths of nine million Soviet citizens through purge, subterfuge, and wanton neglect. Although the Royal Commission on Espionage cleared Ric, suspicions, persecution, negative labeling, and prejudice continued to taunt and haunt him inside and outside the workplace. "Where there's smoke there's fire" is a proverb that appeared to dog him throughout his diplomatic career. However, there may well have been no fire, and the smoke may have been metaphorical dust with distal origins outside his control.

Ric Throssell's alleged espionage played out within the specter of much larger dramas—in Australia the highly public and controversial defection of a Soviet KGB agent and pseudodiplomat, Vladimir Petrov, and in the United States the communist witch hunts, the Hollywood blacklist, and executions of two of the convicted atomic spies, Julius and Ethel Rosenberg. Perhaps for self-serving purposes, Petrov had claimed that Ric was a member of a Soviet spy ring. While just a child, it horrified me to read a 1953 front-page news story in Perth's evening newspaper (now defunct) detailing how long it took for the Rosenbergs to die in the electric chair at Sing Sing Prison in New York State. This was the era of McCarthyism, whose toxicity, malignance, and contagion easily leaped over the Pacific Ocean to permeate Australian politics and social discourse.

Ric's autobiography cast more light on his father's traumatic wartime experience. Not only was Hugo wounded at the Second Battle of Gaza, as well as at Gallipoli, but his beloved brother Eric (Ric), Ric's namesake, died there. Although Hugo Throssell had 13 siblings, his relationship with Eric was of a higher order. Ric likened these fraternal bonds to the devotion shared by David and Jonathan, as told in the Old Testament Books of Samuel—devoid of any analogous homoerotic interpretations of the biblical relationship ascribed by some modern scholars. Ric also mentioned in his autobiography that the executor of his father's will was Charles Merry. A genial giant, "Charlie" Merry and his wife Betty were good friends of my parents. Merry introduced me to the concept of beef steak. I say "concept" because my parents considered his gift of steak for a barbeque at our home as a luxury, which would be wasted on a child. Indeed, many years elapsed before I tasted one.

As another personal note on the Throssell saga, Hugo's nephew Gerald (Gerry) was my father's best friend through their childhood and youth and a recipient of mentions in the Throssell and Prichard biographies and Ric Throssell's autobiography. Gerald wrote me a sparkling letter following my father's death in 1977. Cheerfulness and warmth radiated, and he wrote as if he knew me. I welcomed his gentle amiability and familiarity. Unfortunately, geography and timing prohibited me from ever meeting him. If they were still alive, I would have many questions for Gerald Throssell and my father.

Suicide is complex and persistently painful for the bereaved

My exploration of Hugo Throssell's suicide began with a scintilla of knowledge about the event and ignorance of its precursors, its sequelae, and his name. Throughout most of my life, I have known that this tragedy emotionally scarred my father. However, the story only unfolded and crystallized for me in 2023 and 2024. Complexity smothered the suicides of Hugo and his other family members, and I posit that the same holds for the large majority of (perhaps all) suicides.

I am formally trained as an epidemiologist, demographer, and sociologist, with nods to an undergraduate history degree and a postgraduate diploma of education. These specialists study groups, not individuals, although they frequently analyze individual-level data, as I have done in two of my suicide studies. Although my science is impersonal, I acknowledge that suicides are deeply personal—informed most intimately by my experience of losing loved ones to this manner of death. Family and friends of suicide decedents endure immense pain and grief, as do the devoted fans of such celebrities as Ernest Hemingway, Sylvia Plath, Anne Sexton, Freddie Prinze, Kurt Cobain, Robin Williams, Naomi Judd, Anthony Bourdain, and Kate

Spade, who all died by suicide. I venture to say that such losses touch most readers. I inject personal reminiscences throughout much of the book in the interest of humanizing my topic, and suicide prevention is a crucial motivator for me in writing about data quality.

NOTES

1. He also killed seven enemy soldiers during the battle.

2. My father, Hildreth Rockett, a graduate of the Melbourne University School of Medicine, published one academic article in his career. Coincidentally, given Hugo Throssell's medical history, it was on meningitis and appeared in the year of Throssell's death (Rockett, 1933). This case study preceded the availability of such effective therapies as antibiotics or sulfonamides.

3. At age 14 Yakov Dzhugashvili, Joseph Stalin's son, allegedly tried to end his own life. He potentially fell victim to "suicide-by-guard" during his time as a Nazi prisoner of war. Stalin's second wife died by suicide, to whom Yakov was close (see Barker, 2023). "Suicide-by-guard," a variant of "suicide-by-cop," is a victim-precipitated homicide; in this case, Yakov may have mimicked an escape to provoke a guard to shoot him fatally.

1

Historical Questioning of Suicide Detection

Émile Durkheim

The reliability of a measure refers to its degree of reproducibility or consistency over time and space, and validity refers to the degree to which this measure captures what it purports to measure. My historical starting point in questioning the reliability and validity of suicide rates is research conducted by French sociologist Émile Durkheim. In *Suicide*, a seminal book published in 1897, Durkheim viewed suicide and differential suicide rates as outcomes of social factors and relationships (Durkheim, 1897/1951). He implacably opposed psychological or clinical reductionism and consequently discounted the mental state of individual decedents in explaining group or geographic differentials. Durkheim assumed that mental illness distributed randomly across populations and subpopulations, a spurious assumption, especially when the mental health domain incorporates alcohol and other drug dependence or misuse. Thus, although Durkheim readily accepted the role of psychological factors in accounting for suicide on a personal level, he rejected them as determinants of group differentials in suicide rates. He hypothesized that variable social integration or group connectedness and the nature of shared norms and values explained differentials between Protestants and Roman Catholics.

In one test of his integrationist hypothesis, Durkheim analyzed suicide data for the period 1867–75 on the population aged 15 years and older in the Bavarian provinces, a Germanic state. He inferred that weaker social ties and the prioritization of individualism, together with valuing free inquiry over group values, explained the higher observed suicide rates among Protestants. However, even if Durkheim had deemed the Bavarian suicide rates sufficiently valid to justify sociological investigation, an ecological fallacy may have marred his interpretation through an erroneous attribution of group characteristics to individuals. For example, just because one observes a correlation or association between individuals who wear jeans and the prevalence of suicide, it does not automatically follow that the relationship is causal. Durkheim studied grouped or aggregated data, not individual-level data. Post-Durkheimian follow-up research showed, for example, that suicides in the predominantly Protestant provinces were more likely to have occurred among the minority Catholics (Ward et al., 2012), perhaps because of normlessness or anomie, to adopt a Durkheimian concept.

Whether an ecological bias has undermined Durkheim's interpretation of the religious rate gap, systematic underreporting or differential misclassification of suicide—a bias that is the core motivation for my research—may pose a greater threat to the validity of his study. Whereas countries across the world stigmatize suicide, Japan is likely one outlier. Stigma depresses suicide counts and rates by inhibiting provision and collection of corroborative evidence. If stigma is greater among some groups than others, it plausibly affects their suicide data quality to a greater degree. Thus, families of Roman Catholic suicide decedents and other sympathetic survivors in Bavaria may have been even more inclined than corresponding Protestants to conceal or destroy pivotal evidence of suicide, such as a suicide note or the means and the method. Moreover, officials in predominantly Catholic provinces, empowered to assign manner of death, may have been more inclined to categorize the suicides of Catholics than Protestants as nonsuicides.

However, if the medicolegal officials belonged to the religious denomination of the majority population, whether Catholic or Protestant, they may have been more disposed to classify suicide appropriately when the decedent was a member of the minority religious group—a political question likely remaining unanswered for nineteenth-century Bavaria. Illustrating this possibility, qualitative research by a trio at the Queensland Institute of Technology, Gordon Tait, Belinda Carpenter, and Stephanie Jowett (2018), on a nationwide survey of coroners suggests that detection of suicide among Aboriginals in Australia, an indigenous and frequently impoverished group that has suffered persistent discrimination and injustice, is more complete than for the majority European descent population. This suggestion rests on colonialism, paternalism, and observation of their resulting high dependence on government and relative incapacity to resist the imposition of the label of a societally stigmatized and condemned phenomenon, suicide, as the official manner of death. The research finding has adverse implications for suicide accounting in politically and socioeconomically deprived segments of indigenous populations in other countries, such as the Navajo and Cherokee in the United States, First Nations peoples and Métis in Canada, and the Inuit in both.

In *The Social Meanings of Suicide*, sociologist Jack Douglas (1967) extensively critiqued Durkheim's theory of the social causes of suicide. His criticism included concerns about the validity (true positivity and negativity of certification) and reliability (reproducibility) of official suicide rates, concepts I will discuss in detail in the next chapter. Douglas critiqued Durkheim for assuming that adjudicators (e.g., coroners) share common interpretations of the constituents or definition of suicide, within and across jurisdictions, and for ignoring differential concealment of this phenomenon, such as between rural and urban areas and across sociodemographic groups. He hypothesized that there would be greater concealment of suicides by the more socially integrated members of society than by their less integrated counterparts, even if social condemnation of suicide in the two groups were equivalent.

The introduction to *Suicide: An Essay on Comparative Moral Statistics*, published in the United States in 1882, provided an earlier contrast to Durkheim regarding mindfulness of the underreporting of suicide (Morselli, 1882). Authored by Henry (Enrico) Morselli, an Italian medical professor, this book was a revised, abridged, and translated version of the original published in 1879. While his title reflected the stigma and social condemnation characterizing suicide, he assumed that the quality of data was improving because of apparent diminution of many popular prejudices and the increasing standardization of data collection, civic responsibility, and respect for law and liberty. I imagine that the bar for assessing case ascertainment of suicide in nineteenth-century Italy and elsewhere was exceedingly conservative. Durkheim (1897/1951, 160) himself was not immune to the issue of underreporting and singled out England as a country prone to reporting suicides as accidents.

Aided by powerful computers, there has been substantial improvement in data accumulation, integration, and access and statistical analysis since Durkheim's era. His contributions to the study of suicide were still remarkable and exemplified critical thinking in action. Had Durkheim been able to function in the twenty-first-century research environment, or even that of the later twentieth century, he undoubtedly would have refined his questions, approach, and conclusions. Such an opportunity may have elevated his skepticism about suicide data and motivated him to examine variation both within and between his religious groups of interest. For example, Catholics and Protestants in Bavaria or elsewhere would have varied within their own faiths regarding religiosity—church attendance, adherence to doctrine, and prayer—which likely affected their attitudes toward suicide.

Maurice Halbwachs and Suzanne Serin

Although he was an admirer of Durkheim, the French philosopher and sociologist Maurice Halbwachs (1978) adopted a critical posture in reexamining Durkheim's study in a book entitled *The Causes of Suicide*, using newer data. My interest in Halbwachs had to do not with his effort to reconcile differences in sociological and psychological perspectives on suicide, as meritorious as that was, but with his sensitivity to suicide certification and its impediments. He considered the differential concealment of evidence. In minimizing concealment as problematic for detection or case ascertainment, Halbwachs contended that suicide often comes as a surprise or shock to families and friends of the decedent, giving them little time to reconstruct a nonsuicide scenario. However, he allowed that variable capacity to achieve this reconstruction may help account for lower suicide rates among the married than the widowed and unmarried, as well as among married people with children versus those without. I suspect that fear and avoidance of social stigma, stemming from their relationship with the decedent, could provide a powerful motive for family members concealing evidence that medicolegal authorities could use to substantiate suicide (Brossard & Chandler, 2022). Warranting a mention, Halbwachs commented on the difficulty for death investigators to corroborate drowning suicides without witnesses.

In Halbwach's quotation of Suzanne Serin, a French psychiatrist who worked in a Parisian mental hospital, there is a precursor for the application of a procedure that American suicidologists in Los Angeles, California, later labeled a "psychological autopsy":

> This research which (from January 1925) until July 1926 dealt with 307 cases, 420 until October 1926, was conceived in the following way: where completed suicides are concerned, a social assistant, especially trained for this work, pro-

> ceeded immediately to the home of the desperate person and at the setting gathered from neighbors and family all information able to throw light on his previous history, his attitude during the days preceding the suicide, and the motives he may have given for his act. For the others [suicide attempters], we proceeded either to the survivor's home or to a hospital in order to initiate a psychiatric examination. (Halbwachs, 1978, 249)

I will elaborate on the psychological autopsy and its uses in a later section of this chapter and in the next chapter. Tragically, Halbwachs became a victim of the Holocaust and perished in the Buchenwald concentration camp during the waning days of Nazi Germany.

Gregory Zilboorg

Ukrainian-born psychiatrist and psychoanalyst Gregory Zilboorg was among the first scholars in the United States to question seriously the validity of American suicide data. The ensuing commentary from the 1930s encapsulates his views:

> Statistical data on suicide as they are compiled today deserve little if any credence; it has been repeatedly pointed out by scientific students of the problem that suicide cannot be subject to statistical evaluation, since all too many suicides are not reported as such. Those who kill themselves through automobile accidents are almost never recorded as suicides; those who sustain serious injuries during an attempt to commit suicide and die weeks or months later of these injuries or related infections are never registered as suicides; a great many genuine suicides are concealed by families; and suicidal attempts, no matter how serious, never find their way into the tables of vital statistics. It is obvious that under these circumstances the statistical data available cover the smallest and probably the least representative number of suicides; one is justified, therefore, in discarding them as nearly useless in a scientific evaluation of the problem. (Zilboorg, 1936, 1350)

This trenchant critique of official suicide data by Zilboorg was qualitative, impressionistic, and lacking in sound empirical evidence, although likely not far removed from the accounting capacity of the time. His remarkable intuition and compelling logic armed him to throw down a metaphorical gauntlet to suicidologists in the United States, who are committed to the conduct of careful science and identification and reduction of data deficits to facilitate suicide understanding and prevention. Whereas most users of suicide data appear neither overtly aware of nor burdened by these deficits, some have recognized and accepted the challenge of remediation. This is arguably best exemplified by a brilliant quartet of researchers and practitioners affiliated with the Los Angeles Suicide Prevention Center, which I discuss next. I offer one final comment about Zilboorg: he referred to people "committing" suicide. In the third decade of our new millennium, the suicidology community condemns this characterization because it blames the victim. Their recommended language is "died by suicide," a modern convention to which I subscribe.

Los Angeles Suicide Prevention Center

In 1958, Edwin Shneidman, a clinical psychologist, and two of his colleagues, clinical psychologist Norman Farberow and psychiatrist Robert Litman, established the Los Angeles Suicide Prevention Center in California with funding from the US Public Health Service. These core members rapidly emerged as leaders in innovative theory, empiricism, and practice in suicide scholarship, research, and prevention. The mission of the center, which incorporated a 24-hour suicide prevention hotline, specified "four goals": "1. to save lives, 2. to collect and analyze heretofore unavailable data on the serious public health problem of suicide, 3. to serve as a model suicide prevention agency which other communities might adapt to their needs, and 4. to educate and train in the principles of suicide prevention" (Litman et al., 1963, 102).

Canada-born and Canada-educated Theodore ("Ted") Curphey rounded out the quartet of stellar suicide investigators associated with the Suicide Prevention Center. A pathologist who formerly had been chief medical examiner for Nassau County on Long Island, New York, he migrated to California in 1957 to become the first chief coroner of the Los Angeles County Coroner's Office in 1957. The following quotation from Curphey indicates that his arrival was timely and auspicious: "We know that the specialists upon whom the coroner traditionally calls, the pathologist, the toxicologist, the biochemist, etc., can fairly accurately tell the causes of death, but the social scientist is in a pivotal position in cases of equivocal suicidal death to render the most significant information as the difference between suicidal death and death by some other mode is primarily a matter of the victim's intention to kill himself. Intention and motivation are neither chemical nor tissue mat ters; they are psychological in nature. This is where the social scientists can assist the coroner's office" (1965, 112).

During Curphey's early years in Los Angeles, there was a spate of fatal barbiturate overdoses, which included the tragic death in 1962 of the famous actress and media icon Marilyn Monroe. The coroner ruled her controversial demise a suicide. As part of a longer-term collaboration, Curphey referred 100 equivocal or borderline manner-of-death cases to the Suicide Prevention Center for further examination (Litman, 1968). The later in-depth, behaviorally oriented study, spearheaded by Litman, showed that 55% of these deaths involved barbiturates. Indicating the potential for overcounting of suicide, as well as undercounting, the team reassigned 19 accidental deaths as suicide and 11 suicides as accidents. Barbiturates were present in 71% of the 55 equivocal cases that the research team eventually classified as suicide. Additionally, documentation of recent medical attention was more strongly associated with a suicide than a nonsuicide classification. This research underscored the importance of a suicide note for corroborating suicide. In one California city, which registered a suicide rate only approximately one-third that of Los Angeles, an authenticated handwritten note was required for suicide certification. Such a note surfaced in only one-third of Los Angeles suicide cases, and the study found that some relatives of suicide decedents concealed or destroyed notes and other potential corroborative evidence. Los Angeles County certified over twice as many barbiturate deaths as suicide (85%) as some other California counties, likely due in part to greater fastidiousness in their investigations. Germane to access to the means of suicide, physicians in Los Angeles County may have been more prone than physicians in those other California counties to prescribe barbiturates as sedative treatment for insomnia. With adverse implications for detecting suicide, Litman reported that 25% of police reports were unhelpful in the determination of intentionality and that police lost interest in cases once they eliminated homicide as the manner of death.

Traditionally, most or many people might have conceived a suicide note to be a handwritten document prepared prior to death by a decedent. In more contemporary times, it can assume multiple other forms—typed, digital (text, email, social media), video, or audio. Content can also differentiate suicide notes according to the intentions and aims of the deceased: farewell, instructions, accusations, request for forgiveness, and justification (Acinas et al., 2015). Medicolegal death investigators regard verbal declarations as the equivalent of a "suicide note." Irrespective of form or type, suicide notes function as key forensic evidence in the corroboration and understanding of suicide as a manner of death, as I will demonstrate in a subsequent chapter.

Psychological autopsy

In retrospect, I have particularly come to admire and appreciate the Los Angeles Suicide Prevention Center's development and application of the tool or procedure they called a psychological autopsy—a label coined by Shneidman (Weinberger et al., 2018), with origins extending back at least to the work of the French psychiatrist Suzanne Serin. Although not specified as such, the 1963 Litman study employed a psychological autopsy or close facsimile. The psychological autopsy involved team members conducting semistructured interviews with family, neighbors, friends, physicians, and acquaintances of a decedent—key informants—to reconstruct the circumstances, nature, and motivation for the death, whether or not a suicide. The often critical behavioral and experiential components, which the psychological autopsy infused into medicolegal manner-of-death assignment, generally constituted supplemental information. Acquisition of this information ordinarily lies outside the training and expertise of medical examiners and coroners, the officials responsible for both assigning and amending manner-of-death certification in the United States in medicolegal cases.

As an aside, there is a kindred research and administrative tool to the psychological autopsy called the verbal autopsy. Application of this tool closes or narrows gaps in mortality and cause-of-death data not captured in the continuous civil and vital statistics registration systems of low- and middle-income countries. Officials employ verbal autopsies to collect the supplementary data via community surveys. Ordinarily, deployment of verbal autopsies is ad hoc, but optimally they are integrated into the registration systems.

Shneidman (1969, 246–47) outlined the following elements of a psychological autopsy:

1. Identifying information for victim (name, age, address, marital status, religious practices, occupation, and other details).
2. Details of the death (including the cause or method and other pertinent details).

3. Brief outline of victim's history (siblings, marriage, medical illnesses, medical treatment, psychotherapy, suicide attempts).
4. Death history of victim's family (suicides, cancer, other fatal illnesses), age of death, and other death details.
5. Description of the personality and lifestyle of the victim.
6. Victim's typical patterns of reaction to stress, emotional upsets, and periods of disequilibrium.
7. Any recent—from last few days to last 12 months—upsets, pressures, tensions, or anticipations of trouble.
8. Role of alcohol or drugs in (a) overall lifestyle of victim and (b) his death.
9. Nature of victim's interpersonal relationships (including physicians).
10. Fantasies, dreams, thoughts, premonitions, or fears of victim relating to death, accident, or suicide.
11. Changes in the victim before death (of habits, hobbies, eating, sexual patterns, and other life routines).
12. Information relating to the "life side" of victim (upswings, successes, plans).
13. Assessment of intention, i.e., role of the victim in his own demise.
14. Rating of lethality.
15. Reactions of informants to victim's death.
16. Comments, special features, etc.

Concerned about misclassification of manner of death in equivocal intent drug-related cases, Curphey opined that the "ideal approach then is to perform an autopsy and refer the case with the pathological and toxicological findings in [an] equivocal case to the behavioral scientist before certification" (1967, 172). Not only did the psychological autopsy possess enormous postmortem capacity for informing suicide, homicide, and other manners of death, beyond the information obtained via a forensic autopsy and toxicology—particularly for helping resolve manner of death in equivocal intent injury cases—but it also displayed other extraordinary features in implementation by the Los Angeles team. There was a teaching function in learning lessons from the dead to prevent mortality and other harm among the living, mirroring a leading justification for clinical autopsies. Furthermore, the team instructed interviewers working on projects with the Suicide Prevention Center to communicate with bereaved survivors in empathetic and therapeutic ways. Investigators even helped resolve specific problems emanating from the suicides, such as obtaining childcare for children of decedents.

Fast-forward to Los Angeles in the 1980s, when Litman (1989) led a study of 500 consecutive psychological autopsies. The purpose was to inform manner of death in equivocal or undetermined cases that the Los Angeles County Coroner's Office referred to the Suicide Prevention Center over the period from 1977 to 1985. Relative to a comparison group of registered suicides, the decedents were younger, less predominantly male, overrepresentative of drug intoxication deaths, and underrepresentative of firearm deaths. Comprising researchers and deputy coroners, the Litman team drew on additional evidence from the psychological autopsies to reconstruct the circumstances of death in the equivocal cases. They often offered alternative scenarios or explanations of the deaths and found that almost two-thirds of the cases the Coroner's Office had ascertained to be undetermined were suicides and one-third were accidents. Just nine cases retained "undetermined" as their manner of death.

Psychological autopsies helped clarify the correct manner of death based on the most credible scenario and consensus at a staff conference held in the Coroner's Office. Litman and his team found that 5%–10% of suicides were equivocal in the face of deficient corroborative evidence. Although the court guideline for a coroner ruling on manner of death was a preponderance of evidence, they also found that the decision about manner of death often reflected the most credible scenario created from the available evidence. The major challenge in Litman's study of equivocal cases was to distinguish suicides from accidents. Verbal suicidal communication, behavioral communication, strong but concealed efforts to procure the suicide method or injury mechanism, recent stress or loss, and history of significant depression / mental illness and suicide attempts stood out in suicide detection.

Among other notable findings in the Litman study, homicides constituted 1% of these cases after psychological autopsy, a figure unchanged from the original coroner manner-of-death assignment. Important in this original certification of drug cases was toxicologic evidence of the presence of medically prescribed sedatives and high dosage in tissues. Over half of the undetermined cases were drug related, frequently involving multiple substances. The authors concluded that a history of alcohol or other drug abuse better characterized an accident than a suicide classification. This is a controversial issue, one that I will subsequently address when I introduce and apply a new concept, self-injury mortality.

Shneidman, Litman, Farberow, and Curphey formed the intellectual vanguard of American suicide investigators. More relevant today than ever, they laid the foundations for a comprehensive investigation of suicide among drug poisoning and other equivocal manner-of-death cases. So far, society hasn't listened. A testament to lives well lived, the four investigators, researchers, educators, and preventionists displayed remarkable longevity in accumulating their inspirational legacies. Shneidman and Farberow died in their nineties, Curphey at 89, and Litman at 88.

2

Suicide as Second Fiddle in Medicolegal Death Investigations

Detecting suicide in equivocal cases

In their book *Death Investigations*, criminologists James Adcock and Arthur Chancellor allocate a chapter to equivocal deaths, that is, those whose manner appears uncertain. Suicide is a focus in this chapter, unlike in their other chapters, where homicide predominates. The authors view suicide as more problematic than homicide for investigators, while acknowledging that it is highly stigmatized and laden with grief for survivors (and as a lifelong burden, it can be a risk for future suicides): "Detectives are far more likely to encounter deaths from suicide or self-inflicted injuries than homicides, and investigating suicides may take more time, energy, and professionalism than homicide investigations. From the police perspective our investigation of a suicide is fairly limited to ensuring the death was the result of intentional self-infliction and not the result of a criminal act or omission of another" (Adcock & Chancellor, 2016, 368).

Adcock and Chancellor strongly advocate for the conduct of a psychological evaluation or psychological autopsy to help resolve equivocality or uncertainty in ascertaining manner of death. They also oppose the use by "professionals" of "undetermined" as the manner of death to protect the loved ones of suicide decedents from shame and other negative emotions. Truth is the goal. In an appendix, the two authors present a case study of a comprehensive and very complex investigation, which includes a psychological autopsy, of an equivocal (intent) stabbing death of a National Guard captain that appears to justify suicide as the manner of death. This yearlong investigation is a caution for medicolegal officials and outside experts to resist the temptation to rush to judgment with incomplete data, even when incomplete data is all they can access. Over the course of the investigation, there was vacillation between homicide and suicide as the likely manner of death.

Beginning in the mid-twentieth century, the Los Angeles Suicide Prevention Center established the basis for the scientific evaluation of suicide detection in the United States. Their centerpiece was the creation and implementation of the psychological autopsy to enlighten the detection of suicides in drug intoxication and other equivocal intent cases in the absence of critical corroborative evidence. Still true currently, medical examiners, coroners, and ancillary workers rarely interrogate witnesses or survivors as part of their medicolegal death investigations outside homicide investigations.

Taking up the mantle and advancing the utility of a psychological autopsy, two clinical psychologists, David Jobes and Alan Berman, together with a forensic pathologist, Arnold Josselson, investigated its impact on the determination of manner of death by medical examiners in an array of equivocal intent cases (Jobes et al., 1986). Whereas the Prevention Center studies were descriptive and geographically confined to the Los Angeles area, their study furthered the cause of improved suicide data by being analytic and more national in scope. Randomly selecting 195 medical examiners from the membership of the National Association of Medical Examiners, the investigators employed a three-way factorial design in distinguishing 10 factually based cases as either typical or equivocal, with each representing five different types: single car (motor vehicle traffic crash), child, autoerotic, psychotic, and Russian roulette. Medical examiners categorized these cases as typical or equivocal in pilot studies preceding the main study. Information on the cases provided to the medical examiners by the investigators in the Jobes study was medical and circumstantial, or psychological as well as medical and circumstantial. Only the experimental or intervention group of medical examiners received the psychological information, which derived from standardized psychological autopsies. Attesting to its probative value, the addition of the psychological information to the routinely collected medical and circumstantial information influenced manner-of-death determination as suicide, accident, or undetermined in all the equivocal examples except Russian roulette.

Also important in this discussion of equivocal cases is a study conducted by the University of California, San Diego sociologist David Phillips and his colleague Todd Ruth. While not using the psychological autopsy in researching suicide misclassification, they applied an indirect but highly creative approach. Observing that suicide rates peak or heap at symbolic ages, especially decennial ages like 30, 50, and 70 years, the authors analyzed computerized death certificate data from California for the period from 1966 to 1990 (Phillips & Ruth, 1993). Their focus was five experimental groups: suicides, accidental barbiturate poisoning deaths, accidental deaths of drivers in single-car crashes, accidental pedestrian deaths, and deaths that were relegated to symptoms, signs, and ill-defined conditions (ill-defined conditions for short), and also undetermineds. The final five categories have been identified in the literature as susceptible to suicide misclassification or Phillips and Ruth hypothesized they could be. Harboring substantial implications for the magnitude of differential suicide misclassification by cause of death, they reported in their California data that deaths assigned to ill-defined conditions exceeded registered suicides,[1] while undetermined deaths were less frequent. Relatively speaking, undetermined is the most likely manner-of-death category to obscure suicides (Värnik et al., 2012). Phillips and Ruth used two control or comparison groups that comprised multiple car crash deaths and deaths in all disease categories except ill-defined conditions. They only discerned age heaping within the experimental and undetermined groups, in affirmation of their research hypotheses of age rounding at symbolic ages and suicide misclassification. Serious questions can arise about the accuracy of date and time of death of suicides, since suicide is essentially a private phenomenon and most suicides lack witnesses.

To obtain psychological and psychiatric characteristics of the decedent to optimize suicide case ascertainment, especially in equivocal cases, medical examiners and coroners would need to not only conduct psychological autopsies but also consult with psychiatrists or clinical psychologists who are proficient in self-harm assessment (Botello et al., 2013). Unfortunately, there is no specialized workforce to support investigation of suicides and possible suicides in the United States. This absence contrasts starkly with the indispensable role that police play in homicide investigations (US Public Health Service, 2001). Recent mortality data show that the national suicide rate in the United States is two times higher than the homicide rate, 14.8 versus 7.5 per 100,000 population in 2022 (Centers for Disease Control and Prevention, n.d.), despite the much lower bar for homicide case ascertainment. Assignment of homicide as the manner of death by medical examiners and coroners only requires evidence that the death was caused by another who intended fear, harm, or death or manifested complete disregard for the well-being of the victim in his or her actions. On the other hand, as previously stated, a medicolegal suicide assignment usually rests on evidence that the decedent both administered the means and intended to die.

Use of psychological autopsies to enhance suicide certification and reporting in the United States, specifically in ambiguous cases, has largely been limited to California. Even in Los Angeles, their routine application ended in the 1980s with the evaporation of grant funding (Botello et al., 2013). Because of the salience of psychiatric disorders and mental health history to suicide risk, absence of psychological autopsies more generally ensures that medical examiners and coroners will miss some or many true suicides. Moreover, psychiatrists or clinical psychologists with training and expertise in suicidology are not regular participants in teams investigating equivocal cases or regularly involved in contested cases of suicide (Weinberger et al., 2018).

The psychological autopsy has applications beyond its value in enlightening equivocal cases and as an aid or vehicle for research. These include "insurance claims, criminal cases, estate issues and contested wills, malpractice claims, worker's compensation cases, product liability cases, efforts by organizations to prevent suicide [and] promoting understanding and grieving among surviving family members" (Knoll, 2008, 394). But psychological autopsies pose important ethical issues. Whether they are officials, researchers, insurance investigators, or some other kind of agent, people proposing to implement one need to be sensitive to the interviewees regarding honesty, integrity, trust, tact, diplomacy, delivery, and emotional support for bereaved persons (Vasudevan et al., 2020), a complex endeavor. Psychological autopsies can also be therapeutic for the bereaved (Weinberger et al., 2018).

When a contested medicolegal manner of death as suicide triggers a psychological autopsy—normally by family members (Goodin & Hanzlick, 1995)—the onus typically is on finding evidence of a premortem mental health state of the decedent that could be used in court to refute or contradict that assignment and help substantiate accident as an alternative (Botello et al., 2013). There is no expectation or obligation that the implementers seek counterevidence of mental issues consistent with suicide.

Adcock and Chancellor provide some insight into why psychological autopsies are not a routine part of medicolegal death investigations, even in equivocal cases:

> A crucial part of this type of investigation should include a psychological autopsy performed by a forensic psychologist or psychiatrist. In the performance of this task s/he will need to see all investigative data, reports, statements, etc. Those, coupled with interviews of family and others, will enable the professional to assess the victim's suicidal tendency, based on the totality of the circumstances—particularly the mental and behavioral actions and state of mind of the victim. As an example of how complicated and exhaustive this can be, one of the authors was investigating a suicide that might have involved the use of selective serotonin reuptake inhibitors (SSRI's), [medications] typically used in the treatment of depression, anxiety, or personality disorders. The forensic psychologist assessing the case had asked him to conduct the interview of the family members—the wife and two sons. He was just given a 48-page document that contained 127 questions. The interview of the wife took over 8 hours to complete. Needless to say this piece of the puzzle, the psychological autopsy, is critical to a sound determination as to what happened and maybe even why. (2016, 368)

Utilizing psychological autopsies, Johns Hopkins psychiatrist Paul Nestadt led a National Institutes of Health–funded study of firearm suicides among Maryland youth. The interviews with parents, siblings, and friends of the decedents comprised "approximately 30 pages of questions and a written introduction" (Powder, 2023, 32). Averaging three hours in duration, the interviewers conducted the psychological autopsies via Zoom, as an adaptation to the COVID-19 pandemic. Alan Berman had trained the researchers in this "resource-intensive" procedure, as "a dynamic biography." A noteworthy historical connection, Edwin Shneidman had trained Berman to conduct the procedure at the Los Angeles Suicide Prevention Center in the previous century. The focus of the psychological autopsies in the Nestadt study was to enlighten known suicides and not to resolve manner of death in equivocal cases, which was Shneidman's purpose in California.

Even if a single interview in a psychological autopsy could typically be implemented in three hours for a medicolegal death investigation of an equivocal case, not eight hours as reported by Adcock and Chancellor, one assumes that investigators would need three hours each time to question any additional people. Processing the results would magnify the time and costs spent in a comprehensive investigation, further disincentivizing the use of this procedure by medical examiner and coroner offices. Because of deficits in personnel, facilities, and will, toxicologic testing may be another absentee in some equivocal cases. A lost opportunity from not conducting psychological autopsies and toxicology, besides discovering corroborative evidence of suicide, includes identifying unmet need for mental health treatment (Dhossche, 2003).

Traffic suicides and victim-precipitated homicides

Traffic-related suicides are potentially an important group of equivocal medicolegal cases. They can be broadly distinguished as a driver—typically a single occupant—of a motor vehicle who intentionally died in a crash, or a pedestrian who died because of intentionally jumping or lying before a moving object, such as a car, truck, or train. A team at Australia's Monash University Accident Research Center conducted a literature review of traffic suicides and investigated data practices in various cross-national statistical organizations via a survey of 10 countries, as part of a larger study that included natural deaths in traffic crashes (Routley et al., 2003). These study countries were the United States, Canada, Spain (Catalonia), Germany, England, France, Italy, Scotland, Sweden, and Australia. Publishing their results in 2003, the Monash team concluded that traffic suicides represent a tiny component of both motor vehicular fatalities and total suicides. Their determination was heavily reliant on strong corroborative evidence, and such evidence is uncommon. Indemnification of insurance policies may suppress counts, where elected coroners protect survivors. An overview of the literature on single-car crashes and suicidality, led by Maurizio Pompili, also indicated that suicide by this method was very rare; it nonetheless was underreported (Pompili et al., 2012). Speaking to the plausible rarity of traffic suicides, Colin Pritchard and Lars Hansen (2015) made the commonsense but substantive point that transportation deaths are the most intensively investigated "accidental" deaths. Similarly sensible, an in-depth study of the 322 Swedish road traffic fatalities in 2012, conducted by multidisciplinary professionals, supported the value of authorities employing a psychosocial examination to reduce equivocality in identifying suicides and determining the correct manner of death (Andersson & Svensson, 2015).

A special challenge for suicide detection in the United States is victim-precipitated homicide (more colloquially, "suicide-by-cop"; Mohandie et al., 2009), a method with putative provocation that is particularly associated with certain minority populations. It variously commingles with mental illness, alcohol and other drug intoxication, and alleged police brutality involving shootings. True, too, for traffic suicides, victim-precipitated homicides have received comparatively little research attention. This may or may not be commensurate with their importance in the grander scheme of things. One of my high school friends died that way in his fifties or sixties in Western Australia. Perhaps the progenitor in his case was an unprovoked and ferocious attack on him in his early twenties by a Golden Gloves boxing champion, which resulted in a ruptured eardrum and probable brain damage. The venue was a community dance hall in Crawley, adjacent to the campus of the University of Western Australia, and I was a witness and another victim. Fortunately for me, I only sustained a minor hand injury. Right after the attack my friends and I asked bystanders whether the assailant, who had fled into the night, was "drunk." A legal substance for adult use, alcohol was the unchallenged, recreational "drug of choice" for 1960s Australians. Someone identified our assailant and told us he didn't "drink." In retrospect, I suspect he used anabolic steroids to strengthen muscle tissue, enhance body mass, and improve his boxing performance. We plausibly had fallen victim to "roid rage"—a phenomenon then totally alien to me, as in actuality were steroids.

Robert Litman, Irene Ovenstone, and suicide gradation

Medicolegally, diagnosis of a possible suicide as suicide by a medical examiner or its adjudication by a coroner can be viewed as a binary decision from the perspective of suicidology: suicide or nonsuicide. While pragmatic, this choice does not adequately reflect the psychodynamic continuum that leads up to the act of suicide. Drawing on a wealth of empirical research, conducted in collaboration with other members of the Los Angeles Suicide Prevention Center, Robert Litman graded intentionality for suicide or possible suicide (Litman, 1968). He distinguished first-degree suicide as "deliberate, planned, premeditated self-murder"; second-degree suicide as "impulsive, unplanned, under great provocation or mitigating circumstances"; and "third-degree suicide—sometimes called 'accidental' suicide. Here the person puts his life into some jeopardy by voluntary self-injury, but we infer that he does not really intend to die because the method of self-injury is relatively harmless and provisions for rescue are made" (Litman, 1968, 49). Additional categories distinguished by Litman are where the decedent lacked the capacity for "intention," as when psychotic or highly intoxicated, or was self-negligent, for example, ignored medical instructions or drove recklessly, and finally when the suicide was "justifiable" or "appropriate" (Litman, 1968, 50). Litman offers no elaboration or examples of the last-mentioned category, but he comments that it has no "pragmatic importance to coroners." He noted that suicides he deemed first or second degree rarely surfaced as equivocal cases, unlike cases he categorized as third degree, those lacking capacity for intent. Litman further indicated that applying the psychological autopsy, in a reexamination of equivocal cases, led to reclassification of most third-degree suicides as a formal suicide manner of death.

Gradation of suicide measurement manifested as a research issue across the Atlantic Ocean in Edinburgh, Scotland, in the work of psychiatrist Irene Ovenstone. She reexamined selected injury mortality cases from two overlapping sources, the Crown Office and the Scottish Registrar General's Office, to apply a psychiatric approach for improving suicide detection (Ovenstone, 1973). Her study period was October 1969 through March 1971. She selected all suicides; all undetermined intent deaths where suicide was implicated, but with a deficit of corroborative evidence; accidental deaths where the decedents had been patients at the Regional Poisoning Treatment Center or had met with the Samaritans, a voluntary group dedicated to suicide prevention; gas poisonings; accidental deaths where she deemed suicide a possibility; and a random sample of accidental deaths, excluding previously selected cases, as controls. Ovenstone then applied a set of criteria to this group of deaths to make her own assignments of suicide, undetermined, or accident manner of death. Becoming known as the Ovenstone criteria, for justifying a suicide assignment, the criteria allowed for both direct and indirect evidence. Direct evidence includes situations where the person who died left a suicide note, where the person used an obvious method like hanging or shooting, or where a drug-related suicide can be confirmed through postmortem evidence like high dosage or hoarding of pills. Indirect evidence covered circumstances where decedent behavior was consistent with prior documented suicide attempts, or where there was evidence of a severe personal reaction to a stressful situation or problem in adapting to more distal stress. Ovenstone operationalized severe reaction as periodic mood swings leading to depression or to new or excessive use of alcohol and other drugs.

Ovenstone defined suicide as "deliberate initiation of an act of self-poisoning or self-injury which resulted in death, irrespective of whether there was evidence of intent to die" (1973, 16). Her downplaying of the substantiation of decedent intentionality in her suicide definition deviated sharply from the conventional definitions of suicide I provided in the introduction. Nevertheless, she still inferred intentionality of suicide from the psychological/psychiatric data as a medical supplement to the manifest intent essential to any legal determination of suicide. Ovenstone reserved the undetermined intent category for cases where many factors indicated suicide but there was doubt about self-administration of the means. She reserved the accident category for cases lacking both apparent evidence of deliberate self-initiation and direct or indirect evidence supporting a suicide assignment. From a firm empirical footing, in keeping with the thinking of Litman, she allowed for a conceptual gradation of suicides based on degree of certainty: definite, probable, and doubtful.

Using her reclassification of the selected cases as the criterion or gold standard, Ovenstone estimated that the Crown Counsel and the Registrar General underreported suicide in Edinburgh by 41% and 32%, respectively. In a comparison of her classifications with those from the two government agencies, she inferred that the Crown Counsel overcounted undetermined deaths and undercounted suicides and accidental deaths and that the Registrar General also overcounted undetermined deaths but only undercounted suicides. Her reclassification estimated a 50% higher total suicide rate for Edinburgh than reported from the Crown Counsel data. Differentiating age and sex, she found that underreporting peaked among the population 55 years and older, particularly in the female segment. Ovenstone also compared suicides and misclassified suicides on myriad variables in a series of two-way comparisons (bivariable statistical analysis). These variables extended from such characteristics as social class, household composition, employment, residence in substandard housing, debts, and criminal record to previous psychiatric treatment, suicidal behavior, and disease and psychiatric diagnoses.

Focusing on death circumstances, Ovenstone discerned greater intent among the suicides than the misclassified suicides, in keeping with her more comprehensive criteria for case ascertainment than those employed by the medicolegal officials. Drug intoxication was a major variable separating misclassified suicides from suicides. Another was absence of a suicide note. Ovenstone concluded that suicide misclassification occurred among undetermined cases but not among accident cases. In summary, her criteria for establishing suicide melded objective forensic evidence with a more subjective assessment of the psychological/psychiatric history and proximal mental state of the decedent. Ovenstone brought the sensibilities of a psychiatrist/ suicidologist to her graduated conceptualization of suicide. Unsurprisingly, she found much more suicide in Edinburgh than did the medicolegal authorities. However, whereas the determinations of the latter likely deflated the true suicide rate, Ovenstone's psychological approach may have inflated it.

In the United States, during the second decade of the twenty-first century, Adcock and Chancellor (2016) distinguished seven categories of murder/ homicide, ranging from most to least severe regarding penalties or justice for the perpetrators: first-degree murder, second-degree murder, felony murder, voluntary manslaughter, involuntary manslaughter, negligent homicide, and justifiable homicide. Creation of a comparative hierarchy or gradation for suicide, which would have clinical and public health applications, seems destined to remain an unmet challenge for some time. Perhaps it would be infeasible anyway.

The in-depth investigations, which were conducted by the Los Angeles Suicide Prevention Center and the chief county coroner during the middle of the twentieth century, exemplify the use of psychological autopsies to help resolve borderline manner-of-death drug cases. I would argue that optimal detection of suicide in equivocal cases would be contingent on forensic teams having the services of a psychiatrist or clinical psychologist with training and experience in suicidology, augmented by psychological autopsy data. Although the psychological autopsy can be a formidable tool in helping medicolegal death investigators resolve intentionality in equivocal cases—demonstrated most pointedly by the transdisciplinary work of the Los Angeles Suicide Prevention Center—it brings its own biases, including the nature of key informants, their capacity for accurate recall, and absence of a standardized protocol.

Death investigations and medical examiner / coroner systems

American medicolegal death investigations fall within the broad domains of two alternative systems, medical examiner and coroner. Lacking national oversight, administration of these systems ranges from state control under an appointed state medical examiner to county control under an elected coroner or appointed medical examiner (Hanzlick, 2007). A few coroner systems function like a medical examiner system, exemplified by the Los Angeles County Coroner's Office under Ted Curphey. That office converted to a medical examiner system in 1990. In 2020, it assumed the label of the Los Angeles Department of Medical Examiner-Coroner, but the term "coroner" was deleted in 2023. Medical examiner and coroner systems typically differ profoundly in their philosophical underpinnings and approaches to the conduct of medicolegal death investigations (Hanzlick & Combs, 1998).

Evidentiary standards for classifying a death as suicide are conservative, regardless of system type. Medical examiners assign a suicide diagnosis given "reasonable medical certainty," based on an assumption of greater than 50% probability (Timmermans, 2005), and coroners must demonstrate suicidal intent "beyond reasonable doubt" in applying their legal burden-of-proof approach (Atkinson, 1978; Jentzen, 2009). Medical examiners in the United States are appointed by government officials and are physicians who are usually trained in pathology and forensic pathology, with dual board certification. They may serve multiple counties and frequently a whole state. Primarily occupying the lower end of a continuum for professionalism, coroners generally are elected lay county-level officials untrained in medicine, pathology, or forensic pathology. They may even be as young as 18 years old, and election makes them especially vulnerable to pressures from politicians or families of decedents to avert or reverse a determination of suicide. Moreover, coroners are usually much less familiar than medical examiners with medical and toxicologic processes/terminology and have less contact with medical and forensic toxicologists.

I note that postgraduate training in psychiatry or clinical psychology is not a requisite for medical examiners or coroners, which potentially inhibits postmortem inference of decedent intent substantially. As of 2013, "the vast majority of chief medicolegal death investigation system officers are coroners, but most of the American population is served by medical examiner systems" (Hanzlick, 2014, 8), a product of the typically much less urbanized and more rural character of the areas within the jurisdiction of coroner systems. Likely adversely impacting the quality of coroner offices and smaller medical examiner offices more than larger ones, less than 2.5% of the total 2,479 offices were accredited by the National Association of Medical Examiners or the International Association of Coroners & Medical Examiners as of January 2015, and the coroner offices are far less likely than medical examiner offices to be accredited (National Commission on Forensic Science, National Institute of Standards and Technology, 2015).

A provocative question is whether the predominantly more scientific approach of medical examiners makes them more likely than coroners to detect true suicides, particularly in equivocal cases. Around the turn of the twenty-first century, Stefan Timmermans (2005), a sociologist, conducted a qualitative study of suicides and suspicious deaths by immersing himself in the Boston Medical Examiner's Office as a detached observer, documenter, and interpreter of day-to-day operations. Stated more formally, this type of research qualifies as ethnographic, with roots in anthropology. Timmermans suggested that the professionalism of medical examiners may induce conservatism and consequently make them more concerned about getting their diagnosis of suicide wrong than getting it right. Stated more conventionally, false positives pose a greater threat to professional authority than false negatives. I will revisit this issue in an ensuing section on the social construction of suicide rates.

Death types in medicolegal cases

Over 90% of people in the United States, as in a large majority of more developed Western countries, die from natural causes, that is, disease as distinct from injury (Rockett et al., 2011). On average, those dying from disease are much older than those dying from injury (Rockett, 1998a). The former mostly die in unsuspicious circumstances. A practicing physician usually certifies their death certificates. The training of American physicians in death certificate completion is notoriously deficient, to the detriment of clinical medicine, public health, and forensic death investigations (Pritt et al., 2005).

Medical and coroner cases disproportionately represent middle-aged and younger decedents. Past president of the National Association of Medical Examiners and prominent medicolegal scholar Randy Hanzlick enumerated the types of deaths typically mandated across states to be subject to a medicolegal death investigation:

1. Death is known or suspected as having resulted from injury or poisoning (external conditions).
2. Death is sudden, unexpected, and not explained with reasonable medical probability.
3. Deaths of inmates of jails or state institutions, or while in the custody of law enforcement agencies.
4. Death occurs under unusual or suspicious circumstances.
5. Death occurs and there is no physician to complete and sign the death certificate. (2007, 86)

However, acceptance of a case for a medicolegal death investigation is usually at the discretion of medical examiners and coroners.

Immediate circumstances and decedent biography

English sociologist Steve Taylor (1982) reduced the fundamentals of a medicolegal suicide investigation to two elements. The first element was the *immediate circumstances* of the event, where the purpose of the investigation is to reconstruct the final moments of the decedent, with expository evidence derived from various sources, including results from a forensic autopsy, "archeological relics" from the death scene (e.g., a note, bottles, rope, photographs), and testimony from any reliable witnesses. The second critical element of a suicide investigation was the *biography of the decedent*, or documentation of personal incidents and characteristics and circumstances of the death that could be relevant to the ascertainment of suicide. These could include a history of child abuse, being a child of divorce and family dislocation or dissolution, having an unstable work life, prior suicide attempts, and psychological, financial, domestic, and/or legal problems. Taylor acknowledges that the biographical information assumes added importance as corroborative evidence of suicide when the method tends to be equivocal regarding intent, such as drowning, drug poisoning, gassing, jumping from a height or in front of a train, and a single-vehicle traffic crash.

In a nutshell for Taylor, if a death is to be certified as suicide, it must look like one and have known reasons. An authenticated suicide note can be pivotal corroborative evidence regarding decedent motives and intentionality. However, in the United States, certainly, a note is absent in a large majority of cases, and psychological autopsies are rarely conducted to enlighten manner of death. Thus, other physical evidence from the death scene, besides a note, can be crucial in equivocal cases. Using a female drowning case by way of illustration, potentially important corroborative evidence for suicide would be scene orderliness regarding the distribution of hats, handbags, shoes, and clothing. In addition, if the decedent had been wearing a loose-fitting garment at the time of her entry into the water, further evidence could be the weighting down of this garment with stones for modesty and to hasten death.

Readers unfamiliar with this fact may find it interesting that, historically, England was a country where coroners legally adjudicated suicides. They did not diagnose them as in those areas of the United States served by medical examiner systems. In 2019, however, England and Wales changed their standard of proof for the determination of suicide in coronial inquests from "beyond reasonable doubt" to a "balance of probabilities" (Appleby et al., 2019); now a coroner draws a "conclusion" instead of rendering a "verdict." Application of this less stringent standard should reduce the degree of the underreporting of suicide in the official statistics of these two countries. In terms of scientific and forensic support, the English and Welsh medicolegal death investigation system more closely resembles the typical American medical examiner system than rural county-based coroner systems.

Steps in medicolegal death investigation

I consider that the late Randy Hanzlick was the "academic dean" of American medical examiners. He was imaginative, eloquent, diligent, and prolific in educating his peers and much wider audiences about the particulars, responsibilities, and possibilities of his profession, including an important role in public health. In his primary position as the chief medical examiner for Fulton County, Georgia, which encompasses most of metropolitan Atlanta, he identified five steps in a typical American medicolegal death investigation: initial collection of information; death scene investigation; examination of the body, which could be confined to an external examination or extend to a full autopsy; ancillary investigations and information collection; and preparation of the case record and report (Hanzlick, 2006).

Ancillary investigations involve acquisition of information from additional sources, such as reports from a personal physician, police, and child and family service agencies. Integral to medicolegal death investigations are first responders to the death scene, including emergency medical technicians, paramedics, firefighters, and police (Koehler & Wecht, 2006). To reiterate, American police are rarely trained or expected to perform suicide investigations (US Public Health Service, 2001), unlike in some European countries, for example (Värnik et al., 2012). Police do investigate suicides in some jurisdictions in the United States, such as a few counties in Michigan. However, medical examiners or coroners remain responsible for investigation and signing the death certificates in medicolegal cases.

Stephan Timmermans (2005, 316–17) outlined seven main elements of evidence salient to the identification of suicide by medical examiners: witness reports, suicide notes, use of suicide guidelines, previous suicide attempts, testimonials, life crises, and mode of dying. He noted that most suicides are solitary acts, and thus unwitnessed, and that witness accounts can be unreliable. Suicide notes, while important pieces of direct evidence, are not conclusive. Guidelines for implementing suicide are exemplified by Derek Humphry's (2010) *Final Exit: The Practicalities of Self-Deliverance and Assisted Suicide for the Dying*, and adherents may leave behind such critical corroborative evidence as a plastic bag covering their heads and open pages in suicide guidelines detailing how to conduct a suicide. As Timmermans (2005) states, previous suicide attempts may be apparent from medical records or witness testimony. Testimonies of witnesses, from health care professionals who treated the decedents to relatives and friends, are vulnerable to suppression of evidence in addition to their value as corroborative sources. Life crises, such as loss of an intimate relationship, a profound economic or occupational reversal, and severe mental and physical health problems, can be critical pieces of evidence for medicolegal investigators in rendering a suicide determination. Finally, Timmermans observed that these officials can infer suicidal intent from the mode of dying or type of fatal injury mechanism. He differentiates more forensically overt methods of suicide like hanging and shooting from the more equivocal methods of drowning and jumping in front of a moving train. Nonetheless, he allows for ambiguity regarding the identification of the correct manner of death even in the generally more obvious methods of suicide.

Timmermans refers to a 51% rule where suicides, especially those emergent in equivocal cases, are assigned as the manner of death when the pillars of evidence support a "more likely than not" medicolegal opinion. He reports that medical examiners work inductively rather than deductively—the philosophical approach shaping my research. Thus, their line of inquiry proceeds from specific to general observations rather than the opposite. According to Timmermans, medical pathologists are mindful of the deleterious impact of stigma inherent in a suicide determination, a conservative force.

In developing a scoring system for identifying potential suicides, an Italian research team noted that

> evidence collected at the death scene is one of the key points for the early identification of suicides. Three eventualities are reported, sometimes essential in the reconstruction of a suicidal dynamic. The first, and probably the most important, is the discovery of the weapon or of elements necessary for the performance of the hypothetical suicide near the cadaver (for example, firearms, knives,

> empty pharmaceutical confections or substances used for poisoning, a chair or other raised element in case of complete hanging). The second and the most intuitive eventuality is the detection of a suicide note or farewell message, in which suicidal ideation is reported, or the victim apologizes for his action (even if only a minority of the victims, between 3% and 43%, leave suicide notes), or the presence of ordered personal effects of the victim (close to the body or, in the case of drowning or precipitation, in the place where the victim is suspected to have put his idea into practice). The third eventuality is absence of signs of a struggle, or of forced entry in enclosed places. (Visentin, 2019, 149)

The Italian team also noted that there are no detectable injuries in most poisoning cases, further complicating suicide case ascertainment. This would not be true in poisonings from substances other than drugs, however, such as when a pesticide or household cleaner is the means or method. A graphic example is provided in the penultimate chapter.

Suicide is a stepchild in medicolegal death investigations

With a long tradition, medicolegal death investigations in the United States emphasize homicide and criminal justice over public health issues. This tradition is reflected in two important books published in 2009. The first, *Death Investigation in the United States: Coroners, Medical Examiners, and the Pursuit of Medical Certainty*, was written by Jeffrey Jentzen (2009), a former medical examiner in Wisconsin and the director of Autopsy Forensic Services at the University of Michigan. The second book, entitled *Strengthening Forensic Science in the United States: The Path Forward*, was a report on a study commissioned by the US Congress (Committee on Identifying the Needs of the Forensic Sciences Community, National Research Council, 2009). That study involved presentations to the Forensic Science Committee of the National Academies of Sciences by over 60 experts and officials from universities, professional organizations, think tanks, and numerous national, state, and local law enforcement and criminal-justice-related agencies. These US agencies included the Federal Bureau of Investigation and the Departments of Homeland Security, Defense, and Justice.

Suicide received only scant attention in either book. This speaks volumes about the low status of suicide accounting and prevention in American society. Whereas the homicide rate largely trended downward, the suicide rate rose virtually unabated through most of the two opening decades of the twenty-first century. Reversals in these respective rates manifested just prior to and during the COVID-19 pandemic in the United States. I will return to these suicide declines in chapter 9 and speak to their potential artifactual character associated with heavy pressures on infrastructures and scarce resources for medicolegal death investigations.

In understandable contrast to the history of the Department of Justice, which focuses on illegal behavior (and suicide is not illegal in the United States), the Centers for Disease Control and Prevention (CDC) has viewed both suicide and homicide as public health problems for nearly four decades (Rosenberg & Fenley, 1991), as the medical examiner and coroner communities have become increasingly committed to advancing public health (Hanzlick & Parrish, 1996; Hanzlick, 2006). This broadening domain, coupled with concerns about mismatched infrastructures and underresourcing of medicolegal death investigations in the wake of the opioid epidemic, has prompted my forging of strong working relationships with medical examiners and toxicologists. In addition, by including psychiatrists and emergency physicians in my research teams, I have been able to benefit from their focus on the living, as distinct from those charged with postmortem investigations of suspicious and other unexpected sudden deaths. Aided by the inputs of colleagues representing other disciplines such as sociology, economics, and philosophy, the synergies from these multidisciplinary collaborations are palpable. With give-and-take, then, the sum of these efforts has indeed greatly exceeded their parts.

In his treatise *American Suicide: A Psychocultural Explanation*, Howard Kushner (1991), a medical historian, propounded that the burrowing and siloing associated with specialization of professions, along with psychological reductionism, can impede the understanding of suicide. A variant on the converse, my conviction is that multidisciplinary approaches can markedly enhance the understanding of how medical examiners and coroners make a suicide determination, a conviction that had its genesis in the United States with the work of the Los Angeles Suicide Prevention Center (Curphey, 1967).

The *Global Practice of Forensic Sciences* was published in 2015 (Ubelaker, 2015). An edited book, its chapters contain a description of forensic practice in the United States and 27 other countries. As with *Death Investigation in America* and *Strengthening Forensic Science in the United States*, striking to me was how little attention was accorded suicide and public health versus homicide and crime. My back-of-the-envelope content analysis of the index identified 26 mentions of suicide versus 40 of homicide, 28 of crime scene investigation, 48 of criminalistics, and 31 of criminology. Public health received zero mentions. Autopsy, more appropriately termed forensic autopsy, as distinct from hospital or consent autopsy, was mentioned in the index 88 times. For me, conspicuous by its absence was the psychological autopsy. While registered suicides account for approximately twice as many deaths as corresponding homicides do in the United States, this differential is far wider in most other countries represented in the book.

A personal story of homicide

When a person dies in a homicide, locals often have a readily comprehensible fear of the perpetrator until he or she (mainly he) is apprehended by the authorities, convicted, and imprisoned (or executed). While growing up in the state of Western Australia, I experienced fear of homicide on a grand scale during my later high school and early university undergraduate years. Eventually nicknamed the Night Caller, a serial killer by the name of Eric Edgar Cooke terrorized the capital city of Perth—especially the more affluent suburbs—during a prolonged murder rampage between 1958 and 1963. Mainly concentrated on a narrow strip of land that ran 12 miles from the city of Perth to its port of Fremantle, these suburbs lay between the picturesque Swan River and enticing white sand beaches abutting the Indian Ocean. Today, such suburbs are far more geographically dispersed, as the population of Perth has mushroomed fourfold to its current size of over 2 million.

My general practitioner father, Hildreth Rockett, had the horrendous duty of certifying the death of one of Cooke's eight murder victims, none of whom Cooke knew. Gillian Brewer, an heiress to a chocolate manufacturing company, was massacred by Cooke with a tomahawk and scissors in her apartment, which was located just up the road from my father's medical office (surgery) and my first home. I even knew her neighbor from whom Cooke had stolen the tomahawk, and I was acquainted, as an adolescent, with a hearing- and speaking-impaired young man whom the prosecution unjustly convicted of this murder and who languished in prison for many years. He was eventually exonerated, as was another man who had suffered the same injustice following his wrongful conviction in the deliberate hit-and-run death of his girlfriend. I attended high school and university with a person who had lost a coin toss with his roommate for the luxury of sleeping on an outside porch on a hot steamy night, at a time preceding air-conditioned homes. Cooke shot and killed that roommate.

As part of the protracted police investigations into Cooke's serial murders, I was fingerprinted in an ambitious, metro-wide forensic enterprise, which failed to identify the wily perpetrator but presumably eliminated me as a possible suspect. Complicating identification and capture of Cooke and the recognition that the police were dealing with a serial killer was the fact that he employed diverse methods and mechanisms. These included his deployment of the axe, use of a rifle, manual strangulation, and use of a motor vehicle in the hit-and-run murder. This diversity and the misplaced zeal of an ambitious police administrator facilitated the arrest and conviction of the two innocent men in a "rush to justice." Cooke was finally captured by police after a chance discovery by walkers of his rifle hidden in a small Geraldton Wax bush. The police surveilled the site until Cooke returned to reclaim his weapon. In 1964, Cooke became the last person to be executed in Western Australia. Robert Drewe (2000) encapsulated this story of homicidal horror and police and prosecutorial injustice in his well-written memoir, *The Shark Net*, a story recounted much more recently in the four-part film documentary *The Night Caller*. I would be remiss, however, if I failed to mention that in the United States similar stories perpetually and disproportionately abound among its vulnerable populations.

In his 40-year medical career, my father attended numerous bloody scenes of injury and death. Fatal motor vehicle car crashes were all too common in our neighborhood in the days before seat belts, airbags, traffic lights, safety bumps, stringently enforced drunk driving laws, and other protective measures. My father's office occupied the front of my first home on the corner of Stirling Highway and Eric Street. Stirling Highway was then the major artery uniting Perth and Fremantle, a port city, but has since been supplanted by adjoining freeways south of the Swan River. Occasionally, drivers on that road failed to safely negotiate the turn into Eric Street, and my father had only a short distance to traverse to provide help. Two blocks away was the other major artery then and still linking Perth with Fremantle, a railway line. Nearby was the Napier Street level crossing, a crossing then lacking traffic lights and gates. My father was often called to incidents involving pedestrians and vehicle crashes, which were later reported in the print press. However, the only other death scene besides Gillian Brewer's that he ever mentioned to me was the suicide of Hugo Throssell.

Suicide and homicide coverage in the media

Aside from fear of "contagion" and imitation among youth (Niederkrotenthaler et al., 2019), suicide typically casts a much smaller psychological and cultural shadow than homicide on society in everyday life in the United States. Serial killers, incessant mass shootings, fear of unapprehended perpetrators, and fascination with murder mysteries magnify the insidious and enduring stature of homicide in the public imagination. In the United States, serial homicides have no parallel in the suicide domain, and mass homicides seldom do. Prioritizing homicide and crime over suicide and public health in forensic science can be easily rationalized and justified.

Colorado State University's Silvia Canetto, a psychologist, and two of her colleagues conducted a national study of the comparative coverage of suicide and homicide in newspaper and television stories (Canetto et al., 2017). Their chapter in an edited book on media and suicide was entitled "Suicide Stories in the US Media: Rare and Focused on the Young." Findings most germane to this book are that homicide stories in 2002–3, the observation period, were 18 times more common than suicide stories in their newspaper sample and 14 times more common in their television news sample. With a far higher threshold for corroboration, recorded suicides in the United States at that time were almost twice as frequent as corresponding homicides, a margin that is similar now. The researchers found that suicide's profile was elevated in the media reporting of cases of homicide that culminated in the suicide of the perpetrator. The study's observation period well preceded the explosion of digital social media platforms like Meta (formerly Facebook), X (formerly Twitter), TikTok, and Instagram.

Using the resources of the distinguished online Our World in Data publication in 2019, Hannah Ritchie (2019) showed, via personal Google searches and stories from the *New York Times* and England's *Guardian* newspaper, that suicide and homicide are overrepresented in relation to their respective proportions of deaths in the United States. This observation is expected owing to their inherent violence and excessive toll on younger people. Homicide outweighed suicide in the two newspaper searches. In the Google searches, however, the reverse was true—perhaps a function of suicide's greater ubiquity among families and its highly private nature. The searches were almost fourfold higher for suicide than homicide.

In the enlightened words of Ted Curphey, as the chief coroner for Los Angeles County:

> The importance of a complete and accurate investigation of a homicide by the forensic pathologist stands without question and must always carry a high priority in the workload of any active medicolegal office. When one considers, however, that some offices see about 10% of their caseloads as suicides, 25% as accidents of all kinds, about 60% as natural deaths and up to 5% as homicides, the forensic pathologist, in the interest of the community as a whole, must find some means of rendering equally good service in the study of all the types of cases he sees. He must not and should not expend the lion's share of the resources of his department on homicide, simply because of the traditional error (to which, unfortunately, he frequently subscribes) that this is his only responsibility, and in doing so neglect or study only perfunctorily the broad spectrum of cases that comes under his scrutiny because of the pressure of the district attorney and the police and the clamor of the public for his answer to the *Who dunnit*? (1967, 164)

The death certificate

Standardized mortality data from an established vital statistics system, which are timely, uniform, and universal in population coverage, are of critical importance for criminal justice and for public health surveillance, research, policy, planning, resource allocation, prevention, and intervention. A permanent legal record, the death certificate is their core (fig. 2.1). Besides manner of death, the certificate provides for sequential entry of the immediate cause of death, contributing conditions or mental health and disease comorbidities, and finally an underlying cause. The World Health Organization (WHO) defines the underlying cause of death as "the disease or injury initiating the train of morbid events leading directly to death, or the circumstances of the accident or violence which produced the fatal injury" (World Health Organization, n.d.). Variability in training and practice across certifiers, nosologists (clinical or medical coders), administrative officers, clerks, statistical technicians, and other information managers will induce differential reporting and misreporting of the underlying cause of death (Ruiz et al., 2018), including suicide (Claassen et al., 2010), on the death certificate. In the United States, compilation of death certificate data is first and foremost the responsibility of the states. All coding once occurred there,

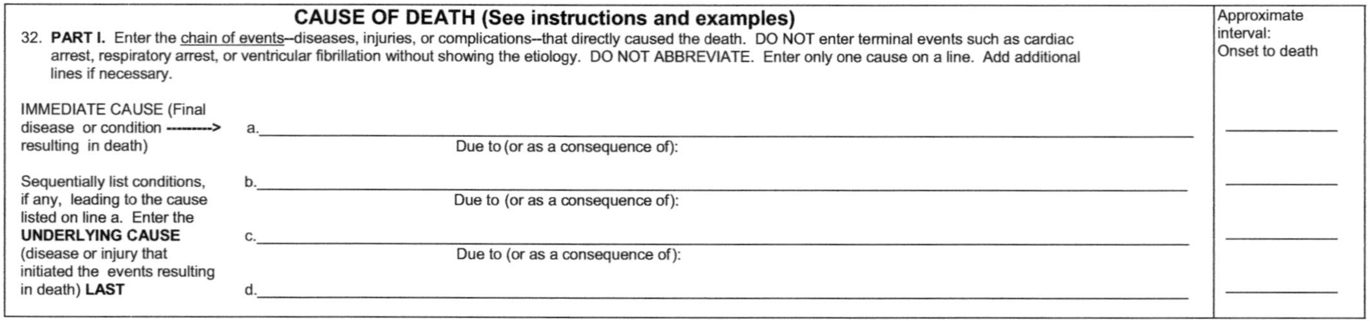

CAUSE OF DEATH (See instructions and examples)

32. **PART I.** Enter the chain of events--diseases, injuries, or complications--that directly caused the death. DO NOT enter terminal events such as cardiac arrest, respiratory arrest, or ventricular fibrillation without showing the etiology. DO NOT ABBREVIATE. Enter only one cause on a line. Add additional lines if necessary.

		Approximate interval: Onset to death
IMMEDIATE CAUSE (Final disease or condition ---------> resulting in death)	a.__________ Due to (or as a consequence of):	______
Sequentially list conditions, if any, leading to the cause listed on line a. Enter the **UNDERLYING CAUSE** (disease or injury that initiated the events resulting in death) **LAST**	b.__________ Due to (or as a consequence of):	______
	c.__________ Due to (or as a consequence of):	______
	d.__________	______

Figure 2.1. Provision for immediate, contributing, and underlying causes on a US standard death certificate.

typically in departments of health. Now this task is confined to difficult cases. To facilitate standardization, minimize error, and expedite processing and public release, states now send the raw data digitally, with some exceptions, to the Division of Vital Statistics at CDC in the Department of Health and Human Services, where coding is automated. However, the system flags inconsistencies and potential errors, and trained nosologists manually conduct the pertinent coding. Depending on the profession of the certifier (e.g., medical examiner, coroner, physician, or funeral director), there are different resources online to assist with the completion of a death certificate (Department of Health and Human Services, 2004; Curtin et al., 2019; National Center for Health Statistics, 2023).

Potential suicide misclassification is associated with errors recorded on death certificates, not only in manner and underlying cause of death but also in entries on contributing conditions or comorbidities, exemplified by various mental health disorders like major depression or alcohol use disorder and such physical diseases as cancer and diabetes. Furthermore, errors in recording any of the other variables on a death certificate, including such decedent demographics as age, sex, marital status, race/ethnicity, occupation, and date and time of death, can increase the likelihood of suicide misclassification (in the United States most suicides are private acts and thus unwitnessed, whereas in some low-income countries and areas they can be social acts; Canetto, 2008). For example, older age at death is associated with multiple medical conditions and morbidities. Without a clinical or forensic autopsy, a certifier might misidentify a drug-related suicide—where prescription painkillers and tranquilizers were the means—as death from cancer or a neurodegenerative disease, for example, amyotrophic lateral sclerosis (aka ALS or Lou Gehrig's disease, my mother's killer), or another chronic disease that had been diagnosed before or after death. Although there may be some compensating errors, misclassification adversely impacts the accuracy of the numerator in a suicide or other type of death rate. Any overestimation or underestimation of the population at risk, the census-based denominator, would respectively deflate or inflate the true or estimated rate.

Reliability of suicide data

Epidemiologists and sociologists are the main users of international suicide statistics for research purposes. Epidemiology emphasizes health-related variables in cross-national rate variation, while sociological interest is driven primarily by the quest for understanding social causation through macroexplanations involving such forces as economic development (Quinney, 1965), industrialization (Barth et al., 2011), urbanization (Shah, 2008), and religion (Stack, 1983).

Two Canadian epidemiologists from Western University in London, Ontario, Mark Speechley and Kathleen Stavraky (1991), identified three empirical approaches that researchers have employed to assess the international reliability of official suicide statistics. Termed experimental, the first approach examines whether medicolegal officials from different countries or jurisdictions varied in assigning manner of death to a common set of cases. A blinded study of respective assignments by Danish and English officials attributed variation in reported suicide rates to different procedures for case ascertainment (Ross & Kreitman, 1975). Discrepant findings between this study and a second study, which compared English and Scottish manner-of-death assignments (Sainsbury & Jenkins, 1982), may have been due to the latter study being confined to cases with an equivocal manner—illustrating an imperative to compare apples to apples for valid inference.

The second approach for assessing international suicide data reliability compares rankings of suicide rates of immigrants in selected countries with the population in their respective countries of origin (Speechley & Stavraky, 1991). Reliability is evaluated by means of a rank-order correlation coefficient as the summary measure. The theoretical boundaries of this measure extend from 0 (no concordance or agreement between the two sets of ranks) to 1 (perfect concordance). A study of American national data, conducted by an English team (Sainsbury & Jenkins, 1982), and an Australian study (Whitlock, 1971) both reported coefficients between 0.8 and 0.9—seemingly attesting to high reliability of international suicide rates. However, any underlying assumption of homogeneity in case ascertainment procedures fails to pass muster in either the United States or Australia. As previously documented, the United States blends medical examiner and coroner death investigation systems, and these systems are varyingly skilled, overstressed, and underresourced (Committee on Identifying the Needs of the Forensic Sciences Community, National Research Council, 2009). At the time of the Australian study, although all states and territories functioned under a coroner system, this was not directly related to how suicide statistics were reported (Cantor & Dunne, 1990). Confounding an assumption of the reliability of international suicide rates for research purposes, as justified by this rate ranking approach, immigrants were unevenly distributed throughout the general population and geographically by ethnic origin in both Australia (Chiswick et al., 2002) and the United States (Massey, 1995). The reliability of official suicide statistics and suicide rates that is being assessed is relative, not absolute. Relative reliability refers to the constancy of the magnitude of error in rates across populations and time.

Speechley and Stavraky (1991) labeled their third approach for assessing the reliability or consistency or reproducibility of international suicide statistics as rate reformulation. Conceptually similar to the second approach, rate reformulation also employs a rank-order correlation coefficient as the summary evaluation measure, with values hypothetically ranging from 0 to 1, with 1 representing maximal reliability. According to magnitude and country, ranked suicide rates are compared or correlated with ranked combined rates of suicide and various causes of death documented in the literature as susceptible to suicide misclassification. English physician-researcher Brian Barraclough (1973) conducted a study of 22 countries in which he compared rankings of the magnitude of their suicide rates with those of rates combining suicides and undetermined intent deaths. This comparison generated a rank-order correlation coefficient of 0.89. In a study of 19 European countries, also conducted by English researchers, the composite comparison rates included accidental drowning and poisoning deaths, as well as suicides and also deaths from other violence, which were a proxy or surrogate for undetermined deaths (Sainsbury & Jenkins, 1982). The associated correlation coefficient was 0.96. Thus, the summary measures from both studies reflected high concordance in respective rate rankings. In turn, they might be used to reinforce an argument or assumption that international suicide data are reliable. However, missing from the respective calculations was the most diffuse and vague cause-of-death category: symptoms, signs, and ill-defined conditions. This residual category may be highly prone to contain misclassified suicides, especially when decedents had multiple morbidities and were elderly. To reiterate, consistent with official classification practices, the suicide research and prevention communities typically view suicide as an acute injury phenomenon. Hence, purported slow methods generally lie outside the purview of their respective domains, although some individuals with self-inflicted wounds who intended to die may have done so only months after the event.

Validity of suicide certification

Patrick O'Carroll (1989), a CDC epidemiologist, adapted methodology from public health and clinical epidemiology pertaining to the evaluation of disease screening programs and therapies to show that the validity of suicide data can be evaluated from two complementary perspectives: specificity and sensitivity. In measuring true negativity—the percentage of deaths that are true nonsuicides—specificity approximates 100%. This is because suicide is not a default, residual, or fallback option for medicolegal officials, and most deaths are patently nonsuicides. Consequently, specificity of suicide certification, and thus overreporting, should not generally be problematic for international, national, or more local suicide research when the data originated in nontotalitarian countries. Other plausible exceptions are certain total institutions like prisons, jails, and maximum-security or forensic psychiatric hospitals (Mitchell & Aronson, 2023). Sensitivity of suicide certification and underreporting are of great concern for research and prevention. Sensitivity measures true positivity, that is, the percentage of correctly certified suicides. Findings from studies that will be presented in the next chapter indicate that there is considerable cross-national variation in sensitivity. In turn, this variation implicates substantial heterogeneity in a constellation of forces, including many already identified: stigma, punitive provisions in life insurance policies, selection of suicide method, duration of dying, sociocultural milieu, nature and training of medicolegal officials and their staffs, and use of forensic autopsies, toxicologic testing, standardized protocols, and psychological autopsies in medicolegal death investigations.

Social construction of suicide rates

In the *Handbook of Suicidology*, published in 1979, Tufts University psychologist Louis Wekstein wrote that "statistics on suicide are synthetic; that is, they are concocted products, and their inaccuracy and unreliability are an open secret. They are contrived by necessity; and variations from country or region may reflect overt or covert underrepresentation" (1979, 38).

Washington State University's Melanie-Angela Neuilly, a criminologist, commented that "death is not solely a physiological and biological event, it is also a social and administrative one" (2022, 233). The social and administrative components loom even larger when the manner of death is suicide. Social constructionists represent a school of thought that critiques the process of how humans create knowledge, such as knowledge founded on measurement and quantification (Burr, 1995). Social constructionism is informed by such factors as education, training, religious beliefs, political ideology, and governance. Lindsay Prior, a sociologist from Queen's University in Belfast, Northern Ireland, stated that "the usefulness of mortality statistics as a resource for epidemiological and sociological research can only be assessed in the light of knowledge concerning their production" (1985, 186).

In 1967, applying social constructionism to suicide as a strongly socially condemned and stigmatized phenomenon, Jack Douglas wrote, "Facts strongly suggest that the relationship between statistical organizations and the suicide rates they produce is subject to the following principle: other things being equal, suicide rates vary directly with the degree of professional medical training of the categorizers, the average rate of man-hours devoted to cause of death categorization, and the independence of the categorizers from interested parties" (1967, 379), and in 1968, Joseph Davis and Joseph Spelman, both of whom once held the presidency of the National Association of Medical Examiners, similarly asserted that "proper diagnosis [or adjudication] of suicidal death rests upon adequate personnel, appropriate legislation, and financial and community support" (1968, 453).

Clear in the conceptual and empirical work I previously cited, generation of official statistics on suicide is a highly complex process riddled with impediments to the attainment of high sensitivity of certification. Beyond compilation of the raw medicolegal data, quality control of suicide statistics falls within the province of a sequence of government bureaucrats, whose competence, dedication, and oversight are plausibly highly variable. In brief, there is an ominous caveat inherent in the social constructionist perspective for any researchers, policymakers, preventionists, and other users who are inclined to accept official suicide data or any official data at face value for that matter.

In the 1980s, sociologist Bernice Pescosolido and economist Robert Mendelsohn tested the relationship between social constructionism and suicide in the United States, using county-level suicide rates for 1970 as their outcome variable (Pescosolido & Mendelsohn, 1986). In their widely cited ecological or correlational study, they employed a two-step multivariable statistical approach to assess whether systematic misreporting of suicide diminished the explanatory power of social causation factors to account for local rate variation. Three variables represented social construction: type of medicolegal death investigation system, selection procedure of responsible officials, and nature of facilities available to them over the course of their investigations. The authors concluded that although there was evidence of systematic misreporting, with elected coroners most prone to undercount suicides, the influence of artifactuality on rate variation was minor. However, very problematic for generalizing research results was the confinement of the study population to Whites. Moreover, the authors omitted decedent age and differences in suicide case ascertainment procedures between medical examiners and coroners as covariates from their statistical analysis of suicide data quality in the United States (Jobes et al., 1987). A covariate is a variable that may be predictive of the research outcome or dependent variable of interest, such as the magnitude of a suicide rate, and whose omission by the researchers as a predictor or control variable may induce misleading or inaccurate results.

The authors of a subsequent ecological study of county variation in suicide rates, which used national data for 1999–2002, concluded that elected coroners were more susceptible than appointed medical examiners and coroners to undercounting suicide (Klugman et al., 2013). Drawing on conventional conceptions, these investigators interpreted the modest rate variation, according to type of death investigation system, as a product of less autonomy and greater political pressure on elected coroners to rule against suicide as the manner of death, emanating from the social stigmatization of suicide and less scientific rigor in the case ascertainment process.

Treading the pathway forged by Irene Ovenstone in the 1970s, three suicidologists in Scotland conducted a limited test of the tenability of social construction in suicide determination in the 1980s (Platt et al., 1988). They examined 1,077 deaths in Edinburgh that had officially been classified as suicides or undetermined deaths during the period 1968–83, to evaluate whether the former differed from the latter regarding the prevalence of prior psychiatric contact. Psychiatric contact covered both inpatient and outpatient treatment at either of two area hospitals, as well as admission to a poisoning treatment center pursuant to an episode of parasuicide. Parasuicide mimics a suicide attempt, but without lethal intent, and essentially functioned in the Edinburgh study as a proxy for mental health variables, such as depression, alcoholism, and social isolation, which are established risk factors for suicide. Under social constructionism, knowledge of psychiatric/psychological history might predispose officials to classify decedents as suicides. The researchers considered evidence of lack of difference between suicides and deaths of undetermined intent as refutation of a related social constructionist hypothesis. Comparing undetermined deaths with suicides on various circumstances and other characteristics could beget invaluable insights on suicide case ascertainment related to observed differences between the two groups of decedents.

Besides prior psychiatric contact, other independent variables for predicting a suicide versus undetermined classification in the Scottish study were decedent sociodemographics (age, sex, marital status, and social class) and method (injury mechanism). The researchers distinguished suicide methods as active (hanging, jumping, firearms, and cutting), passive (poisoning, gassing, and residual passive methods, e.g., jumping from a height, victim-precipitated homicide, and vehicle crash), and drowning. Linguistically, I prefer "more and less behaviorally and forensically overt" to "active" and "passive." Under this alternative terminology, drowning could then be grouped with the researchers' passive methods as a less overt one.

Registered suicides were 66% of their pooled suicide and undetermined deaths in the study. More overt methods were more likely than less overt methods to be associated with a suicide classification, but the proportions were the same by sex. Whereas no statistically significant interaction emerged between prior psychiatric contact and sex or between method and sex, it was observed between age and sex. A higher proportion of deaths of female decedents under age 40 years were classified as suicide, as were a higher proportion of deaths of male decedents aged 40 years and older.

Large sample size was touted as a major strength of the study by the researchers. Benefiting from hindsight, I beg to differ. The study was small, even ignoring the fact that we are now living in an era of artificial intelligence and big data, where I define artificial intelligence as a set of technologies, enabled by computers/machines, that autonomously simulate human intelligence to enhance knowledge in performing such tasks as learning, reasoning, creating, problem-solving, translating, and decision-making. Consequently, the researchers likely missed some substantively important associations. Predictors were few. However, in their discussion, the researchers referenced other putatively important variables, including evidence of a suicide note and/or previous suicide attempts. Although not incorporated in the study, I appreciate their acknowledgment that the accident manner-of-death category contains covert or misclassified suicides. The study was innovative and markedly influenced the design and implementation of some of my later research.

A seemingly egregious example of social constructionism in suicide determination was exposed by the late University of Nebraska–Lincoln sociologist Hugh Whitt (2006) in his study of the declining suicide rate in the New York City borough of Manhattan during the 1980s. Rate decline was not evident in the other four boroughs of Staten Island, Queens, the Bronx, and Brooklyn. Whitt concluded that the Manhattan aberration was an artifact of political, economic, and journalistic pressures that induced medical examiners to assign "accident" wittingly, but surreptitiously, as the manner of death in many true suicide cases. One alternative explanation to deliberate suicide misclassification would be that the misclassification ensued from poorly trained and overstressed staff working in a chaotic environment. Another less plausible explanation involves variable socioeconomic status and suggests that the observed differences in suicide trends are not artifactual. Manhattan is more affluent than the other boroughs.

Strongly implicating an opposite influence from social construction on suicide counts, another study showed increasing not decreasing numbers of suicides among American Black youth from the 1970s through the mid-1990s, which paralleled a decline in their deaths classified as undetermined or accidental drowning, poisoning, fall, or shooting (Best, 2004). Since criteria for medicolegal assignments of deaths as suicide are conservative, this increase was likely partially or wholly a product of improved measurement, or more precisely an increase in the sensitivity of suicide certification for Black youth.

Over time, I have come to embrace "social constructionism" as a label for my orientation or perspective in researching suicide data quality and as reinforcement of my advocacy for better concepts and more accurate and representative data to improve suicide and other self-injury surveillance, research, prevention, and evaluation.

Operational criteria for suicide determination

Mark Rosenberg, a prominent CDC psychiatrist and public health researcher, convened an expert panel to develop operational criteria for determining suicides in the United States toward the close of the 1980s (Rosenberg et al., 1988). With no parallel since, his panel recommended that medical examiners and coroners assign a death as suicide where there was a fatal injury or injuries that involved self-infliction coupled with evidence substantiating an intention to die and specified criteria. To establish the self-infliction of means, medicolegal death investigation teams must focus on proximal behavioral evidence collected postmortem and analyzed through toxicology and autopsy, as well as refer to police reports and any supplementary psychological evidence. Often very contentious, because most acts of suicide are unwitnessed and the subjects are deceased (De Leo et al., 2006), substantiation of intent puts the focus much more squarely on premortem psychological/psychiatric factors.

In 2007, originating from the work of the panel, CDC enumerated the types of information that can serve as evidence of suicide:

1. There is evidence that death was self-inflicted. Pathological (autopsy), toxicological, investigatory, and psychological evidence, and statements of the decedent or witnesses, may be used for this determination.
2. There is evidence (explicit and/or implicit) that at the time of injury the decedent intended to kill [him- or her]self or wished to die and that the decedent understood the probable consequences of his or her actions:
    a. Explicit verbal or nonverbal expression of intent to kill self
    b. Implicit or indirect evidence of intent to die, such as the following:
        i. Expression of hopelessness
        ii. Effort to procure or learn about means of death or rehearse fatal behavior
        iii. Preparations for death, inappropriate to or unexpected in the context of the decedent's life
        iv. Expression of farewell or desire to die, or acknowledgment of impending death
        v. Precautions to avoid rescue
        vi. Evidence that decedent recognized high potential lethality of means of death
        vii. Previous suicide attempt
        viii. Previous suicide threat
        ix. Stressful events or significant losses (actual or threatened)
        x. Serious depression or mental disorder. (Department of Health and Human Services et al., 2007, 21–22)

No research blueprint

The pre-1990s conceptual thinking and empirical research reported in this and the previous chapter could have served as a blueprint for the bulk of my research and scholarship, which I will present over most of the remainder of this book. However, reality was quite different. Some of that material I had carefully read before embarking on my incremental journey into medicolegal determination of suicide and suicide data quality—particularly that assessing the reliability of suicide rates using rank-order correlation coefficients. Other material I had read only cursorily, and much not at all. An example of my ignorance, I only uncovered "Methodological Strategies in Suicide," published in 1986, in March 2024 (Robins and Kulbok, 1986). This article highlighted how various epidemiologic research designs could be more or less effective in the investigation of suicide outcomes. Of particular interest to me was the authors' cognizance of how artifacts in measurement could contribute to observed differences in suicide rates across such variables as space, time, autopsy and toxicology prevalence, heterogeneity in suicide case ascertainment criteria, race, political pressure, and religion. In naming religion, they invoked the research of Émile Durkheim.

My own work did eventually position me to prepare my background chapters on suicide data quality with far more insight and appreciation than I could have summoned at the beginning of my journey over three decades ago. Nonetheless, deficits in my reading may inadvertently have led me to reinvent wheels. As an offset, when this was the case, reinvention transpired in a new context with very different data. This is most profoundly exemplified by the overlapping suicide and opioid mortality epidemics that continue to afflict the United States, although both were overshadowed temporarily, but likely exacerbated, by the COVID-19 pandemic. In addition, my methods frequently varied from those of prior researchers who studied suicide data quality. I now launch into an account of my evolution as a suicidologist and data skeptic and my gradual conversion from a pessimist to an optimist about effecting change in how society and government agencies view suicide and other fatal self-injury.

NOTE

1. The proportion of deaths in a country assigned to ill-defined conditions and unknown causes serves as a crude indicator of the quality and coverage of that country's

cause-specific mortality. Less than 3% of deaths are so assigned in high-income countries, whereas the prevalence (proportion or percentage) tends to be much higher in low-income ones, according to Our World in Data (n.d.) (https://ourworldindata.org/). With temporal reporting differences, which were slight compared to the magnitude of the prevalence gaps, the United States posted a prevalence of 1.4% in 2021, compared to 10.4% in Poland in 2020 and 22.7% in Thailand in 2019. Many low-income countries did not report this information to the WHO, the global health data repository. In all countries using the *International Classification of Diseases, Tenth Revision*, nosologists (medical coders) employ "ill-defined conditions and unknown causes," formerly labeled "signs, symptoms, and ill-defined conditions," as a residual cause-of-death category.

3

American Suicide Data Quality in International Perspective

Two cross-national injury mortality studies

During the mid-1980s, I worked as an injury epidemiologist at the Rhode Island Department of Health. Ignorant of the specialty at hire, I rapidly benefitted from the orientation and guidance that internal and external experts offered me. My primary focus was motor vehicular traffic trauma, for which I designed and implemented a statewide hospital emergency department study and conducted two seatbelt use surveys. Almost concurrently, I embarked on a series of cross-national injury mortality studies, thanks in part to the courtesy of an enlightened and lenient boss.

The first three studies examined comparative patterns. They variously included seven countries: the United States, the United Kingdom, France, West Germany, Japan, Australia, and New Zealand. By the time of publication, I had secured employment as an epidemiologist at the University of Tennessee, Knoxville. In each study, I had a coauthor, New Zealander Gordon Smith, who was a fellow injury epidemiologist, then serving as an epidemiologic intelligence service (EIS) officer at the Centers for Disease Control and Prevention (CDC) headquarters in Atlanta, Georgia. An EIS officer is a trainee in field epidemiology who learns his/her craft through classes and participating in teams responding to public health threats domestically and overseas, especially in less developed nations. My introduction to Smith came through a 45-minute phone call in which he was very generous in giving me an overview of injury epidemiology.

Following a first article on cross-national premature injury mortality (Rockett & Smith, 1987), which appeared in the *American Journal of Public Health*, our second article reported the findings from a five-country study in the same journal (Rockett & Smith, 1989). That article marked the entry of suicide into my research domain. The data were age-, sex-, and cause-specific mortality tabulations for populations aged 15 years and older in 1980, and their source was the World Health Organization (WHO). Although children and younger teens can die by suicide, such cases are extremely rare. Consequently, their suicide rates are unstable and difficult to study statistically. Among notable findings from our second study, only the United States showed a female suicide rate peaking at younger middle age. I later learned anecdotally that this middle-aged peaking also existed in Canada and some Scandinavian countries. In France, West Germany, Japan, and the United Kingdom, the four other countries in the study, female suicide rates emulated those of all country-specific males in peaking among the elderly. A second notable finding was that elderly Japanese females registered by far the highest suicide rates for their sex.

Consistent with most population-based records and related epidemiologic research, the variable sex in this book is a binary distinction, male or female, derived from assignation at birth according to a visual anatomic assessment. Although biological sex is frequently used interchangeably with gender in population-based research, they are different concepts. See chapter 10.

Questioning elderly Japanese female drownings

The preceding cross-national research was followed by an article marking my debut in the realm of suicide undercounting (Rockett & Smith, 1993). This study examined drowning suicides among the Japanese female population as an intriguing outlier. Its genesis sprang from my serendipitous perusal of a series of graphs I had previously prepared on age-, sex-, cause-, and country-specific injury mortality data. In an "aha" moment, what caught my attention was similarity in patterns between the suicide rates and the accidental or unintentional drowning rates among Japanese females. This similarity prompted me to question whether drowning was a common suicide method for this group. Unfortunately, the question could not be answered from the WHO data, which were an aggregation of country mortality datasets. However, the Japanese Ministry of Health and Welfare graciously and expeditiously honored my request for the requisite data, in English translation (fortuitously for me). Their rapid response was a vote of confidence for the importance they accorded suicide research. The data for 1980 showed that drowning was indeed a common method of suicide in Japan, especially for females. Confirmation followed when my research assistant, Chise Kumano, translated an earlier Japanese article that reported drowning as the method in 1 in 7 female suicides, versus 1 in 19 male suicides (Chikazawa, 1974).

The Japanese study was the first in which I calculated ratios, employing some manner- and cause-specific categories that potentially contained misclassified suicides, to address suicide data quality. In this instance, the categories were undetermined intent and accidental drowning. With advancing age, drowning became a much more common suicide method for Japanese females than males. At ages 15–24 years, for example, the respective ratios of accidental drownings to undetermined deaths for females and males were 0.2 and 2.3, and at 75 years and older they were 13.9 and 2.7. The accidental drowning mortality rates and drowning suicide rates increased markedly with age for both sexes. After ages 15–24, there was an inverse relationship between age and magnitude in the ratio of accidental drownings to drowning suicides. However, the trend was much more pronounced among females, where the ratio declined from 5:1 at ages 25–34 years to less than 1:1 at ages 75 and older. It remained under parity for males across the age spectrum. Respective declines in that ratio were 81% for females versus 49% for males.

My ex post facto explanation for the finding that elderly Japanese women appeared highly prone to suicide misclassification, within the accidental drowning category, rested on age-sex differentials in the ratio of drowning suicides to "accidental" or unintentional drownings and speculation that implicated the effects of timing—when they died and when they were born, as well as their age at death. These women had matured prior to the post–World War II American occupation of Japan, when suicide was unstigmatized and even glorified, but died in 1980, during an era when suicide faced increasing social stigma as Western values were being superimposed on, if not displacing, traditional ones. Moreover, at their time of death most of these decedents likely had been living alone, as the nuclear family was replacing the extended family as the basic household unit. There was a large sex gap in life expectancy at birth in favor of females, and females typically married at younger ages than their husbands. Adherence to traditional values, coupled with sensitivity to new or modified ones, may have motivated some elderly Japanese women to conceal from their progeny stresses, crises, and, ultimately, suicide as an elected manner of death. Perhaps their motive was altruistic—not wanting to burden their children.

Needing further scientific investigation, drowning may still be more problematic than poisoning for suicide data quality in Japan and some European countries than in the United States. A comparative study of suicide methods in Japan and the United States, using data for 1999, showed that drowning stood out as a method for Japanese women, except in comparison with American Black women (Ojima et al., 2004). Even as a suicide method for Japanese women, however, drowning was much less common than hanging and jumping from a high place, especially at a scenic spot—historically representing a beautiful death. Hanging, a forensically overt method, was dominant in accounting for 60% of their official suicides. To reiterate, the Japanese study arose from serendipity, a revelation from a welcome and most unanticipated insight. An unanswered question, given the data limitations, was the extent to which the females drowning by suicide had done so in bathtubs, swimming pools, streams, rivers, lakes, or oceans. Salient to prevention and restriction of means, for example, did they have easier access than the general public to large bodies of water? If so, did this impact the choice of method? Among more equivocal suicide methods, I had viewed drowning as of greater consequence in the United States than drug intoxication and other poisoning through much of the opening decade of the twenty-first century. However, the slow realization that I was living amid an opioid epidemic led me to downgrade my subjective ranking for this country.

In concluding my discussion of the Japanese drowning study, I note that a newer study, which examined mortality data for 47 prefectures between 1995 and 2016, indicated that Japanese suicide data are of high quality (Matsubayashi & Ueda, 2021). One enduring lesson from my fascinating Japanese interlude was the importance of being receptive to unexpected research opportunities, coupled with a willingness to follow through. I have been fortunate to have experienced other such "aha" moments as a researcher. Apropos, I believe, is this quote from Louis Pasteur, the renowned French chemist and microbiologist: "Dans les champs de l'observation le hazard ne favorise que les esprits prepares" (Where observation is concerned, chance favors only the prepared mind). Unfortunately, economic constraints increasingly dictate that new scientists and scholars adhere to pragmatic and conservative pathways as they doggedly pursue the money to support their research. "Eat what you kill" has become a universal slogan in this grant-grab, publish-or-perish world of twenty-first-century academia.

As a not rare companion and muse on my own research journey, I am enchanted by the mystery and power of serendipity, a chance happening with beneficial outcomes. For readers wishing to delve deeper into this phenomenon in action, I enthusiastically recommend Morton Meyers's *Happy Accidents: Serendipity in Modern Medical Breakthroughs* (2007). The author references the late Nobel laureate theoretical physicist and media personality Richard Feynman, who observed that the demands for publishing science as a polished article and maintaining professional dignity allow no room for admitting the role of serendipity in discovery. Regrettably, my own articles are no exceptions, save my obscure, brief, and little-cited research autobiography in the *International Review of Modern Sociology* (Rockett, 2017). That article—one I immensely enjoyed writing—addressed biological sex (misstated as gender) and suicide misclassification. I was pleasantly surprised to find out that it was "discovered" and cited in a global suicide study in one elite medical journal, *The Lancet* (GBD 2017 SDG Collaborators, 2018), and in a CDC report on female suicide (Crosby et al., 2021).

Another serendipitous story, which also featured in *Happy Accidents*, involved a hometown hero of mine, Barry Marshall. While a medical resident in training at Royal Perth Hospital in the early 1980s, Marshall, along with Robin Warren, a pathologist at the same hospital, hypothesized that *Helicobacter pylori* (*H. pylori*) caused peptic (gastric and duodenal) ulcers. Later affirmed, their hypothesis rested on laboratory observations by Warren and painful self-experimentation by Marshall. One common notion was that peptic ulcers ensued from the overconsumption of spicy foods. However, whereas spicy foods may aggravate them, they are not the initiators. Although a leading suicide determinant, stress was long mistakenly considered by the public and many physicians as the primary cause of ulcers. Being the spokesperson for the *H. pylori* research, Marshall endured years of ridicule from stubborn foes in the scientific establishment for alleged naivety and lack of training in the scientific method. Ultimate vindication came for Marshall and Warren, however, when they received the 2005 Nobel Prize in Physiology or Medicine. No longer was Perth an Antipodean outpost—or, adopting the jocularity of Morton Meyers, Western Australia was no longer "the wrong end of the wrong place."

Conventional wisdom asserted that bacteria could not survive in the acidic environment of the stomach. This was incorrect, as *H. pylori* produced their own protective alkaline environment. Superseding primitive treatments or pseudotreatments like gastric freezing, effective therapy for stomach ulcers is typically a course of two antibiotics and the administration of a proton pump inhibitor, which suppresses acid accumulation. Later research determined that *H. pylori* causes gastric cancer and non-Hodgkin lymphoma. These diseases have a far longer latency period than ulcers.

Ratios and evaluation of cross-national suicide data quality

My application of ratios to suicide rates was expanded in a paper I delivered in 1994 at the National Institutes of Health in Bethesda, Maryland, as part of the inaugural conference of the International Collaborative Effort (ICE) on International Injury Statistics (Rockett & Smith, 1995). This paper combined a literature review of issues that I deemed important in researching suicide data quality and the results of a suicide study of 29 countries, including the United States. Data were cause-specific mortality statistics for 1990 from the WHO. The first of two sets of ratio calculations incorporated three categories I had identified in the literature as most susceptible to suicide misclassification: accidental drowning, accidental poisoning, and undetermined intent—although data inaccessibility necessitated use of the residual "other violence" category as a proxy for undetermined deaths. The ratio of these combined deaths to suicides extended from 0.1 for Austria to 4.1 for Mexico. Results indicated minimal potential for suicide misclassification in those three alternative categories in Austria, Hungary, and the Netherlands (Holland)—perhaps due to having unified health systems and routine surveillance—and high potential in such countries as Romania, the Union of Soviet Socialist Republics, Portugal, and Malta, as well as Mexico. The addition of symptoms, signs, and ill-defined conditions to the second set of ratio calculations produced a range from 0.2 for Austria and Hungary to 16.8 for Greece. I inferred that the Austrian and Hungarian data were of extremely high quality because the ratios were low, and I deemed it a reasonable assumption that few of the nonsuicide deaths were misclassified suicides. Expressed colloquially, there was little wiggle room for nosologists in Hungary and Austria to get it wrong. By contrast, combined rate ratios exceeding 6.0 cast serious doubt on the quality of the suicide data from Uruguay, Mexico, Portugal, and Greece. I speculate that religion and economics played a role in their outcomes.

The purpose of using ratios to generate a comparative picture of suicide data quality, for countries with the requisite data, was to highlight major discrepancies, not small differentials. I knew that most of the deaths in the nonsuicide categories were not misclassified suicides. This cognizance also pertained to my second international study, as well as to subsequent related research on the United States. In this study, I calculated annual-averaged sex-, age-, and cause-specific rates based on mortality data for the period 1988–90 and the population aged 15 years and older from the WHO for 20 countries (Rockett & Thomas, 1999). My coauthor and I first assessed data reliability by computing rank-order correlation coefficients for suicide rates and the combined suicide, accidental drowning, accidental poisoning, and other violence (a proxy for undetermined) mortality rates by age and sex. With 1.00 the cap, coefficients ranged from 0.93 to 0.97, indicating that suicide data would be more than sufficiently reliable to justify their use in epidemiologic and sociological research. The sensitivity of the suicide data was much more problematic. We estimated the sensitivity, that is, the true positivity of suicide certification across the countries, expressed as a percentage, with the suicide rate as the numerator and the combined rates as the denominator. Hungary was not in the study, but the results again yielded confidence in the high quality of the Austrian suicide data, irrespective of sex or age, with sensitivity mainly occupying the narrow 80%–90% range. At the other end of the quality spectrum lay suicide case ascertainment for Israeli, Greek, and Irish females aged 75 years and older, with estimated sensitivity concentrated in the range of 39%–43%, and that for Israeli males aged 15–24 years, with estimated sensitivity at 38%. We concluded that the general quality of American suicide statistics was good—second tier—but not excellent, and we were concerned about the quality for female seniors, where sensitivity was only 55%. In the discussion section of the article, we noted that American decedents aged 65 years and older had an autopsy rate one-third that for those aged 15–64 years and only one-fifth that of their Austrian counterparts.

Israeli vindication of the indirect methodology

In between the ICE paper and the last-mentioned study, I was fortunate to be asked to present a paper at the second ICE conference, which took place in Melbourne, Australia, in 1996. At the conference, I casually and a bit facetiously remarked to Vita Barell, a distinguished injury epidemiologist, that Israeli suicide data had serious deficits. To my utter astonishment, she readily concurred and told me about an in-depth investigation that she and colleagues had conducted concerning underreporting of suicides among Jewish males aged 18–21 years in Israel (Barell, 1995). Focusing on accidental firearm deaths only, she and her team had discovered major misclassification of suicide. I later wondered how many more missed suicides they may have discovered had they investigated fatal accidental poisoning and drowning cases. Barell's motivation for the study was that the males in question were likely preoccupied with military conscription and service. Adopting a broader conceptual focus but a narrower geographic one, a psychotherapist/psychopathologist and colleagues subsequently drew attention to areas of concern about suicide detection or case ascertainment in Tel Aviv, Israel (Bakst et al., 2016). A valid criticism of my research on suicide data quality is its indirect nature. However, the results of our second international study, considered in conjunction with those from the Israeli field investigation, bolstered my confidence about making inferential leaps when apparent discrepancies in suicide rates across countries and decedent demographic characteristics are large.

Life table analysis and premature mortality

My paper at the second ICE conference was a life table analysis of the impact of the hypothetical elimination of injury mortality on life expectancy at various ages in the American population and those of eight other countries (Rockett, 1998b). The population-based life table is a versatile tool with a long history dating back to late seventeenth-century England and the avocational calculations of astronomer Edmond Halley (of Halley's Comet fame) on mortality data from the Germanic state of Breslau—now Wroclaw, Poland (Love, 2023), following its de-Germanization after World War II. Demographers, actuaries, and epidemiologists employ this tool to estimate life expectancy at birth and other ages for a designated population and to project the years of life lost by the total population and the decedents themselves.

The life table also allows researchers to estimate potential gains and losses in life expectancy as an outcome of specific diseases, exposures, other events, and interventions. In my study, estimated gains in life expectancy at birth in the United States were 2.08 years for males and 0.81 years for females. Taking the data at face value, elimination of suicide would have accounted for 21% of those gains among males and 15% of the female gains. Gains were far more substantial for the subpopulations whose deaths would have been hypothetically averted had injury mortality been eliminated. The "saved" males and females would have averaged 31.4 and 26.6 additional years of life, respectively. This line of research becomes highly relevant in chapter 8, where I share findings from a comparative analysis of self-injury and disease mortality. In terms of public health and prevention, the implications of death are not equal given that people dying younger have lost many more years of potential life than those dying at older ages. Worth consideration by health planners and policymakers, the two major summary death rates, the crude rate and the cause-specific rate, obscure the unequal force of premature mortality. However, comparative measures of years of life or health lost captured it.

Estimating upper and lower limits for suicide rates

Employing a similar methodology to that I had used previously, I published (with colleagues) ratio estimates for the United States and 27 European countries circa 2006 (Rockett et al., 2011; see table 3.1). Our data source for the United States was CDC's Wide-ranging Online Data for Epidemiologic Research database, and for the remaining countries we used the WHO's European Health for All database.

We first calculated the ratio of the undetermined death rate to the suicide rate, the basis for a lower-limit estimate of the true suicide rate and associated upper-limit estimates of the sensitivity of suicide certification. These ratios ranged from lows of 0.02 for Spain, 0.03 for Italy, and 0.04 for France and Hungary to highs of 0.43 for Poland, 0.53 for the United Kingdom, and 0.55 for Estonia. Adopting a more conservative approach, we then calculated the ratio of the combined undetermined intent and ill-defined conditions and unknown cause death rates to the suicide rate. Signifying high-quality suicide data, the Hungarian ratio only increased to 0.10. Suggesting data of moderately high quality, the American ratio rose from 0.15 to 0.58. By contrast, the ratio for Spain rose from 0.02 to 2.42, that for Poland from 0.43 to 4.45, and that for Cyprus from 0.10 to 18.26. Also noteworthy, the ratio for the Netherlands increased from 0.06 to 3.01. Within- and across-country discrepancies in range and magnitude in the two sets of ratios give pause concerning the interpretation of international variation in

Table 3.1. Ratio of undetermined injury intent and ill-defined conditions and unknown cause mortality rates to suicide rates for selected countries, circa 2006

Country	Suicide rate per 100,000	Ratio of undetermined injury intent mortality rate to suicide rate	Ratio of combined undetermined injury intent and ill-defined and unknown cause mortality rates to suicide rate
Cyprus	2.4	0.10	18.26
Portugal	9.6	0.60	7.07
Poland	14.3	0.43	4.45
Latvia	19.3	0.36	4.07
Bulgaria	10.5	0.18	3.36
Netherlands	8.7	0.06	3.01
Denmark	10.6	0.26	2.93
Estonia	18.7	0.55	2.58
Spain	6.6	0.02	2.42
France	15.4	0.04	2.30
United Kingdom	6.5	0.53	2.13
Norway	11.2	0.00	2.10
Germany	9.8	0.22	1.93
Italy	5.2	0.03	1.75
Sweden	12.0	0.23	1.57
Slovakia	11.9	0.40	1.50
Luxembourg	13.1	0.09	1.48
Switzerland	14.9	0.06	1.30
Malta	6.0	0.07	1.20
Lithuania	28.9	0.46	1.03
Czech Republic	12.2	0.34	0.97
Slovenia	22.8	0.16	0.80
USA	11.2	0.15	0.58
Austria	13.4	0.12	0.57
Romania	11.9	0.11	0.45
Ireland	9.1	0.16	0.40
Finland	19.0	0.08	0.32
Hungary	23.2	0.04	0.10

Source: Rockett, I.R.H., Kapusta, N.D., Bhandari, R., "Suicide misclassification in an international context: Revisitation and update," *Suicidology Online* 2011;2:48–61.

Note: All data are for 2006, except those for Estonia, Hungary, Slovakia, and Spain (which are for 2005) and those for Portugal (which are for 2004).

official suicide rates. They further justify an argument that the magnitude of the rate variation between countries at least partially reflects an artifactual component or social construction.

Later, using the same data, I calculated lower and upper estimates of suicide rates for the same 28 countries (Rockett & Kapusta, 2015). The lower rate estimates were calculated by dividing respective country-specific suicide rates by the combined suicide and undetermined mortality rates, and the upper estimates also included the death rate for ill-defined conditions and unknown causes in the denominator. The comparisons factored in the rates for ill-defined conditions and unknown causes. Thus, whereas the first value supports a claim that the cross-national data are highly reliable, the second indicates high unreliability. Indicating the least misclassification, Hungary's official suicide rate was 24.1 per 100,000 population, and its upper limit factoring in ill-defined conditions and unknown causes only increased to 25.5. In contrast, the official suicide rate for Cyprus was 2.4 per 100,000 population, and its upper limit rose 19-fold to 46.2. Corresponding rates for the United States were 11.2 and 17.7 per 100,000 population. None of these calculations, however, factored in accidental drowning and poisoning, two other cause-of-death categories strongly implicated in suicide misclassification.

Multiple causes of death and psychiatric documentation

Research opportunities occasionally materialize serendipitously from cyberspace, a variant on the spark for my study of drowning suicides among elderly Japanese females. An example of this occurred when I learned via email of an article by a Columbia University biostatistician on the virtues of multiple-cause-of-death analysis, which can allow for all of the causes listed on the death certificate and not just the underlying cause (Wall et al., 2005). Shortly thereafter, I uncovered an Australian multiple-cause-of-death study on suicide classification (Ruzicka et al., 2005). Its purpose was to examine associations between psychiatric and physical disease comorbidity (accompanying medical conditions) on the death certificate and classification of death as suicide versus accident, as the control or comparison group. This study used multivariable logistic regression analysis, a statistical procedure with a dichotomous dependent or outcome variable, which can accommodate more than one independent variable or correlate. The analysis showed associations for schizophrenia, depression / mood disorders, and cancer. Preparatorily to reporting their statistical findings, the authors of the Australian study presented prevalence data on the various comorbidities listed on the death certificates, disaggregated by age and sex.

Figure 3.1 shows the portion of a standard American death certificate

To Be Completed By: MEDICAL CERTIFIER

CAUSE OF DEATH (See instructions and examples)

32. **PART I.** Enter the chain of events--diseases, injuries or complications--that directly caused the death. DO NOT enter terminal events such as cardiac arrest, respiratory arrest, or ventricular fibrillation without showing the etiology. DO NOT ABBREVIATE. Enter only one cause on a line. Add additional lines if necessary.

Approximate interval: Onset to death

IMMEDIATE CAUSE (Final disease or condition ---------> resulting in death) a. ______ ______

Due to (or as a consequence of):

Sequentially list conditions, if any, leading to the cause listed on line a. Enter the **UNDERLYING CAUSE** (disease or injury that initiated the events resulting in death) **LAST**

b. ______ ______

Due to (or as a consequence of):

c. ______ ______

Due to (or as a consequence of):

d. ______ ______

PART II. Enter other significant conditions contributing to death but not resulting in the underlying cause given in PART I

33. WAS AN AUTOPSY PERFORMED?
□ Yes □ No

34. WERE AUTOPSY FINDINGS AVAILABLE TO COMPLETE THE CAUSE OF DEATH? □ Yes □ No

35. DID TOBACCO USE CONTRIBUTE TO DEATH?
□ Yes □ Probably
□ No □ Unknown

36. IF FEMALE:
□ Not pregnant within past year
□ Pregnant at time of death
□ Not pregnant, but pregnant within 42 days of death
□ Not pregnant, but pregnant 43 days to 1 year before death
□ Unknown if pregnant within the past year

37. MANNER OF DEATH
□ Natural □ Homicide
□ Accident □ Pending Investigation
□ Suicide □ Could not be determined

38. DATE OF INJURY (Mo/Day/Yr) (Spell Month)

39. TIME OF INJURY

40. PLACE OF INJURY (e.g., Decedent's home; construction site; restaurant; wooded area)

41. INJURY AT WORK?
□ Yes □ No

42. LOCATION OF INJURY: State: City or Town:
Street & Number: Apartment No.: Zip Code:

43. DESCRIBE HOW INJURY OCCURRED:

44. IF TRANSPORTATION INJURY, SPECIFY:
□ Driver/Operator
□ Passenger
□ Pedestrian
□ Other (Specify)

Figure 3.1. Causes and manner of death and other selected characteristics on the death certificate.

pertaining to autopsy status and the manner of death, as well as the immediate, contributing, and underlying cause-of-death information. Among other data provisions, also shown are the date, location, place, and circumstances of any injury, including whether it occurred at work or implicated transportation.

I decided to replicate the Australian multiple-cause-of-death study for the United States, using annual-averaged data for the period 1999–2003 from the National Center for Health Statistics—recognizing that the United States and Australia shared an identical suicide rate (at 11 per 100,000 population), democratic governance, and a similar level of socioeconomic development (Rockett et al., 2007). Age in the study was delimited to 15 years and older. There was no a priori reason to believe that Australians dying by suicide were more physically or mentally ill than their American counterparts. In referring to both studies for a cross-national comparison, Australia appeared to capture more comorbidity than the United States did among suicides on its death certificates. Despite the very similar associations between mental and physical comorbidities and a suicide versus an accident classification for Australia and the United States, one-quarter of Australian male suicides and one-third of Australian female suicides had at least one mental disorder or physical disease listed on their death certificates. This compared to just one-seventh and one-fifth of corresponding American decedents. The prevalence gap in registered comorbid mental and behavioral disorders between the two countries was striking. American death certificates only registered about one-third of the corresponding comorbidity prevalence reported on Australian death certificates for both sexes. The size of the comorbidity gap between Australian and American death certificates may suggest that Australian death investigators are more fastidious in accumulating evidence—benefitting from less fragmented health data collection systems—or, alternatively, in reporting accessible evidence. On the other hand, this gap may simply reflect differences in the training of the medicolegal death certifiers in Australia and the United States, which in turn may be a function of variable budgetary allocations.

Take, for example, firearm cases with cause of death being gunshot wound to the head, manner of death being suicide, how injury occurred being shot self with revolver, mental health diagnoses of major depressive disorder and alcohol use disorder, and augmenting social diagnoses of poverty and homelessness. For economic reasons, it would be understandable if American certifiers were trained to omit both the mental health and social diagnoses from the death certificate. However, even if Australian death certificates better capture psychopathology and circumstances from pertinent medicolegal records than American counterparts, they also appear deficient in documenting comorbidities as important evidence for corroborating suicides.

4

Are Black Suicide Rates Really Lower than White Rates?

A racial paradox and minority health data disparities

Untenable as biological constructs (Winker, 2008), race and race/ethnicity are social constructs that alternately generate adverse and beneficial social, economic, political, and health consequences in the United States (Krieger, 2000). Differences are most evident in large health disparities separating non-Hispanic Blacks from non-Hispanic Whites. Blacks manifest lower life expectancy at birth (Levine et al., 2001; Kochanek et al., 2019). Their disparities are consistent with their status as a vulnerable minority whose lives are characterized by racial oppression, discrimination, segregation, political gerrymandering, and voter suppression and nullification by the White majority population, as well as concomitant gross socioeconomic inequality, barriers to health care, medical exploitation, excess incarceration, willful distortion and erasure of public records, misappropriation of property, and associated profound stigma and stress dating back to the inception of slavery in the American colonies during the early seventeenth century (Moynihan, 1965; Myrdal, 1969).

Violent atrocities perpetrated by Whites against Black populations are myriad and far beyond tragic through present times. In the twentieth century, examples include the Tuskegee Syphilis Study; the murders of Emmet Till, Medgar Evers, and Martin Luther King Jr.; the Birmingham Church bombing that killed four young girls; and the bombing and shooting annihilation of the thriving Greenwood neighborhood of Tulsa, Oklahoma, also known as Black Wall Street. Exemplifying White-on-Black savagery and atrocities in the twenty-first century are the mass shootings in a Black church in

Charleston, South Carolina, and in a supermarket in Buffalo, New York, predominantly patronized by Blacks.

Initially overlooking earlier research on differential suicide misclassification by race conducted by Mary Ellen Warshauer and Mary Monk (1978) from Johns Hopkins University, I observed that American Blacks recorded a suicide rate less than half that of American Whites across most of the age spectrum. I wondered whether this differential was partially or wholly artifactual. In pondering the racial suicide paradox, I knew of no other manner or major cause of death where Blacks registered lower rates than Whites. My investigation of this paradox sensitized me to the very real possibility that racial health disparities are measured conservatively because the underlying calculations disregard what I term (minority) health data disparities, as conceptually distinct from health disparities. There is an extensive literature on health disparities, much related to differential access to health care. However, problematic access means that there will also be differential diagnosis and documentation of medical and mental health disorders by such population characteristics as race/ethnicity and socioeconomic status. In turn, these data gaps have adverse implications for medicolegal records. Before presenting and discussing my own research on suicide-related data disparities, I deem it essential to acknowledge prior work of others.

Warshauer and Monk's (1978) seminal study, conducted in New York City in the 1970s, provided direct evidence of a connection between race and differential suicide misclassification. Their study compared city health department records of suicides with corresponding records in the office of the medical examiner. The two researchers used medical examiner suicide cases as their criterion or gold standard. Besides cases signed out to the health department (definite suicides), they included cases medically diagnosed as suicide but where corroborative evidence would not meet legal standards (assigned, but not reported as suicides) and cases missed by the city health department because it had not requested final case disposition. Following the introduction of classification codes for injury of undetermined intent under the *International Classification of Diseases, Eighth Revision*, Warshauer and Monk found that Black suicide cases were almost twice as likely to be undercounted as White cases in the health department records. A higher prevalence of jumping from a height among Blacks compared to Whites complicated detection of their suicides. Easy access to means facilitated use of this method, since skyscrapers and many other high-rise buildings have long characterized New York City. The study also preceded the abundance of firearms, as a method more amenable than jumping to suicide detection.

In a study I discussed in chapter 2, David Phillips and Todd Ruth (1993) found indirect evidence of suicide undercounting among Blacks and women. Another study, which adapted their methodology to a study of suicide trends among the younger American population for the period 1979–94, reported excess undercounting for Blacks that peaked among Black male youth (Mohler & Earls, 2001). The authors concluded that systematic underreporting of suicide did not substantially affect the direction of trends in youth suicide.

Some scholars have speculated that the observed lower suicide rate for Blacks can be explained by the combination of greater social cohesion and religiosity (Utsey et al., 2007) and excess resilience in combatting relentless adversity, or by direction of anger and frustrations outward through homicide rather than inward through suicide (Henry & Short, 1954). By contrast, an eminent team of suicidologists from the University of Rochester asserted that there is no research explaining how being Black in the United States protects against suicide (Knox et al., 2004)—a rationale for my first study of the racial suicide paradox (Rockett et al., 2006b).

I extracted the underlying cause-of-death data used in my study from the Centers for Disease Control and Prevention's (n.d.-c) publicly accessible, query-based Web-based Injury Statistics Query and Reporting System (WISQARS). Examined cross-sectionally, these data covered the period 1999–2002. The demographic characteristics tapped were race (Black/White), age, and sex, with the study population further restricted to the age group 15 years and older. Suicide rates were annual averaged to minimize data instability. Nosologists precoded the causes of death according to the *International Classification of Diseases, Tenth Revision* (World Health Organization, 2004). Included manners or causes were suicide, sequelae of intentional self-harm, undetermined (injury intent), accidental or unintentional poisoning and exposure to noxious substances, and drowning. The literature identifies the three final categories as all being highly susceptible to suicide misclassification (Snowdon, 2023). I estimated lower and upper limits for the reported suicide rates by age, sex, and race using respective combinations of suicides plus undetermined deaths and suicides plus undetermined and accidental poisoning and drowning deaths. Only at ages 45–54 years was there rate crossover by race, where the combined rates for Blacks exceeded those

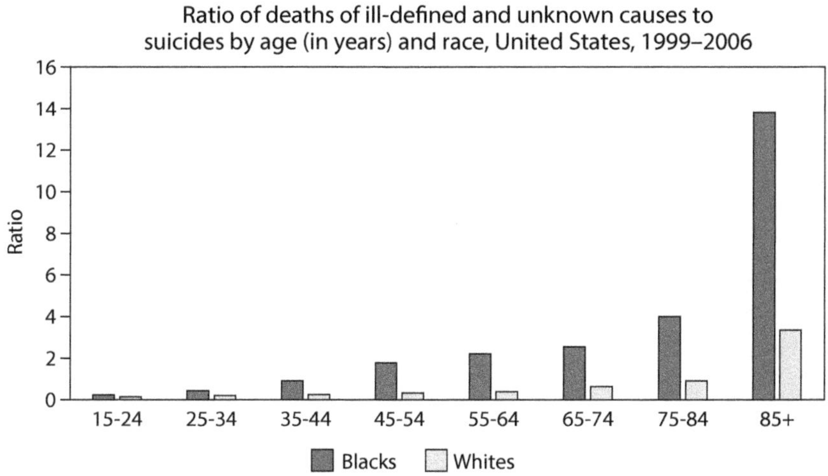

Figure 4.1. Ratio of deaths of ill-defined and unknown causes to suicides by age (in years) and race, United States, 1999–2006. Source: Centers for Disease Control and Prevention, *Wide-ranging Online Data for Epidemiologic Research (WONDER)*, underlying cause-of-death data, 1999–2020 (https://wonder.cdc .gov/ucd-icd10.html), and compressed mortality files, 1979–98 (https://wonder .cdc.gov/cmf-icd9.html).

for Whites. Crossover only occurred for males within the upper limit scenario. Nonetheless, particularly in that scenario, there was marked shrinkage of the racial suicide rate gaps by sex. The WISQARS data did not include many variables that might plausibly impact case ascertainment of suicide, such as death circumstances, psychiatric history, disease comorbidities, autopsy status, toxicology, and type of medicolegal death investigation system.

Originally, the upper rate estimates for suicide rates in the study also incorporated ill-defined conditions and unknown causes—a category even more imprecise and vague than undetermined—further closing the racial suicide gaps and enhancing rate crossover. However, I deleted the category from the calculations in complying with an editorial fiat, a regrettable demand given its proneness to suicide misclassification (Phillips & Ruth, 1993; Jougla et al., 2002). Previously unpublished, figure 4.1 illustrates enormous potential for differential suicide misclassification between American Blacks and Whites associated with the ill-defined and unknown causes of death—a differential that widened with increasing age. Researchers in Australia revealed undercounting of suicide within the ill-defined, undetermined, and accident manner-of-death categories (De Leo et al., 2010), findings included in a persuasive body of evidence that motivated a full-scale investigation of suicide and suicide data quality by officials of the Australian Senate. The ensuing report was entitled *The Hidden Toll: Suicide in Australia* (Senate Community Affairs Committee Secretariat, 2010). There is an urgent need for a similar investigation in the United States, where suicide reports have ignored or downplayed misclassification and undercounting. Even the Institute of Medicine's *Reducing Suicide: A National Imperative*, an otherwise thorough, expert-driven exposition of suicide and its challenges as of the beginning of the twenty-first century, dismissed these problems as an immutable fact of life: "Official suicide statistics are fraught with inaccuracies. Undetermined cases and open verdicts and under-reporting [diminish] their strength" (Goldsmith et al., 2002, 55). Moreover, this report showed no cognizance of health data disparities by race or race/ethnicity.

I prepared a table with sensitivity estimates from a prior study that strongly argue suicide certification for Blacks of both sexes and White females is inferior to the certification for White males (table 4.1). Overall estimated sensitivity of suicide certification for White males was 64.3% versus only 54.9%, 52.3%, and 26.7% for Black males, White females, and Black females, respectively. Generally, Black females showed the lowest sensitivity across age, with potential for gross suicide misclassification at ages 85 years and older. By contrast, White males manifested minimal susceptibility at the older ages. Great susceptibility to suicide misclassification was apparent at ages 35–54 years for Black males and at ages 25 years and older for Black females.

I used multiple cause-of-death files from the National Center for Health Statistics to conduct two studies in my quest to comprehend the racial paradox of White suicide rates exceeding those of Blacks. It was a simple leap for me to replicate the American study disaggregating race/ethnicity as non-Hispanic White, non-Hispanic Black, and Hispanic and using the same observation period, 1999–2003 (Rockett et al., 2009). There was no a priori evidence that Whites dying by suicide were more physically or mentally ill than minority counterparts, irrespective of sex. Yet, at 10.5%, comorbid mental and behavioral disorders were 27% more prevalent on the death certificates of White females than those for Black females and 39% more prevalent than those for Hispanic females (table 4.2). At 7.8%, they were 51% more prevalent for White males than for Black males and 60% more prevalent than for

Table 4.1. Estimated sensitivity of suicide certification by age, sex, and race: United States, 1999–2002

Age (years)	Black male (%)	White male (%)	Black female (%)	White female (%)
15–19	55.5	66.7	68.5	63.8
20–24	66.4	62.3	55.6	51.0
25–34	54.0	59.3	34.6	50.5
35–44	32.2	53.3	20.2	45.3
45–54	23.1	60.3	18.8	52.2
55–64	34.7	78.6	33.8	63.7
65–74	56.5	86.0	42.7	66.0
75–84	63.9	88.1	28.7	57.4
85+	41.0	85.5	11.1	44.0
Total	54.9	64.3	26.7	52.3

Source: Centers for Disease Control and Prevention, *Web-based Injury Statistics Query and Reporting System (WISQARS)*, https://www.cdc.gov/ncipc/wisqars.

Note: Sensitivity is estimated as the number of suicides divided by the combined number of suicides and deaths classified as other violence and accidental/unintentional drowning and poisoning multiplied by 100.

Table 4.2. Characteristics of prevalent comorbid conditions among United States suicides by sex and race/ethnicity

	Male			Female		
Medical condition (*ICD-10*)	White	Black	Hispanic	White	Black	Hispanic
Mental/behavioral disorders:						
Average mentions[a]	1.22	1.21	1.14	1.21	1.30	1.20
Percentage of total mentions	43.9	35.4	30.0	42.8	39.0	39.6
Percentage of total suicides	7.8	3.8	3.1	10.5	7.7	6.4
Physical disease:						
Average mentions	1.67	1.44	1.49	1.79	1.85	1.57
Percentage of total mentions	56.1	64.6	70.0	57.2	61.0	60.4
Percentage of total suicides	7.3	5.7	5.5	9.5	8.5	7.4
Total disorders/diseases:						
Average mentions	1.44	1.35	1.37	1.49	1.59	1.40
Percentage of suicides with 1 mention	15.1	9.5	8.6	20.0	16.2	13.8
Percentage of suicides with 2+ mentions	6.7	3.3	3.2	9.7	9.5	5.5

[a] Average = arithmetic mean.

Source: Rockett, I.R.H., Lian, Y., Stack, S., Ducatman, A.M., Wang S., "Discrepant comorbidity between minority and white suicides: A national multiple cause-of-death analysis," *BMC Psychiatry* 2009;9.

Table 4.3. Logistic regression analysis of the association of comorbidities listed on the death certificate with a suicide versus accident manner-of-death classification for three racial/ethnic groups: United States, 1999–2003

Medical condition (*ICD-10*)	Odds ratio[a]	95% CI (Wald)	
	Whites		
Mental/behavioral disorders:			
Organic (F00–F09)	0.11	0.089	0.129
Alcohol use (F10)	0.47	0.447	0.487
Other substance use (F11–F19)	0.18	0.171	0.196
Schizophrenia (F20–F29)	2.27	1.929	2.661
Depression / mood disorder (F30–F39)	31.34	29.273	33.561
Other mental health (F40–F99)	1.63	1.404	1.898
Physical disease:			
HIV (B20–B24)	0.88	0.636	1.220
Other communicable (A+B residual)	0.20	0.178	0.231
Cancer (C00–C99)	2.04	1.911	2.187
Nervous system (G00–G99)	0.72	0.686	0.758
Circulatory (I00–I99)	0.23	0.218	0.234
Respiratory (J00–J99)	0.21	0.200	0.222
Digestive (K00–K99)	0.61	0.562	0.656
Other diseases (D, E, H, L–R)	0.32	0.312	0.337
	Blacks		
Mental/behavioral disorders:			
Organic (F00–F09)	0.27	0.130	0.566
Alcohol use (F10)	0.31	0.259	0.376
Other substance use (F11–F19)	0.12	0.091	0.147
Schizophrenia (F20–F29)	4.13	2.701	6.322
Depression / mood disorder (F30–F39)	61.80	43.353	88.101
Other mental health (F40–F99)	1.12	0.550	2.291
Physical disease:			
HIV (B20–B24)	0.53	0.279	0.996
Other communicable (A+B residual)	0.29	0.195	0.438
Cancer (C00–C99)	1.88	1.388	2.535
Nervous system (G00–G99)	0.87	0.713	1.059
Circulatory (I00–I99)	0.22	0.191	0.255
Respiratory (J00–J99)	0.25	0.198	0.310
Digestive (K00–K99)	0.54	0.394	0.746
Other diseases (D, E, H, L–R)	0.36	0.315	0.420
	Hispanics		
Mental/behavioral disorders:			
Organic (F00–F09)	0.21	0.075	0.567
Alcohol use (F10)	0.30	0.254	0.366
Other substance use (F11–F19)	0.12	0.090	0.157
Schizophrenia (F20–F29)	4.01	1.985	8.108
Depression / mood disorder (F30–F39)	36.05	24.202	53.706
Other mental health (F40–F99)	2.60	1.240	5.437

Table 4.3. Continued

Medical condition (*ICD-10*)	Odds ratio[a]	95% CI (Wald)	
	Hispanics, continued		
Physical disease:			
HIV (B20–B24)	1.44	0.642	3.223
Other communicable (A+B residual)	0.26	0.152	0.431
Cancer (C00–C99)	1.26	0.811	1.943
Nervous system (G00–G99)	1.52	1.286	1.786
Circulatory (I00–I99)	0.26	0.216	0.304
Respiratory (J00–J99)	0.31	0.240	0.399
Digestive (K00–K99)	0.55	0.428	0.709
Other diseases (D, E, H, L–R)	0.40	0.342	0.470

[a] Odds ratios adjusted for age and sex. Unintentional injury decedents served as the referent or comparison group.

Source: Rockett, I.R.H., Lian, Y., Stack, S., Ducatman, A.M., Wang, S., "Discrepant comorbidity between minority and white suicides: A national multiple cause-of-death analysis," *BMC Psychiatry* 2009;9.

Hispanic males. Patterns of statistical associations between various comorbidities on the death certificate and a suicide versus accident manner-of-death classification were very similar by race/ethnicity (table 4.3).

Emphasizing the salience of psychiatric history for accurate suicide case ascertainment, a prior Tennessee record-based study of adult enrollees in TennCare, a Medicaid waiver, public assistance program, found that serious mood disorders among Black suicide decedents and possible suicide decedents were grossly underdiagnosed or undertreated relative to corresponding Whites (Ray et al., 2007). Possible suicides were operationalized as deaths from injury of undetermined intent, and no subjects had a record of chronic psychosis or serious medical illness. Only 29% of the Black subjects used prescription antidepressants in the year prior to death, compared to 51% of White subjects. A study conducted in Fulton County, Georgia, utilizing medical examiner data found that Black suicide decedents were 37% less likely than corresponding Whites to have previously reported depression (Abe et al., 2006).

Tangential to psychiatric/psychological determinants, but portentous for differential suicide misclassification by race or race/ethnicity, the Tennessee investigators reported that Black suicide decedents were 67% less likely than White suicide decedents to have left a suicide note (Ray et al., 2007). As forensic evidence, the suicide note becomes the focal point of research I will report on in the next chapter, although not in the racial/ethnic context.

Media dissemination

In April 2009, the results of my previous study were reported in a story in *HealthDay News* and other popular news outlets under the title "Death Certificates Incomplete for Suicide Victims." Although brief, this story captured the essence of this research, where I stated that "death certificates are vital to an understanding of suicide because they provide frontline data in terms of suicide surveillance. We need detailed and accurate information [for designing, targeting, and evaluating interventions] to help get our suicide rates down. We can't track this when reporting is casual, sloppy, or nonexistent" (Thomas, 2009). I also said that deficient death certificates hamper policymakers in creating prevention strategies amid data disparities for Blacks and Hispanics.

Penetrating the racial paradox

Lessons learned from my two previous multiple-cause-of-death studies informed an analytic study I designed, which aimed to penetrate the enigma of the American racial or racial/ethnic suicide paradox from a social constructionist perspective (Rockett et al., 2010b). Representing the period 2003–5, the data were national and derived from the de-identified multiple-cause-of-death files released for public use by the National Center for Health Statistics. The study population comprised pooled or combined undetermined intent deaths and suicides and was confined to non-Hispanic Whites, non-Hispanic Blacks, and Hispanics owing to heterogeneity and small numbers among other racial/ethnic groups. Small numbers further limited this population to the age group 15 years and older. The outcome or dependent variable was death of undetermined intent, as a proxy for a misclassified or possible suicide, versus classification as a (definite) suicide. Alternately expressed, the outcome variable measured potential suicide misclassification. I operationalized the undetermined category as deaths from injury of undetermined intent or sequelae and suicide as deaths from self-harm. As an aside, the United Kingdom combines registered suicides and "open" verdicts (undetermined deaths) in their official suicide rates, a modification that increases the British suicide rate by about 20% (Palmer et al., 2015).

My third multiple-cause-of-death study sought to enlighten the racial suicide paradox by addressing three questions pertaining to the existence or degree of differential suicide misclassification between Blacks and Whites.

First, do the death certificates of Black suicides and possible suicides show less comorbid psychopathology than those of corresponding Whites? Second, is lack of psychiatric documentation associated with potential suicide misclassification? Third, do Blacks appear more susceptible than Whites to suicide misclassification, after adjusting for sociodemographic characteristics and psychiatric documentation on the death certificate? Motivating these questions was my suspicion that differential knowledge of the proximate mental health status of Black and White decedents, on the part of medical examiners and coroners, could influence the respective tipping points where they diagnosed or ruled deaths as suicides and thus precipitate differential suicide misclassification. Virtually an afterthought in this study was a fourth critical question: was susceptibility to differential misclassification affected by the suicide method, or more generally by the mechanism or mode of fatal injury?

In applying the full statistical model for predicting an undetermined versus suicide manner-of-death classification, this study included six variables: four sociodemographic variables together with documentation of comorbid psychopathology (yes/no) and mode of injury. Exemplifying less forensically overt modes of injury were poisoning and drowning. Firearm, hanging, and cutting exemplified more overt modes. Table 4.4 presents the results of our statistical test of the social constructionist hypothesis that Blacks have higher odds than Whites of an undetermined classification. Odds and odds ratios have popular application to horse racing and other forms of gambling. For example, if the horse you laid a bet on at the Kentucky Derby had odds of seven to six, this would mean that with a victory your horse would return you seven dollars for every six dollars you wagered.

In presenting results from the study, my coauthors and I cumulatively introduced four models, with the first containing race/ethnicity as a sole predictor. The univariable logistic regression analysis showed that Blacks had 2.4 times higher odds than Whites of an undetermined classification. Supporting our research hypothesis, this association persisted through incorporation of the sociodemographics, then the psychiatric documentation, and finally injury mode.

Noteworthy, whereas Blacks were more than twice as prone as Whites to have their pooled suicides and undetermined deaths classified as undetermined, both their official crude and age-adjusted suicide rates were less than half those of the Whites during the 2003–5 observation period—5.2

Table 4.4. Logistic regression models of the association between race/ethnicity, other individual characteristics, and potential suicide misclassification, United States, 2003–5

Characteristic	Model 1 (n = 105,946) OR (95% CI)	Model 2 (n = 105,946) OR (95% CI)	Model 3 (n = 105,946) OR (95% CI)	Model 4 (n = 105,946) OR (95% CI)
Race/ethnicity:				
White (referent)	1.00	1.00	1.00	1.00
Black	2.38 (2.25, 2.52)	2.26 (2.13, 2.39)	2.28 (2.21, 2.36)	2.38 (2.22, 2.57)
Hispanic	1.08 (1.00, 1.16)	1.00 (0.93, 1.08)	1.28 (1.24, 1.32)	1.17 (1.07, 1.28)
Sex:				
Male (referent)		1.00	1.00	1.00
Female		2.36 (2.27, 2.45)	2.29 (2.25, 2.34)	1.01 (0.97, 1.06)
Age (years):				
15–34 (referent)		1.00	1.00	1.00
35–54		1.40 (1.34, 1.46)	1.37 (1.34, 1.40)	0.88 (0.84, 0.93)
55–74		0.61 (0.58, 0.66)	0.85 (0.82, 0.87)	0.52 (0.49, 0.57)
75+		0.44 (0.40, 0.48)	1.47 (1.42, 1.52)	0.51 (0.46, 0.57)
Education (years):				
0–8		1.82 (1.66, 2.00)	1.82 (1.75, 1.90)	2.34 (2.10, 2.62)
9–12		1.51 (1.45, 1.58)	1.43 (1.40, 1.46)	1.66 (1.58, 1.74)
13+ (referent)		1.00	1.00	1.00
Unknown		1.84 (1.70, 1.99)	1.37 (1.32, 1.43)	2.08 (1.89, 2.28)
Psychiatric documentation:				
Yes (referent)			1.00	1.00
No			6.56 (6.16, 6.99)	3.12 (2.78, 3.51)
Mode of injury:				
More overt (referent)				1.00
Less overt[a]				46.33 (43.32, 49.55)

Note: Potential suicide misclassification was operationalized as a binary outcome measure of manner of death: undetermined intent (1) and suicide (0).

[a] Deaths classified under *ICD-10* X60–69, X71, X75–77, X79, X81–84, Y10–19, Y21, Y25–27, Y29, and Y31–34. Residual injury deaths were classified as more active.

Source: Rockett, I.R.H., Wang, S., Stack, S., et al., "Race/ethnicity and potential suicide misclassification: Window on a minority suicide paradox?," *BMC Psychiatry* 2010;10:35.

and 5.3 per 100,000 for Blacks versus 12.2 and 11.9 for Whites, respectively. Hispanics, a second vulnerable minority, manifested higher odds than Whites of an undetermined classification in the application of models 3 and 4. However, inference of artifactuality or social construction with regard to the outcome was weaker for them than for Blacks. It is remarkable that these racial/ethnic differentials persisted after inclusion of injury mode. The odds of an undetermined versus suicide classification were over 46 times higher for decedents in the less versus the more forensically overt category. Predictably, drug and other poisoning deaths predominated among the less overt group.

Conducted by Nathalie Huguet and associates, a subsequent analysis used the restricted access data from the National Violent Death Reporting System (NVDRS; see box 1). In the case of Whites, they found that among pooled suicide and undetermined intent deaths, the odds of poisoning deaths were 66 times higher than those of firearm deaths to be classified under undetermined intent (Huguet et al., 2012). For African American Blacks, however, the odds were 229 times higher—a striking racial/ethnic difference. The restricted access data contain detailed information on the circumstances of manner of death and life history of decedents not available in the underlying and multiple-cause-of-death public use files.

Furthermore, using the NVDRS restricted access data, Texan researchers conducted an interstate study entitled "Suicides and Deaths of Undetermined Intent by Poisoning: Reexamination of Classification Differences by Race/Ethnicity and State" (Choi et al., 2020). They referenced our 2018 finding that suicide notes were critical corroborative evidence for a suicide classification in comparing suicide versus undetermined intent deaths (Rockett et al., 2018a). However, they excluded suicides accompanied by an evidentiary suicide note. Among their important findings were that the five states with the largest proportion of undetermined deaths had 7–10 times higher odds of an undetermined classification than other states participating in the NVDRS and that the corresponding odds for non-Hispanic Blacks were double those of non-Hispanic Whites. Their racial/ethnic finding aligned with both prior and co-occurring findings (Rockett et al., 2006b; Rockett et al., 2010b; Rockett et al., 2020b).

Although not subjected to formal hypothesis testing, there are other observations from our study that are informative about the impact of artifactual influences on the relative odds of an undetermined versus suicide

Box 1. The National Violent Death Reporting System

Administered by the Centers for Disease Control and Prevention (CDC), the National Violent Death Reporting System (NVDRS) is a state-, territory-, and incident-based surveillance system that uses public health informatics to link data from multiple sources, principally death certificates, law enforcement records, and medical examiner and coroner reports. The last reports include toxicologic data. Among optional supplemental data sources for this system are hospital records and crime laboratory reports. The NVDRS generates detailed individual-level data about suicides, homicides, undetermined intent deaths, and other selected violent deaths. Data are disaggregatable to the county level. To preserve privacy, CDC de-identifies these microdata prior to their release. They include geographic location, circumstances of death and its investigation, and the sociodemographic characteristics of the decedents. Data collection for the NVDRS commenced in six states in 2003 but is now universal.

CDC sets requirements for people wishing to use the microdata, since there is potential for inadvertent or deliberate identification of individual decedents. Users must be government employees or have an advanced degree and hold an academic appointment with a research institution, or work under the mentorship of a qualified person who would serve as the principal investigator. Access requires application to use the data that includes describing the nature, methods, and anticipated publications and public health benefits of the proposed project; specification of any links to other databases; and plans for managing and protecting data confidentiality. Permission for use rests with a scientific review committee within the NVDRS.

classification associated with decedent sex, age, and educational attainment. Under the full model, females align with males, but in the application of models 2 and 3 they have 2.3 times higher odds than males of an undetermined classification. This gap could reflect an excess propensity of females to use softer and less lethal methods of suicide, especially drug poisoning. Whether this excess reflects greater concern than males with postmortem appearance and rescue potential, less access to more lethal means, and other factors, these methods tend to be a larger impediment than violent and overt methods to suicide detection by medical examiners and coroners. Tangentially, a European study found not only that females tend to use less lethal methods of suicide than do males but also that when they use identical methods their outcomes are less likely to be fatal (Mergl et al., 2015).

In our study, all older age groups exhibited lower odds than the reference or comparison group, 15–34 years, of an undetermined classification under the full model. This finding supports the notion that medical examiners and coroners are more conservative in assigning suicide as the manner of death when decedents are young, perhaps in deference to protecting families from social stigma. All less educated groups show higher odds of an undetermined classification than their comparison group, the most educated. Those whose educational attainment is unknown resemble the least educated in the analysis, the group with eight or fewer years of schooling.

Quantitative researchers, irrespective of topic, face the sometimes very formidable problem of how to handle missing information. Commonly, they either omit missing cases or reallocate them according to the known distribution of a given variable across its categories—a type of statistical imputation. The education results of this study, in conjunction with the high magnitude of missing data, argue for retention of unknowns as a separate category in such instances. Even more important than information on education, regarding missing data, decedents without psychiatric documentation had over three times higher odds than documented counterparts of an undetermined classification. My research to this juncture prompted Diego De Leo to invite me to publish an editorial in the journal *Crisis*, an opportunity I deeply appreciated (Rockett, 2010).

Among other results from a previously cited NVDRS study, Blacks had a higher prevalence than Whites of missing data in 11 of the 16 states in the dataset—evidence of health data disparities that are problematic for accurate case ascertainment of suicide (Huguet et al., 2012). When considered with our results, there is strong, although indirect, evidence that the lower suicide rates for Blacks than Whites—the racial suicide paradox—are at least partially an artifact of differential misclassification. Later in the book, I reevaluate this paradox in the context of self-injury mortality, an enhanced category of fatal self-injury.

Complicating suicide accounting among Blacks, this population may stigmatize suicide even more than Whites do. In early 2005, I presented my preliminary research on discrepant reporting of suicide by race as part of an internal seminar series in the health sciences center at West Virginia University. In attendance was James "Jack" Frost, a former president of the National Association of Medical Examiners and a recently retired medical examiner who had overseen medicolegal death investigations in West Virginia's north and north central regions. Starting with a spirited debate between us that carried on in an adjacent space after the seminar, he became a valued collaborator and fast friend until his death in 2016. Frost became the first of three medical examiners who have graciously worked with me on various projects. Once I earned his confidence, he shared an experience he had with a Black family who had lost a female member to suicide. In vain, they protested vociferously at his determination, and one exclaimed that "Blacks don't kill themselves." In contrast to this belief, Henry Morselli, writing in the nineteenth century, referenced "the extraordinary propensity [of American Blacks] to suicide" (1882, 133). Sadly, no substantial demographic groups are spared the risk of suicide, except infants and toddlers.

A black swan

In retrospect, I believe that the suicide rate for Blacks is less than half that for Whites, astonishing considering the pervasiveness, potency, and persistence of minority health data disparities (Purnell et al., 2016; Shi & Stevens, 2021; Dawes et al., 2023), and that only a part of the observed rate gap is an artifact of these disparities. I view the remainder of the differential as a black swan, a metaphor for an unlikely happening (Taleb, 2010). However, this metaphor is a source of amusement to me since black swans are native to Australia. Initially unaware of white swans, black swans were part of my childhood in my home state of Western Australia. The natural and first major artery linking the capital city of Perth with its port of Fremantle is the Swan River. Moreover, the black swan is the state bird and official emblem of Western Australia and occupies pride of place on the coat of arms of my alma mater, the University of Western Australia.

5

Surging Opioid Mortality Complicates Suicide Detection

Leading causes of injury mortality: Bucking convention

In 2012, I published an article with multidisciplinary colleagues on national rate trends in five categories of injury mortality: suicide, homicide, and accidental motor vehicle traffic crash, poisoning, and falls. I had accessed the data from the Web-based Injury Statistics Query and Reporting System (WISQARS; Rockett et al., 2012) of the Centers for Disease Control and Prevention (CDC). Our observation period was 2000–2009. For background, we presented trend data for injury and disease mortality rates encompassing the period 1980–2009 (fig. 5.1). While the age-adjusted disease mortality rate trended downward through the latter period, the corresponding injury mortality rate reversed a downward trend beginning in 2001, a change in trajectory that could not be accounted for by the shift from the 9th to the 10th revision of the *International Classification of Diseases*.

In their annual rankings of the leading causes of death in the United States by age and sex, CDC distinguishes suicide, homicide, and accidental (unintentional) deaths using the mandated injury manner-of-death classification. Their categorization, however, is potentially problematic for health planning and policymaking because it mixes apples and oranges. My logic for this assessment is as follows: On the first cut, CDC employs one umbrella category, unintentional injury, which subsumes all accidental deaths by cause, whereas they dichotomize intentional injury deaths into suicides and homicides. In their rankings, they similarly disaggregate natural causes, the disease manner-of-death category. Considering these inconsistencies, we broke with convention by selecting three categories of accidental mortality—motor vehicle traffic crash, poisoning, and fall deaths—for a direct compar-

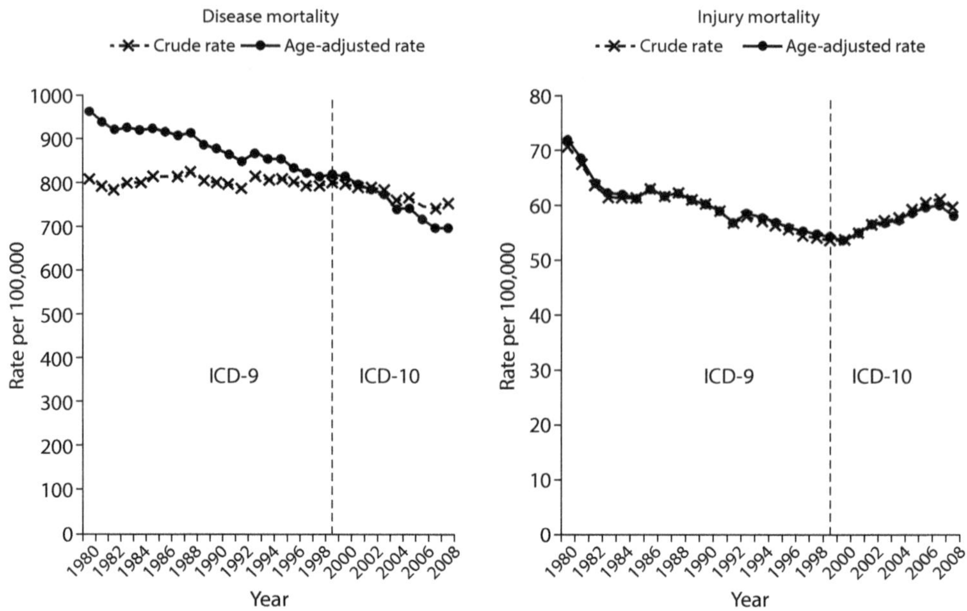

International Classification of Diseases (World Health Organization). The vertical dashed line demarcates the transition between these two revisions.

Figure 5.1. Annual crude and age-adjusted mortality rates from disease and injury: United States, 1980–2008. Source: Rockett, I.R.H., Regier, M.D., Kapusta, N.D., et al., "Leading causes of unintentional and intentional injury mortality: United States, 2000–2009," ***American Journal of Public Health*** **2012;102(11): e84–92.**

ison with suicides and homicides. We could then report that suicide had surpassed motor vehicle traffic crash trauma in 2009 to become the leading cause of injury death in the country (fig. 5.2). This finding attracted widespread media interest. However, I readily concede that motor vehicle traffic death rates had been declining from the later part of the twentieth century through the early twenty-first century because of the implementation of evidence-based safety interventions targeting individuals, vehicles, roads, bridges, tunnels, and the adjacent environment. This success story provides a model with lessons for suicide prevention.

Several significant findings emerged from the American injury mortality study besides our observation that suicides nationally had surpassed motor vehicle traffic crash deaths. Most relevant to this book, we reported that accidental drug and other poisoning mortality registered large absolute in-

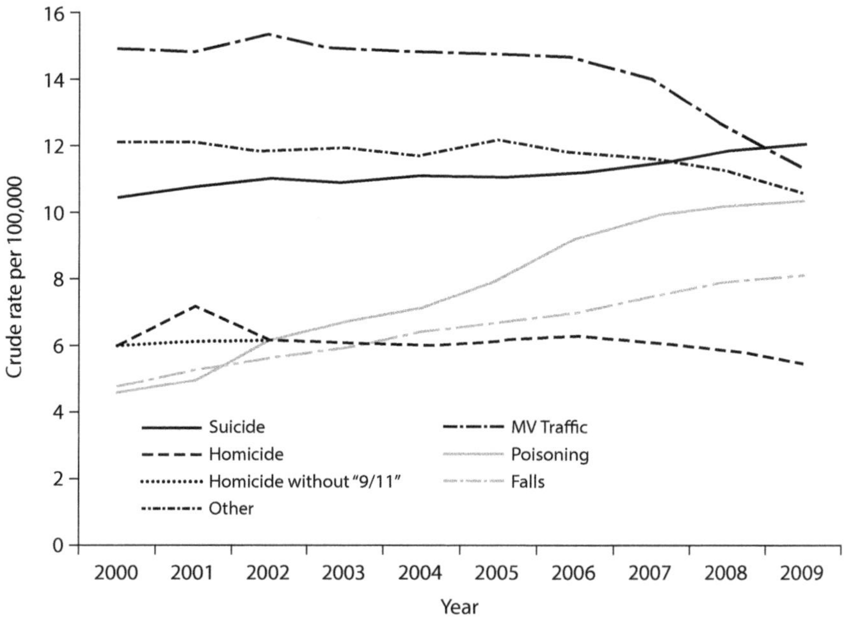

Figure 5.2. Rates for leading causes of total unintentional and intentional injury mortality: United States, 2000–2009. Note: MV equals motor vehicle. Source: Rockett, I.R.H., Regier, M.D., Kapusta, N.D., et al., "Leading causes of unintentional and intentional injury mortality: United States, 2000–2009," ***American Journal of Public Health*** **2012;102(11):e84–92.**

creases among the middle-aged, females, and Whites between 2000 and 2009, with rates of poisoning and suicide mortality rising by 128% and 15%, respectively. A departure from most of my studies, we accepted the suicide and other injury mortality rates at face value, with no evaluation of the likelihood that the true suicide rates were appreciably higher than the official rates.

In a sober assessment, a Norwegian group sounded a caution about researchers departing from conventional categorization of leading causes of death for political and funding purposes (Gjertsen et al., 2019). Of particular concern for them was suicide, and their article subtitle offered a provocative question: "Uncover Facts or Misrepresent Statistics?" While not dismissing the importance of this question, in most instances I think that suicide, as a highly stigmatized phenomenon, warrants special concern because of its susceptibility to undercounting and the typical lack of concern about the accuracy of its reporting from familial to societal levels. The Norwegians are correct that suicide is rare, for example, relative to death from heart disease and cancer, although perhaps not as rare as they suggest. Ranking leading causes of death is based on death counts. Worth mentioning from a public health perspective, suicide disproportionately impacts the young, like most causes of injury mortality (Rockett, 1998a). We all die, but public health workers have the minimization of premature mortality as their goal. Conventional rankings of leading causes of death overlook that fact, which itself has critical implications for politics, funding, and therefore the prioritization of treatment and prevention. I note that the Norwegians' article acknowledges potential merit in research conducted by my colleagues and me, which questions the continuing value of registered suicides serving as the sole representative of fatal self-injury, a topic that will become ascendant in this book.

Are rising accidental poisoning and suicide mortality rates separate phenomena?

Two studies conducted by other researchers informed and buoyed my suspicion that the rising accidental poisoning and suicide mortality rates in the United States in the twenty-first century were intercorrelated and possibly causally related. The first study was an analysis of National Violent Death Reporting System (NVDRS) data for 13 states (Breiding & Wiersema, 2006), and the second used a procedure called classification and regression tree analysis to reassign undetermined poisoning deaths in Utah to the suicide and accident manner of death categories (Donaldson et al., 2006). I was slowly becoming aware that opioid intoxication deaths (especially those attributable to oxycodone and hydrocodone, both prescription analgesics; Warner et al., 2009) were beginning to dominate the undetermined and accidental poisoning mortality categories.

Colleagues and I evaluated whether the suicide and unintentional/accidental poisoning trends were independent in a study I also designed and led, which was published in 2010 (Rockett et al., 2010a). Our data source was WISQARS, and the observation period extended from 1987 to 2006. We disaggregated the mortality data by age and sex, as well as by two selected manners of death, suicide and undetermined, and one underlying cause of death, unintentional/accidental poisoning. Rates for undetermined mortality

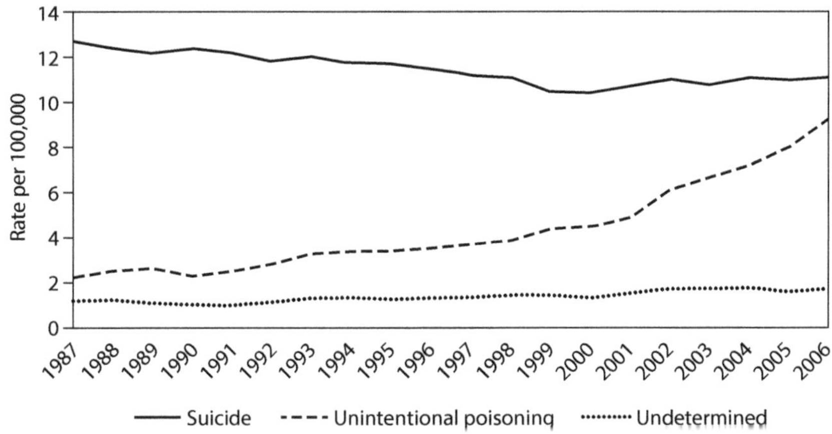

Figure 5.3. Crude death rates of suicide, unintentional/accidental poisoning, and undetermined intent, United States, 1987–2006. Source: Rockett, I.R.H., Hobbs, G., De Leo, D., et al., "Suicide and unintentional poisoning mortality trends in the United States, 1987–2006," *BMC Public Health* 2010;10:705.

were both low and relatively stable over the entire observation period. The basis for my concern about serious suicide undercounting in unintentional/accidental poisoning mortality was evident after the mid-1990s. Respective unintentional/accidental injury mortality rates rose sharply, while changes in the corresponding suicide and undetermined injury death rates were minimal (fig. 5.3), and the suicide and undetermined poisoning death rates remained flat relative to the rapid upward trajectory of the unintentional/accidental poisoning death rate (fig. 5.4). This last finding invited skepticism on my part that people dying by suicide were not increasingly turning to drug poisoning as a method given obviously easier access to this means. Regardless of sex, the age group 65 years and older recorded the only sustained decline in age-specific suicide rates between 1987 and 2006 (data not shown). This finding suggests that suicide misclassification, which mainly implicates drug poisoning, appears less problematic for the elderly.

A subsequent English study (Gunnell et al., 2013) and a Canadian replication of my 2010 trend study (Skinner et al., 2016), in which I participated, also implicated growing suicide misclassification within upward trends in unintentional/accidental poisoning mortality rates. The Canadian research was later updated and expanded with greater drug specification (Snowdon

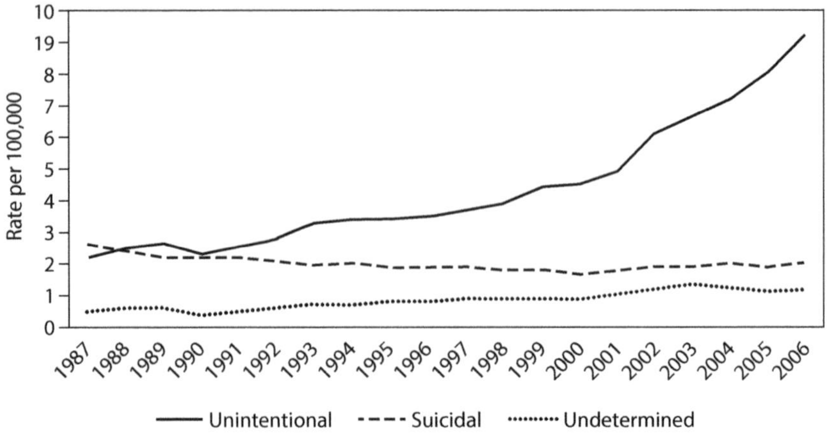

Figure 5.4. Crude poisoning mortality rates by intentionality, United States, 1987–2006. Source: Rockett, I.R.H., Hobbs, G., De Leo, D., et al., "Suicide and unintentional poisoning mortality trends in the United States, 1987–2006," ***BMC Public Health*** **2010;10:705.**

& Choi, 2022). The update incorporated ill-defined conditions and unknown causes of death in the mix.

As an aside, a 2020 study by health economist Ted Miller and associates demonstrated the importance of distinguishing drugs by class or type with respect to their poisoning suicide lethality (Miller et al., 2020). Relative to all other classes, opioids were 5.2 times more deadly regarding suicide completion, versus 4.3 times more for barbiturates, 3.2 for antidepressants, 2.6 for antidiabetics, and 1.9 for alcohol. An Australian comparison of poisoning-related and non-poisoning-related suicides found an excess of antidepressants, benzodiazepines, nonopioid analgesics / anti-inflammatory drugs, and opioids among the poisoning cases (Lim et al., 2023). Alcohol intoxication (ethanol ≥ 0.9 grams/100 milliliters of blood) did not differentiate. There was an excess of amphetamines and cannabinoids among the non-poisoning-related cases, and multiple drugs commonly manifested in the toxicology for the poisoning group.

Collectively, the trend studies indicate increasing unreliability of international suicide statistics, which is associated with rising drug poisoning mortality, particularly during the twenty-first century. They begged new questions, several of which were addressed in a series of studies my colleagues and I subsequently conducted.

A suicide survivor's reaction to undercounting

Anna Mehler Paperny (2019), a Reuters reporter in Toronto, Canada, wrote a lively, frank, and engaging, but disturbing, narrative of a chronically suicidal person and suicide survivor— herself—entitled *Hello I Want to Die Please Fix Me*. Clinical depression dominated her life. Mention of personal drug misuse was minimal but tinged with regret. Her book was published in 2019. Some three years earlier, she had telephoned me to discuss my research on suicide data deficits, as part of her quest to better understand not only her own history but also the larger picture. She colorfully summarizes her frustration at battling chronic and stigmatizing depression and her quest for enlightenment: "No one wants this crap illness that masquerades as personal failing. I had no desire to plumb its depths. The struggle to function leaves me little capacity to do so. But, in the end, I had no choice. I approached this enemy I barely believed in the only way I knew how: as a reporter. I took a topic about which I knew nothing and sought somehow to know everything. I talked to people in search of answers and mostly found more questions" (Paperny, 2019, xiv).

From reading Paperny's book and perusing the index, it was clear to me that she had consulted an impressive who's who of experts in suicidology. In retrospect, since my research on undercounting had hovered on the fringe of the suicide literature, I was flattered and honored that she contacted me. Her book indicated that a number of my research concerns resonated with her, including suicide undercounting associated with declining autopsy rates, differential autopsy rates favoring homicide over suicide cases, and excess susceptibility to undercounting among marginal populations, such as the United States' two largest "vulnerable" minorities, Blacks and Hispanics. The minority discrepancy partially implicated the nexus between relative inaccessibility to the health care system and sparse psychiatric histories.

In the vibrant language of Paperny, "The consequences of [suicide] underreporting extend beyond public health nerds who get off on accuracy. [Undercounting] suggests something is less of a problem than it is and therefore less deserving of our attention and our dollars. Which is convenient, given how icky suicide makes us feel in the first place. Finding fewer suicides can make it less of an issue." She then quoted me: "If you think about it, society hasn't been that invested in suicide prevention. If you more accurately portray self-injury deaths and say this is mental health, there's potential for rather more resources to be directed toward the problem" (Paperny, 2019, 74). My statement alludes to the new category that expands fatal self-injury beyond registered suicides, which I expound on in the next chapter.

Tennessee Hospital Emergency Room Drug Study

Our suicide and poisoning mortality study indicated that the elderly seem less prone than younger counterparts to poisoning suicide misclassification, especially drug poisoning. This likelihood provides what I consider a natural transition for me to describe and discuss a statewide hospital emergency department study that Sandra Putnam—a medical sociologist and my wife—and I conducted in the mid-1990s. Hospital emergency departments are a front line for identifying people in trouble with drugs. As a stand-alone nationally, the Tennessee Hospital Emergency Room Drug Study was unique in a set of five survey research studies that her Community Health Research Group, at the University of Tennessee, Knoxville, conducted during the 1990s on behalf of the United States Center for Substance Abuse Treatment. However, the other four studies replicated research implemented outside Tennessee: the Drug Use Forecasting Substance Abuse Need for Treatment Assessment studies of juvenile and adult arrestees, a household survey, and a social indicators study. I designed and directed the Tennessee Hospital Emergency Room Drug Study.

In our first article from that study, we estimated the prevalence of alcohol and other substance use and the need for treatment of dependence (Rockett et al., 2003). To my knowledge, this research remains the only statewide, population based study of unmet substance abuse treatment need among adult emergency department patients ever conducted in the United States. Patient sampling was a two-stage process. Sandra Putnam and I used probability sampling first to select seven representative hospitals from those with an annual minimum patient volume of at least 10,000 emergency department visits and then to select patients from each sample hospital. Enhancing research generalizability, we attained a participation rate of 79%. As study director, and facilitating the attainment of this high rate, I met with the chief executive officers of the seven hospitals and the medical directors of their emergency departments to explain the nature of the study and its goals. Our data were obtained through self-reported behavior and toxicologic screening of use of alcohol and a range of other drugs, including marijuana, cocaine, opioids, barbiturates, stimulants, and benzodiazepines. We validated the use of alcohol by means of a saliva test and that of other drugs through urine testing.

Our primary research question in the Tennessee Hospital Emergency Room Drug Study was how criteria for assessing substance abuse treatment need, which combined objective toxicologic data with subjective self-report data, increased the magnitude of estimated need prevalence relative to that based on self-report alone—including the subset of information conforming to the definition of current drug dependence enumerated in the *Diagnostic and Statistical Manual of Mental Disorders, Fourth Edition* (*DSM-IV*; American Psychiatric Association, 1994). To accommodate a comprehensive definition of treatment need, as well as more limited ones, we assessed this need according to whether a patient met at least one of the following 14 criteria: (1) currently in drug treatment, (2) wanted treatment, (3) currently drug dependent according to the *DSM-IV* criteria, (4) self-diagnosed current dependence, (5) past treatment / current use, (6) past treatment / test positive, (7) past treatment / test refusal, (8) *DSM-IV* lifetime dependence / current use, (9) *DSM-IV* lifetime dependence / test positive, (10) *DSM-IV* lifetime dependence / test refusal, (11) self-diagnosed lifetime dependence / current use, (12) self-diagnosed lifetime dependence / test positive, (13) self-diagnosed lifetime dependence / test refusal, and (14) declared nonuse / test positive. Under *DSM-IV*, drug dependence covered tolerance, withdrawal, frequent excessive use, persistent desire, failed attempts to curb use of drugs, prolonged time and effort to obtain them, disruption of important activities in order to use, and continuance of use despite awareness of adverse physical and psychological consequences.

Under our comprehensive case definition, we estimated the point prevalence for substance abuse treatment need among the Tennessee emergency department patients at 27%. Illustrating the power of social construction, this prevalence contrasted with the 4% under the *DSM-IV* definition and the mere 1% if we had been forced to base our estimate on the information available in the medical records of the participating hospitals. Our estimate of the prevalence of unmet need was also 27%, showing how few patients were receiving substance abuse treatment. Heavy excess need for treatment manifested in all younger age groups of the adult patients in the study relative to the elderly, patients aged 65 years and older. This finding assumed added interest for me when I considered it in conjunction with the findings for the elderly from our 2010 suicide and poisoning mortality trend study. A reasonable inference from these two streams of research is that few patients who are in trouble with alcohol and other drugs earlier in their lives reach age 65 in the absence of treatment. This is not to say, however, that the elderly are largely immune from substance misuse and dependence. To the contrary, since most of them are afflicted with many diseases and disabilities, as well as preventable conditions, they are consequently users of an increasing array and doses of prescription drugs, including antidepressants and painkillers. Moreover, their multiple physical conditions may mean that mental problems, beyond dementia, can be overlooked during standard medical care. It is a sign of progress that, as a senior citizen myself, I am invariably asked whether I am depressed during routine medical care visits.

Accompanying our article was a supportive editorial penned by a prominent Yale University emergency physician, Gail D'Onofrio (2003), entitled "Treatment for Alcohol and Other Drug Problems: Closing the Gap." We had extrapolated from our Tennessee sample in estimating a range of 3–22 million emergency department patients nationwide who needed drug treatment. She reasoned that our upper estimate likely better approximated the true total and stated that even patients in relapse should not be viewed differently than other chronic disease patients by the health care system. They, too, require continuity of care. While the opioid epidemic remained somewhat under the radar, D'Onofrio anticipated rising numbers of patients in need and gave an example of a successful brief intervention program that refers patients to specialized treatment programs.

We shifted our focus in the second article from the Tennessee Hospital Emergency Room Drug Study to an examination of health care utilization associated with unmet substance abuse treatment need (Rockett et al., 2005). Utilization differentiated physician visits for primary care, hospital emergency department visits, and hospital admissions. Consistent with our expectation, we observed excess utilization of care from the two hospital-based measures but not for that of primary care services, which afford people more discretion about access because their health problems are less severe. We also estimated costs of these excesses.

In our third article, we scrutinized declared and undeclared alcohol and other substance use (Rockett et al., 2006a). Toxicologic results from the saliva and urine screening served as the criterion or gold standard against which to compare self-reported use in order to measure undeclared use. We reported corrected use estimates for alcohol and the seven other drugs or drug groups that our testing could accommodate. Predictably, self-reported use of alcohol was most accurate, as a legal drug in Tennessee for people aged 21 years and older, followed by marijuana. Of course, legalization of marijuana is becoming increasingly common in the United States for medical and nonmedical use. The main drugs of concern at the time of our study were marijuana, opioids, stimulants, benzodiazepines, and barbiturates, based on a combination of the magnitude of use prevalence and that of the prevalence gap between self-reported use and test positivity as a validation check.

Elderly patients manifested not only the lowest prevalence of substance abuse treatment need but also the lowest prevalence of substance use. This finding was somewhat surprising given their usual multimorbidity and related excess ingestion of prescription pharmaceuticals. Originally, we planned to use the term "denied use" rather than "undeclared use" in the third article. We converted to "undeclared use" following a prudent recommendation by Konrad Jamrozik, an Australian epidemiologist, who, after informally reading a draft of the manuscript, pointed out that polypharmacy among the elderly may make them especially prone to ignorance about the particulars of their medications. When the elderly die suddenly, without suspicion of trauma or drug poisoning, and are under regular medical care with documented potentially fatal conditions, they are the least likely age group to be autopsied. Moreover, multiple disease diagnoses mean that physicians will almost invariably attribute such deaths to natural causes, that is, diseases. To reiterate, an inference I informally draw from the Tennessee Hospital Emergency Room Drug Study is that it is difficult for younger individuals addicted to drugs to reach age 65, or to reach that age in good health.

We provided further details on our methodology in the Tennessee study, together with additional results, in the three resultant journal articles. Although we found a high prevalence of need and unmet need for substance abuse treatment among the patient participants, we conducted our survey in 1996, when the American opioid epidemic was only in its incipient phase. Thus, need prevalence may be considerably higher in the 2020s. During study design and data collection, through publication of the manuscripts, I sensed no link between the emergency department study and my research on suicide data quality. Seemingly, the twain never meet. But this proved not to be true, as borne out by time and my growing awareness of the interconnectedness of the suicide and poisoning mortality epidemics.

Two Tennessee media stories on our report of the high prevalence of unmet need for substance abuse treatment among the adult emergency department patients illustrated ambivalence in public perceptions about how to address drug problems. The first story, published in a Nashville newspaper, *The Tennessean*, blamed the victims and likely further fueled stigmatization of drug dependence. The second story, published in the University of Tennessee, Knoxville, student newspaper, stressed the importance of the findings as a call to action to address treatment need. The headline for the first story was "Drug Users a Burden on ER Services," and that for the second one was "Info from ER Could Aid Drug Abusers." Regrettably for prevention, the perspective of the first reporter is generally more prevalent owing to societal resistance and inertia in confronting alcohol, opioid, and other drug problems nationally and locally.

While the second media story on the Tennessee Hospital Emergency Room Drug Study is much more enlightened than the first, the reporter's use of the term "abuser," from the vantage point of contemporary times, could be viewed as problematic because of its connotations of victim blaming. One of my collaborators, philosopher John Kleinig, advocates for a substitute, "active substance user," where persons are "habituated, addicted, or dependent" on psychoactive drugs and disinclined to stop using (2012, 596). Ethically, this substitution makes good sense to me. Ideally, however, my preference would be to describe active users as nondetoxified rather than view them as conscious users, whose conditions are not being treated—with treatment exemplified by taking medications like disulfiram (Antabuse) for alcohol use disorder and buprenorphine for opioid use disorder—and/or whose recovery is not being managed through a regimen like cognitive behavioral therapy or continuing participation in 12-step self-help programs, typified by Alcoholics Anonymous and Narcotics Anonymous. A final mass media article on the Tennessee Hospital Emergency Room Drug Study, published in the *Knoxville News Sentinel*, was balanced and included authoritative comments from Gail D'Onofrio and a spokesperson for the American College of Emergency Physicians, Larry Alexander (Mansfield, 2003). Reflecting the era, "drug abuse" featured in the title.

I turn now to another hospital emergency room study, an analysis of the 2007 Nationwide Emergency Department Sample (NEDS; Xiang et al., 2012). This study suggested that poisoning suicides were profoundly underestimated in the United States. Officially, only 8% of opioid and other drug poisoning deaths nationally in 2007 were classified as suicides, 6% as undetermined deaths, and 1% as homicides. The rest were classified as accidents. By contrast, in focusing on morbidity, the NEDS study found that 41% of the 161,000 drug-related emergency department visits attributed to painkilling drugs reflected suicidal intent, 40% were accidental or unintentional, and the remainder were undetermined—bearing in mind a caveat that visits do not equate to individual patients, as they will also include multiple visits by the same patients ("frequent flyers" through the revolving emergency room door). Germane to suicide misclassification and undercounting of suicide, assessment of intentionality among NEDS patients involved psychiatric evaluation, a process with no effective analogy in suicide ascertainment in the United States owing to a dearth of forensic psychological autopsies or close facsimiles being conducted at the behest of medical examiners and coroners.

Autopsies, toxicology, and differential suicide rates

The forensic or medicolegal autopsy is a systematic gross and microscopic physical examination of bodily organs, tissues, and fluids conducted by a forensic pathologist involving postmortem laboratory investigations and related toxicology to provide medical examiners or coroners with physical information on a given death to help them determine both its cause (disease or injury) and its manner or circumstances (natural, suicide, homicide, or accident). A clinical autopsy is a corresponding procedure that is typically conducted in a hospital by a pathologist on a deceased patient to diagnose the underlying and contributing disease and/or injury causes of the death. Although forensic autopsies are important diagnostically for identifying mechanism of injury and ascertaining disease and injury comorbidity, they do not invariably enlighten decedent intentionality (Vanatta & Petty, 1987; Sorenson et al., 1997). Nonetheless, they may be an important marker or surrogate for the fastidiousness of medicolegal death investigations (Shojania et al., 2003).

Implying less fastidiousness in suicide versus homicide accounting, 97% of American homicides in 2007 were autopsied, compared with just 60% of suicides and 81% of undetermined intent deaths (Hoyert, 2011). By comparison, Finnish medicolegal authorities conducted forensic autopsies in 99% of suicides, 98% of homicides, and 97% of undetermined intent deaths for the period 2000–2003 (Lunetta et al., 2007). A low national autopsy rate (combined clinical and forensic autopsy rates) was reported as problematic for the quality of Danish cause-of-death statistics (Larsen & Lynnerup, 2011).

During the period 1998–2007, Finland had an annual-averaged suicide rate of 20 per 100,000 population as compared to 12 for Denmark (Kapusta et al., 2011). Corresponding national autopsy rates (combined clinical and forensic), however, were 31% in Finland against just 8% in Denmark. This large autopsy rate differential may at least partially account for the suicide rate gap between these two countries. Also speaking loudly for the possibility that Finnish suicide data are of higher quality than the Danish data was a 2014 study reporting 13 times higher odds of a death being coded under ill-defined conditions and unknown causes in 2010 in Denmark (Ylijoki-Sørensen et al., 2014). Moreover, whereas a forensic autopsy was performed in 88% of these deaths in Finland, only 3%–4% of them in Denmark were investigated with the aid of either a forensic or clinical autopsy.

Combined forensic and consented clinical autopsy rates in the United States and other countries declined through the later part of the twentieth century. In the United States, the rate fell by over 50% between 1972 and 2007 (Hoyert, 2011). This decline may have depressed the quality of suicide data. Pertinent to this issue, I was invited to participate in an important international study that examined the association between autopsy and suicide rates (Kapusta et al., 2011). The lead author was Nestor Kapusta, an Austrian psychiatrist and suicidologist at the Medical University of Vienna, with whom I have enjoyed multiple and ongoing collaborations in research projects conducted at his institution and mine. For this longitudinal and cross-sectional ecological study, he obtained data for 35 Eurasian countries from the World Health Organization's European Health for All database that covered three decades and enabled calculation of autopsy rates.

The Austrian study included the following manner-of-death categories: suicide and undetermined; it also included the following cause-specific mortality categories: symptoms, signs, ill-defined conditions, and unknown causes. Unfortunately, the database did not permit separation of forensic from clinical autopsies, including clinical autopsies that were followed by a forensic autopsy. A longitudinal multivariable logistic regression analysis of the association between the autopsy and suicide rates, adjusted for the undetermined death rate, unemployment rate, and degree of urbanization, showed that a 1% increase in the autopsy rate across all 35 countries in the study was associated with an increase of 0.42 suicides per 100,000 population. Cross-sectionally, a 1% difference in the autopsy rate was associated with a difference in the suicide rate of 0.49 suicides per 100,000. These findings made an essential contribution to the conception of our research on suicide case ascertainment that utilized data from the NVDRS, which I will report on in a later section. The Eurasian autopsy/suicide study expanded a study of four Nordic countries: Denmark, Finland, Norway, and Sweden (Reseland et al., 2008).

For readers interested in detailed accounts of the conduct of medicolegal death investigations, I can recommend four books that greatly expanded my knowledge of the topic: *Cause of Death: A Writer's Guide to Death, Murder and Forensic Medicine* (Wilson, 1992), *Death Investigation: The Basics* (Randall, 1997), *Postmortem: Establishing the Cause of Death* (Koehler & Wecht, 2006), and *Death Investigation: Systems and Procedures* (Hanzlick, 2007). The last-mentioned book was written by Randy Hanzlick, who reported on the status of medicolegal death investigations in the United States in 2013 (Hanzlick, 2014). He identified marked heterogeneity in practices across states, which in turn portends very uneven quality. The proportion of medical examiner and coroner cases that were autopsied ranged from 21% to 73%, although some states with lower autopsy rates may have compensated to a degree by conducting larger numbers of external exams and partial autopsies. Hanzlick commented that a survey of state medical examiners had revealed a serious shortage of forensic pathologists to assist in medicolegal death investigations, a situation that is presumably direr in many, if not most, of the areas under decentralized county coroner systems.

A study of the NVDRS and WISQARS data reported wide variation in the percentage of violent deaths classified as undetermined manner of death in the 13 states in NVDRS for 2003 and 2004 (Breiding & Wiersema, 2006). Accidental deaths, except those attributed to firearms, are excluded from the NVDRS database. In 2003, the range for the percentage of undetermined manner deaths extended from 0.4% in New Jersey to 60% for Massachusetts. Another NVDRS study of the same states reported toxicologic testing results for suicide decedents in 2004 (Karch et al., 2010). These states then represented slightly less than one-quarter of the total US population, and their testing rates varied widely from 26% to 98%.

At a time when the American opioid epidemic was on the eve of exploding with the entry of illicit fentanyl, a 2013 analysis of mortality data from the National Vital Statistics System for 2008–10 described the injury manner-of-death distribution for drug intoxication deaths across all 50 states and the District of Columbia (Warner et al., 2013).[1] This analysis was conducted by Margaret Warner from the National Center for Health Statistics and colleagues, one of whom was Kurt Nolte, a former chief medical examiner of New Mexico and a frequent and highly valued collaborator of mine. They classified 87% and 40% of drug intoxication deaths in Maryland and Utah, respectively, as undetermined; homicide classifications were negligible at less than 1%. In 11 states, undetermined deaths composed 4% or less of drug intoxication deaths. The wide discrepancies in percentage of undetermined deaths, which varied from 1% in Wyoming to 85% in Maryland, likely imply large differentials in the capture of true drug intoxication suicides by state. Elevating this likelihood is the fact that substance use disorders are an important risk factor for suicide (Wilcox et al., 2004), and researchers have implicated opioid use disorder itself in suicide misclassification (Cantor et al., 2001; Bohnert et al., 2013).

The Warner study also reported some interstate variation in the specification of at least one drug on the death certificate of drug decedents (Warner et al., 2013). Specification was higher in states with a centralized state medical examiner system (92%) than in states whose medicolegal death investigations were administered under a decentralized county coroner system (62%) and in states with a hybrid of decentralized medical examiner systems and decentralized county corner systems (73%). These differentials may reflect variable fastidiousness by system type in the investigation of suicide and other manners of death in drug intoxication cases, or a lack of training of the coroners and medical examiners who work in these smaller offices. A county-level study from Harvard University and the University of Rochester compared medical examiner and coroner systems in their respective capacity to specify fatal drug overdoses (Denham et al., 2022). The authors found that the drug deaths in counties with coroner systems were almost four times as likely to be unclassified as counterparts occurring in counties with medical examiner systems. An interesting follow-up question would be whether accreditation by the National Association of Medical Examiners or the International Association of Coroners & Medical Examiners was associated with variation within medicolegal death investigation type.

The Warner study was the source of the two predictors or analytic variables we adopted in a national ecological study of drug intoxication deaths (Rockett et al., 2015): type of medicolegal death investigation system, and citation of at least one drug on the death certificate. States variously have a centralized medical examiner system, a decentralized county coroner system, or a hybrid system. We also used cross-sectional data for 2008–10 from the National Vital Statistics System in evaluating our hypotheses that the odds of a nonhomicide drug intoxication death being classified as suicide is a function of both drug citation and death investigation system type, as a test of partial artifactuality in suicide case ascertainment.

For our ecological study, we first calculated annual-averaged rates by state of nonhomicide drug intoxication deaths, distinguished by manner of death, and the percentage of death certificates citing at least one drug, distinguishing medicolegal death investigation system type (table 5.1). We then mapped the percentage of nonhomicide drug intoxication deaths classified as suicide by state and region (fig. 5.5). Strongly indicating variable potential for suicide misclassification in these deaths by state, the range extended from a low of 6% in Louisiana to a high of 29% in South Dakota.

Drug citation, death investigation system type, and suicide classification

In a multivariable logistic regression analysis, to evaluate our two hypotheses, we factored five state-based covariates into our models: age, sex, urbanization rate, poverty rate, and US region (West, Midwest, South, and Northeast). This statistical analysis showed that drug citation was positively associated with the odds of a nonhomicide drug intoxication death being classified as suicide versus accident or undetermined (table 5.2). Type of medicolegal death investigation system showed no association. We concluded that interstate variation in the classification of drug intoxication suicides was a partial function of variation in the application of forensic practices, in turn suggesting variable potential for suicide misclassification. The odds of a suicide classification were lowest in the South, as a distinct regional outlier. Southern medicolegal death investigations disproportionately fall within the domain of decentralized county coroner systems. Worthy of in-depth, population-based research is the impact of the sociocultural milieu on suicide case ascertainment, over and above the technical capacity of medical examiners and coroners to conduct their medicolegal death investigations.

Our study was constrained by its ecological or correlational research design, which precluded us from making causal inferences. Moreover, since it was state based, it lacked such important personal, individual-level data as death circumstances, psychological history, and autopsy status. Nevertheless,

Table 5.1. Annual-averaged rates for selected cause-specific manners of death and specific drug citation by state and death investigation system type: United States, 2008–10

State	Nonhomicide drug intoxication death rates by manner (per 100,000)[a]				Drug intoxication deaths with 1+ specific drugs cited on the death certificate (%)[b]
	Suicide	Accident	Undetermined	Total	
United States	1.7	1.0	9.5	12.2	75.1
		Centralized medical examiner			
Alaska	1.9	1.7	12.7	16.3	95.5
Connecticut	1.2	0.5	8.9	10.7	76.8
Delaware	2.1	1.3	1.8	15.1	79.3
Maine	2.1	0.3	9.3	11.8	89.7
Maryland	1.0	9.9	1.2	12.1	98.6
Massachusetts	1.3	0.6	10.1	12.0	97.0
New Hampshire	2.1	0.9	8.5	11.5	99.1
New Mexico	3.7	1.2	18.5	23.4	68.7
North Carolina	1.9	0.5	9.8	12.3	92.9
Oklahoma	1.8	1.1	15.3	18.3	97.2
Oregon	2.4	1.4	9.0	12.7	91.2
Rhode Island	2.3	0.3	13.6	16.2	97.3
Utah	2.5	6.6	7.8	16.9	94.2
Vermont	2.3	0.9	6.9	10.1	98.9
Virginia	1.6	0.3	6.3	8.2	92.7
West Virginia	1.3	1.9	18.4	21.5	99.4
		Decentralized county coroner			
Arkansas	1.9	2.9	7.4	12.2	76.7
Colorado	2.7	1.3	10.5	14.6	70.4
Idaho	2.3	1.7	6.6	10.6	59.6
Indiana	1.7	2.2	9.7	13.7	45.8
Kansas	1.5	0.9	6.9	9.3	58.8
Louisiana	0.8	1.6	11.1	13.5	34.8
Nebraska	0.9	0.6	4.3	5.8	69.4
Nevada	3.3	0.6	16.6	20.4	97.7
South Carolina	1.7	0.2	11.6	13.5	59.8
South Dakota	1.7	1.2	3.1	6.1	88.8
Wyoming	1.8	0.8	10.8	13.4	64.8
		Decentralized medical examiner (DME) or combined county coroner / medical examiner			
Alabama	1.1	1.0	10.4	12.5	45.0
Arizona (DME)	2.5	1.2	11.7	15.4	80.2
California	1.8	0.4	8.5	10.8	73.1
Florida (DME)	2.5	0.5	13.3	16.3	68.8
Georgia	1.2	0.4	8.7	10.4	71.4
Hawaii	1.3	2.0	6.9	10.1	83.1

Table 5.1. Continued

State	Nonhomicide drug intoxication death rates by manner (per 100,000)[a]				Drug intoxication deaths with 1+ specific drugs cited on the death certificate (%)[b]
	Suicide	Accident	Undetermined	Total	
Decentralized medical examiner (DME), continued					
Illinois	1.3	0.4	8.7	10.4	86.5
Iowa (DME)	1.8	0.7	4.8	7.4	96.1
Kentucky	1.4	1.7	16.6	19.6	64.8
Michigan (DME)	1.9	2.2	9.5	13.6	65.8
Minnesota	1.5	0.9	5.1	7.6	82.4
Mississippi	1.1	1.1	8.6	10.8	43.4
Missouri	1.8	0.8	12.0	14.6	79.3
Montana	3.0	1.8	8.5	13.4	69.9
New Jersey (DME)	0.8	0.2	5.9	7.0	59.3
New York	1.2	0.7	6.5	8.4	94.0
North Dakota	0.6	0.2	4.0	4.8	87.9
Ohio	1.5	0.6	11.8	13.9	71.4
Pennsylvania	1.7	0.7	12.4	14.9	45.0
Tennessee (DME)	1.8	1.2	12.8	15.7	77.8
Texas	1.2	0.3	7.7	9.2	74.7
Washington	2.2	0.9	11.5	14.6	92.6
Wisconsin	2.1	0.8	8.1	11.0	85.9

[a] Spearman's rank-order correlation coefficient (Rho) for drug intoxication suicide rates and combined accident and undetermined intent drug intoxication death rates = 0.38 ($p \leq 0.01$).

[b] Includes drug intoxication homicides. Source: Warner, M., Paulozzi, L.J., Nolte, K.B., Davis, G.G., Nelson, L.S., "State variation in certifying manner of death and drugs involved in drug-intoxication deaths," *Academic Forensic Pathology* 2013;3(2):231–37.

Source: Rockett, I.R.H., Hobbs, G., Wu, D., et al., "Variable classification of drug-intoxication suicides across US states: A partial artifact of forensics?," *PLOS One* 2015;10:e0135296.

the findings helped guide our multilevel (individual and contextual or county) research that utilized the enriched, restricted access database from the NVDRS, the core material in the next chapter.

A recovering addict's response

With the passage of time, I refined my view of poisoning mortality to home in on poisoning deaths attributable to drug intoxication—in recognition that drug overdose deaths mainly implicated prescription and nonprescription opioids, or a lethal combination of these painkillers and benzodiazepines (tranquilizers). Our prior interstate study (Rockett et al., 2015) was referenced in a 2016 story in *VICE* magazine (Szalavitz, 2016). The author

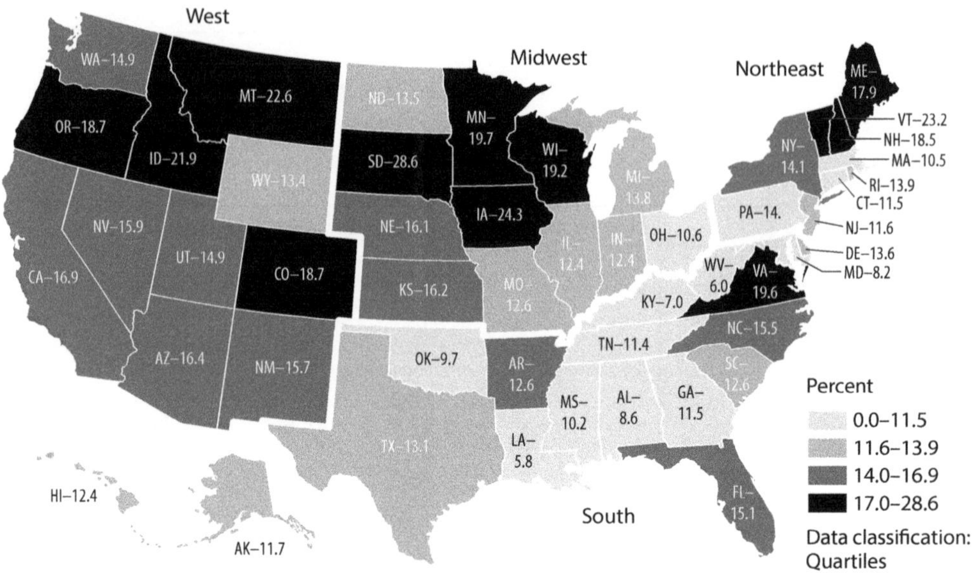

Figure 5.5. Percentage of nonhomicide drug intoxication deaths classified as suicide in quartiles by state and region, United States, 2008–10. Source: Rockett, I.R.H., Hobbs, G., Wu, D., et al., "Variable classification of drug-intoxication suicides across US states: A partial artifact of forensics?," *PLOS One* 2015;10: e0135296.

was Maia Szalavitz, a recovering heroin addict and a perceptive and provocative writer and tweeter/blogger. She subscribed to our suspicion that large discrepancies in the proportion of the overdoses that were classified as suicides reflected an artifactual component beyond true differences in drug suicide rates. She voiced our speculation that suicide may be more stigmatized in the South than in the Mountain states and that the latter may have more resources to dedicate to the investigation of suicide. Indeed, we had found that specificity of drug testing on the death certificate was positively associated with the suicide rate, while dying in the South showed a negative association. Szalavitz (2016) opined that

> discovering suicidal intent is of particular concern for pain patients, who are now reporting [awful] experiences of [not being able to get] needed opioids as doctors and pharmacists become more cautious and suspicious. The rate of suicide in this group is already high—and intractable pain due to denial of medication is [one cause]. In our rush to prevent deaths from addiction, we need to be

Table 5.2. Predicting the odds of a nonhomicide drug intoxication death being classified as suicide versus accident or undetermined intent

Characteristic	Beta	Odds ratio	95% CI Lower	95% CI Upper	Probability
	Single risk factor model				
Drug citation[a]	0.526	1.051	1.011	1.093	0.015
Region:[b]					
West	0.460	1.584	1.234	2.035	0.001
Midwest	0.448	1.565	1.212	2.021	0.001
Northeast	0.313	1.368	1.035	1.809	0.033
South (referent)		1.000			
Death investigation system type:					
Decentralized county coroner	0.128	1.137	0.841	1.537	0.409
Combined[c]	−0.007	0.993	0.773	1.275	0.954
Centralized medical examiner (referent)		1.000			
	Multivariable model				
Drug citation[a]	0.630	1.062	1.016	1.110	0.011
Region:					
West	0.358	1.430	1.115	1.836	0.007
Midwest	0.341	1.407	1.072	1.846	0.018
Northeast	0.289	1.335	1.014	1.756	0.045
South (referent)		1.000			
Death investigation system type:					
Decentralized county coroner	0.298	1.347	0.956	1.899	0.096
Combined[c]	0.104	1.110	0.852	1.446	0.444
Centralized medical examiner (referent)		1.000			

[a] Assuming a 10% increase in citation of one or more specific drugs on the death certificate.
[b] Age, sex, urbanization, and poverty; the other four preselected sociodemographic covariates were not significant predictors of suicide classification.
[c] Comprises decentralized medical examiner states and states with hybrid county coroner/medical examiner systems.

Source: Rockett, I.R.H., Hobbs, G., Wu, D., et al., "Variable classification of drug-intoxication suicides across US states: A partial artifact of forensics?," *PLOS One* 2015;10:e0135296.

> sure that we aren't increasing suicides in pain patients who are benefiting from medication. Suicide has gone practically unmentioned in most discussions of the overdose problem, whether they focus on pain treatment or on addiction. And this isn't actually surprising when the conversation is focused on or led by families who have suffered such great pain.

Interviewed for the story, I made the case that we need better ways of classifying overdose deaths, arguing that a category called "death by drug self-intoxication" (DDSI) would help distinguish between people who took the wrong dose and those who clearly wanted to get high, suicidal intent notwithstanding. I also said that some CDC officials have expressed interest in the classification.

Szalavitz (2016) added that she thought "the CDC should embrace this idea—and other ways of encouraging medical examiners and coroners to look more closely at the possibility of suicide in overdose cases. In order to spare other families from heartbreak, we need better data on just how bad the suicide problem is among people who overdose—and what's making so many people feel their lives aren't worth living."

As an addendum, among my multidisciplinary colleagues who collaborated with me on the DDSI article (Rockett et al., 2014b) were the chief medical examiner for Fulton County, Georgia, Randy Hanzlick, and a future chief medical examiner of New Mexico, Kurt Nolte. They provided invaluable on-the-ground information for me about suicide detection, as did my clinical colleagues who observe and treat high-risk populations in emergency departments and other hospital settings.

CDC panels on deciphering manner of death in drug cases

Scientific interest in suicide misclassification in the United States in the new millennium is most strongly associated with opioid and other drug poisoning deaths. My own research aligned perfectly with the topic of a panel convened in 2015 by CDC—entitled "Deciphering Suicide and Other Manners of Death Associated with Drug Intoxication" for the summary report (Stone et al., 2017)—which probably was no coincidence. In response to invitations facilitated by Eric Caine and in the spirit of research translation, I had previously conducted two webinars for the Self-Directed Violence Prevention Workgroup at CDC's National Center for Injury Prevention and Control in April and June 2014. I delivered my first webinar, titled "Suicide

Misclassification and Poisoning: Journey into a Cause for Concern and Action," via a laptop from a cramped and dark living room in a small rustic cottage located on the Provincetown end of Cape Cod, Massachusetts, but I imagined that my audience at CDC had assembled in a more formal setting. My second webinar was shorter and more specific: "Death from Deliberate Self-Intoxication (DDSI): Introducing a New Mortality Concept."

I welcomed the invitation to participate on the panel, which was organized and coordinated by CDC epidemiologist Deborah Stone. Membership was diverse in terms of disciplines and training, as well as expertise and experience. Panel members were affiliated with academia, state and federal government health agencies, a private foundation, the American Association of Suicidology, and both medical examiner and coroner offices. A rarity, one member was a policeman who conducted suicide investigations in a Michigan county. Another member was Michael Peck, a physical anthropologist who began working at the Los Angeles Suicide Prevention Center in 1963. Drawing on his personal perspective, Peck reinforced my admiration for the consummate professionalism and dedication to suicide research and prevention that characterized the center. The panel was the first at CDC to address suicide measurement issues since the panel led by Mark Rosenberg in the late 1980s, which proposed a set of uniform criteria for the medicolegal determination of suicide in the United States (Rosenberg et al., 1988). The 2015 panel identified three problem areas that were inhibiting the creation of a uniform manner-of-death classification related to fatal drug intoxication: (1) "ambiguous evidence at the death scene or the circumstances leading to the deaths," (2) "missing or incomplete information because either no death scene investigation (DSI) took place or information was not obtained or only partially obtained during the DSI," and (3) "heterogeneous DSI practices" (Stone et al., 2017, 1234).

Panel proceedings covered many of the issues I had been studying in the seven or so years preceding the meeting, as well as revisiting in detail the basics of suicide and other manner-of-death investigations outlined in chapters 1 and 2. Besides identifying barriers to uniform classification of drug intoxication deaths, extending from individual- and system-level to place-based factors, the panel offered a series of potential solutions. These solutions included continuing education, training, and certification; standardization of practices; creation and adoption of best practices for both toxicology and forensic autopsies; documenting issues arising from research and surveillance and investigating their impact on manner-of-death classification and injury prevention; researching the impact of place-based heterogeneity; and standardization of definitions and establishment of a new definition: DDSI. The origins of DDSI and its application to an enhanced category of self-injury mortality, which transcended registered or known suicides, are key components of the subject matter addressed in chapters 7 and 8.

There was a follow-up panel in which I participated in an initial face-to-face meeting hosted at CDC in 2017, although I did not participate in its subsequent interactions, as they moved well beyond my technical expertise. This panel addressed technology that would improve data collection and utilization, and CDC published a report of the proceedings in 2021 (Mercado et al., 2021). I will elaborate on their findings in chapter 10, since these are much more salient to the future than to the past.

NOTE

1. The National Center for Health Statistics published *A Reference Guide for Completing the Death Certificate for Drug Toxicity Deaths* (National Center for Health Statistics, 2019). This guide provides very comprehensive assistance to certifiers, including presenting scenarios of varying complexity—from single drug cases to cases with mixed toxicity involving contributions from numerous drugs—and examples of cases where significant health conditions also impacted a drug poisoning death.

6

The Importance of Supplemental Information

Enlightening suicide classification through the National Violent Death Reporting System

Formal acknowledgment by their respective professional communities that medicolegal death investigation systems (Committee on Identifying the Needs of the Forensic Sciences Community, National Research Council, 2009) and emergency health care systems in the early twenty-first-century United States were severely stressed and underresourced (Institute of Medicine, 2006a, 2006b) helped shape my research questions about possible associations between drug overdoses and suicide misclassification. In this chapter, I will describe and discuss two complementary multilevel (individual/county), multivariable studies I conducted with my collaborators that analyzed data from the National Violent Death Reporting System (NVDRS; Rockett et al., 2018a, 2018b). My overriding goal for these studies was to enlighten detection of drug poisoning suicides relative to suicides involving more overt methods, particularly gunshot wound and hanging, the two leading methods of suicide nationally. This hypothesis-driven research was delayed for three years owing to arbitrary allocation of an injury research center grant funded by the Centers for Disease Control and Prevention (CDC), and then by personal illness.

During the complete observation period for the two studies, 2011–13, the NVDRS encompassed 17 states: Alaska, Colorado, Georgia, Kentucky, Maryland, Massachusetts, New Jersey, New Mexico, North Carolina, Ohio, Oklahoma, Oregon, Rhode Island, South Carolina, Utah, Virginia, and Wisconsin. Notable omissions were the four most populous states: California, Florida, New York, and Texas. Now the NVDRS is universal in the United States, and there are analogous databases in some other countries, for example, the National Coronial Information System for Australia and New Zealand (Bugeja et al., 2016).

Suicide notes, psychiatric history, and drug poisoning suicides

The suicide note was central to both NVDRS studies. This research will attest that most suicide cases are not accompanied by an authenticated suicide note and that its importance, as corroborative forensic evidence, is not uniform across methods. The suicide note has long been established as pivotal evidence in corroborating suicide in a medicolegal death investigation. In the early 1960s, Robert Litman mentioned an anonymous California city where a death would not be classified as suicide in the absence of such a note (Litman et al., 1963)—which could be colloquially expressed as "no note, no suicide." The book *Postmortem: Establishing the Cause of Death* reported a case study that involved a young, part-time refrigerator repairman who died from asphyxiation due to Freon toxicity (Koehler & Wecht, 2006). Two competing manners of death arose during the investigation. The lack of a note tilted the balance away from an assignment of suicide and toward an assignment of accident. In *Cause of Death: A Writer's Guide to Death, Murder and Forensic Medicine*, one chapter was devoted to distinguishing homicide from suicide by cause (Wilson, 1992). Mechanisms of injury death discussed by the author were gunshot wound, hanging, stabbing, and drowning. In each instance, a criterion for suggesting suicide was the presence of a suicide note.

In the first of our two NVDRS studies, the study population comprised decedents in two manner-of-death categories: intentional self-harm, that is, registered suicides, and undetermined deaths (Rockett et al., 2018a). Excepting firearm deaths, accidental deaths are not part of the NVDRS. However, not only is the undetermined manner-of-death category most susceptible to suicide misclassification, but it can also provide a window into the nature of misclassification of suicides within the much larger accident category. The study population, which numbered 40,581, was limited to decedents aged 15 years and older, since fewer than 1% of known suicide decedents in the United States were younger. All decedents in this study had a known state and county of death. We used what is called a generalized linear mixed model (UCLA Advanced Research Computing, n.d.) in statistically testing five hypotheses, which were stated as follows: "Among our pooled suicide and undetermined cases, medical examiners and coroners are more likely to classify a death as suicide when (1) the injury mechanism/cause was gunshot wound or hanging/suffocation (as more overtly violent methods of suicide), versus drug intoxication (poisoning); and there was documentation of (2) a suicide note, (3) a prior suicide attempt, or (4) a primary diagnosis of major depression or bipolar disorder. (5) Any observed associations, pertaining to hypotheses 2 through 4, are stronger among drug intoxication than gunshot/hanging cases. The dependent or outcome variable was suicide versus undetermined death" (Rockett et al., 2018a, 5).

Elaborating, the individual-level variables in our multilevel models were forensic overtness of selected injury mechanisms/causes (gunshot and hanging/suffocation vs. drug intoxication), suicide note (yes vs. no or unknown), prior suicide attempt (yes vs. no or unknown), and primary mental diagnosis (depression or bipolar disorder vs. none or unknown). Engendering a conservative bias in internal comparisons, when variables were dichotomous (yes/no), the NVDRS data would not permit us to distinguish a clear negative response from the missing data—a deficit that needs to be minimized (Logan et al., 2009). With the same restriction, other individual-level covariates were autopsy status, current mental health treatment, crisis in past two weeks, number of intimate partner or legal or job or financial or school problems, blood alcohol concentration (grams of alcohol per deciliter of blood), number of other specified drug positives, physical health problem, age, sex, race/ethnicity, marital status, and education.

Linked to the individual-level data, our multivariable models also included two county-level medicolegal variables: selection mode and accreditation status. Selection mode of the chief medical examiner or coroner was either appointed or elected, and the accreditation status / type of death investigation system was accredited medical examiner, accredited coroner, unaccredited medical examiner, or unaccredited coroner. We obtained the data for the selection mode from the CDC website (Centers for Disease Control and Prevention, n.d.-a), and the sources for status/type were the websites of the two respective accrediting agencies, the National Association of Medical Examiners (n.d.) and the International Association of Coroners & Medical Examiners (n.d.). In instances where we had outstanding questions to resolve, we contacted the relevant state, district, or county offices by email or telephone. Adding an extra degree of refinement over the analytic capacity of our correlational study, we could factor into the analyses down to the county level the two medicolegal variables, together with a third contextual variable, namely, urbanicity or urban living. Suicides are overwhelmingly private and local phenomena, as I have previously mentioned. Urbanicity functioned as a proxy for external forces that might help or inhibit the death investigations (Waldhoer et al., 2003). We operationalized urbanicity across five ranked categories (large metropolitan, small metropolitan, adjacent metropolitan, micropolitan or adjacent, rural), a reduction from the more refined but statistically cumbersome 12 categories that constituted the 2013 Urban Influence Codes. The *County Area Health Resource File* for 2014–15 was the data source (Health Resources and Services Administration et al., 2015).

Since our NVDRS data represented only 17 states out of the total 50, an important question is whether generalizability of findings would be severely compromised as a result (Rockett et al., 2018a). In addressing this question, we profiled the NVDRS population and the national population according to various mortality and population characteristics (table 6.1). The remarkable similarity of the two profiles, given that the NVDRS population was less than one-third the size of the national population, greatly assuaged any concern I had about the representativeness of the study—that is, its external validity or generalizability. When I discuss our second study, I will reinforce the case for generalizability, based on the experience of the 17 states then participating in the NVDRS during our observation period.

A second set of profiles compared decedents by sociodemographics, death circumstances, and death investigation characteristics according to their assigned manner of death as suicide or undetermined (table 6.2). Consistent with our first hypothesis, the injury mechanism was gunshot or hanging in 68% of the suicide cases, compared to 11% for drug intoxication. Among the undetermined, the prevalence of drug intoxication cases was 55%, compared to 4% for gunshot/hanging. Consistent with our second hypothesis, 31% of the suicides were accompanied by an evidentiary suicide note, whereas the prevalence was only 1.5% for the undetermined cases. The prevalence data provided preliminary support for the suicide attempt hypothesis as well. There was documentation of a previous suicide attempt in 18% of the suicide cases versus 12.5% of the undetermined cases.

The preliminary data offered only partial support for our fourth hypothesis about the association between documentation of an affective disorder

Table 6.1. Selected population characteristics: 17 National Violent Death Reporting System (NVDRS) states and the United States, 2012

Characteristic	Percentage	
	NVDRS states (*n* = 95,297,084)	United States (*n* = 314,112,078)
Age (years):		
0–14	19.5	19.5
15–34	27.2	27.5
35–54	27.3	27.0
55–74	20.1	19.9
75+	5.9	6.1
Sex:		
Male	49.1	49.2
Race/ethnicity:		
Non-Hispanic White	69.0	63.9
Non-Hispanic Black	15.3	12.9
Hispanic	10.4	16.9
Other	5.3	6.3
Manner of death:		
Homicide	0.62	0.67
Suicide	1.66	1.62
Accident	5.33	5.12
Undetermined	0.23	0.19
Natural causes	92.15	92.40
Death rate (per 100,000 population):		
Crude all cause	819.6	810.2
Age-adjusted all cause	756.6	732.8
Crude suicide	13.4	12.9
Age-adjusted suicide	13.0	12.6
Crude undetermined	1.9	1.5
Age-adjusted undetermined	1.8	1.5

Source: Rockett, I.R.H., Caine, E.D., Connery, H.S., et al., "Discerning suicide in drug-intoxication deaths: Paucity and primacy of suicide notes and psychiatric history," *PLOS One* 2018;13:e0190200.

and a suicide classification. Prevalence of depression was higher among suicide cases but lower for bipolar disorder. Suicide cases were underrepresentative of the age group 15–54 years, females, minorities, the single, those with 9–12 years of education, and those who had resided in a large metropolitan area. There was proportionately higher representation among the suicide cases of decedents who were not in receipt of mental health treatment or whose treatment status was unknown, or who had a recent crisis or personal problems. There also was higher representation among those cases where the official charged with administering the death investigations, the chief

Table 6.2. Profiling suicide and undetermined deaths by demographics, precipitating circumstances, and investigation characteristics: National Violent Death Reporting System states, 2011–13

Demographics	Manner of Death (%) Suicide (n = 36,190)	Manner of Death (%) Undetermined (n = 4,391)
Age (years):		
15–34	28.5	32.0
35–54	38.9	45.4
55–74	25.3	19.7
75+	7.2	2.9
Sex:		
Male	77.8	61.7
Female	22.2	38.3
Race/ethnicity:		
White non-Hispanic	84.4	79.1
Black non-Hispanic	5.7	7.4
Hispanic	3.4	4.2
Other	6.5	9.3
Marital status:		
Single	33.4	40.9
Married	35.3	24.8
Widowed/divorced/separated	30.0	31.6
Unknown	1.3	2.7
Education (years):		
0–8	3.3	3.0
9–12	4.9	7.8
13+	76.3	78.0
Unknown	15.6	11.2
County urbanicity:		
Large metropolitan	42.6	57.6
Small metropolitan	36.0	27.3
Adjacent metropolitan	17.5	12.3
Adjacent micropolitan	1.8	1.7
Rural	2.0	1.1

Circumstances
Prior suicide attempt:
Yes
No/unknown
Mental diagnosis:
Depression
Anxiety disorder
Bipolar disorder
Other
No/unknown
Mental treatment:
Yes
No/unknown
Recent crisis:
Yes
No/unknown
Personal problem:
0/unknown
1
2
3+
Physical health problem:
Yes
No/unknown

Manner of Death (%)			Manner of Death (%)	
Suicide (n = 36,190)	Undetermined (n = 4,391)	Investigation	Suicide (n = 36,190)	Undetermined (n = 4,391)
		Chief ME/C selection:		
		Elected	37.7	18.7
18.0	12.5	Appointed	62.3	81.3
82.0	87.5			
		System accreditation/ type:		
		Accredited coroner	5.2	4.5
28.4	23.2	Medical examiner	25.2	45.0
1.7	2.7	Unaccredited coroner	32.4	14.2
3.8	4.8	Medical examiner	37.2	36.3
		Mechanism/cause:		
2.3	2.6			
		Gunshot/hanging	68.1	4.3
63.8	66.7			
		Drug intoxication	11.5	55.3
		Specified other	9.3	8.2
		Unspecified	11.0	32.1
29.7	32.6			
		Suicide note:		
70.3	67.4			
		Yes	30.9	1.5
		No/unknown	69.1	98.5
10.4	6.2			
		Autopsy:		
89.6	93.8			
		Yes	51.2	83.1
		No/unknown	48.8	16.9
		Blood alcohol con-		
55.2	82.4			
		centration (g/dl):		
31.5	14.2			
		0.00	32.9	44.7
10.3	2.8			
		0.01–0.07	5.7	8.8
3.0	0.6			
		≥0.08	15.1	16.8
		no test/unknown	46.4	29.7
		Other drug positive:		
19.2	21.1			
		0/unknown	74.6	30.4
80.8	78.9			
		1	15.0	29.4
		2	6.8	24.8
		3+	3.6	15.5

Source: Rockett, I.R.H., Caine, E.D., Connery, H.S., et al., "Discerning suicide in drug-intoxication deaths: Paucity and primacy of suicide notes and psychiatric history," *PLOS One* 2018;13:e0190200.

Note: ME/C = medical examiner or coroner; g/dl = grams of alcohol (ethanol) per deciliter of blood.

Table 6.3. Adjusted odds ratios and 95% confidence intervals for suicide versus undetermined manner-of-death classification according to injury mechanism/cause and documentation of a suicide note and other selected psychological/psychiatric characteristics: 17 National Violent Death Reporting System states, 2011–13

Characteristic	Odds ratio (95% CI)	*n*
Mechanism/cause:		
Gunshot/hanging	41.14 (34.43, 49.15)	24,848
Specified other	3.60 (3.08, 4.21)	2,642
Unspecified	0.40 (0.35, 0.46)	5,389
Drug intoxication	1.00	7,702
Suicide note:		
Yes	33.90 (26.11, 44.05)	11,263
No/unknown	1.00	29,318
Prior suicide attempt:		
Yes	2.42 (2.11, 2.77)	7,045
No/unknown	1.00	33,536
Mental diagnosis:		
Depression	1.61 (1.38, 1.88)	11,295
Bipolar disorder	1.41 (1.10, 1.81)	1,575
Anxiety disorder	0.83 (0.60, 1.16)	718
Other	1.39 (1.03, 1.86)	966
No/unknown	1.00	26,027

Source: Rockett, I.R.H., Caine, E.D., Connery, H.S., et al., "Discerning suicide in drug-intoxication deaths: Paucity and primacy of suicide notes and psychiatric history," *PLOS One* 2018;13:e0190200.

Note: Adjusted for autopsy status, blood alcohol concentration, specification of one or more drugs, selection mode of chief medical examiner/coroner, accreditation status/type of medicolegal death investigation system, mental treatment, recent crisis, number of personal problems, physical problem, age, sex, race/ethnicity, marital status, education, and county urbanicity.

medical examiner or coroner, was elected; where the death investigation system type was unaccredited coroner, or autopsy status was unknown; and where there was no toxicologic testing for alcohol and other drugs, or testing status was unknown.

Our full model comprised the four associated predictors for the multivariable testing of our first four hypotheses (table 6.3). The statistical analysis adjusted for the impact of 15 other variables that represented the sociodemographic composition of the decedents, their death circumstances, and characteristics of the medicolegal death investigations. With drug intoxication cases serving as the comparison group or referent, decedents who died by gunshot/hanging had 41 times higher odds of a suicide versus undetermined manner-of-death classification—potent support for the first hypothesis. There also was strong support for our second hypothesis. Where deaths were accompanied by an evidentiary suicide note, decedents had 34 times higher odds of a suicide classification than those for which there was no note or note status was unknown. The third hypothesis, too, was affirmed by our analysis. Decedents with documentation of a previous suicide attempt had two times higher odds of a suicide classification than those without such evidence. The fourth hypothesis, which concerned a primary diagnosis of an affective disorder, was also affirmed. Cases where there was documentation of a primary diagnosis of major depression or bipolar disorder had 1.6 and 1.4 times higher odds, respectively, of being classified as suicide relative to their opposites.

Buttressed by the enriched data from the NVDRS, this study affirmed that prior research indicated that detection of drug intoxication suicides is much more problematic than that of suicides by the much more lethal and overt means of gunshot/hanging. To better specify the nature of these difficulties, we distinguished the two groups for a stratified analysis where we were able to compare the relative impact of our respective hypothesized associations of evidence of a suicide note, a prior suicide attempt, and a primary diagnosis of an affective disorder and a suicide classification. Table 6.4 profiles drug intoxication and gunshot/hanging deaths separately in terms of their manner-of-death classification, suicide or undetermined. The respective prevalence of an evidentiary suicide note or a prior suicide attempt was higher among suicide decedents, independent of injury mechanism, and similarly for documentation of a primary diagnosis of major depression. However, a primary diagnosis of bipolar disorder was not more common among gunshot/hanging cases that were suicides versus those that were undetermined deaths.

The multilevel, multivariable statistical analysis of the data, stratified by or distinguishing injury mechanism as drug intoxication or combined gunshot/hanging, supported the original hypotheses with two exceptions (table 6.5). There was no association between a prior suicide attempt and a suicide classification in gunshot/hanging cases, and there was no association for either drug intoxication or gunshot/hanging cases when there was documentation of a primary diagnosis of bipolar disorder. However, consistent with evidence that indicated the problematic nature of case ascertainment of drug intoxication suicides and our fifth and final hypothesis, the

Table 6.4. Prevalence of a suicide note and other selected psychological/psychiatric characteristics documented in drug intoxication and gunshot/hanging suicide and undetermined death cases: 17 National Violent Death Reporting System states, 2011–13

	Drug intoxication (%)		Gunshot/hanging (%)	
Characteristic	Suicide (n = 4,175)	Undetermined (n = 2,430)	Suicide (n = 24,657)	Undetermined (n = 191)
Suicide note:				
Yes	42.2	1.3	29.4	4.2
No/unknown	57.8	98.7	70.6	95.8
Prior suicide attempt:				
Yes	34.5	14.0	14.9	10.0
No/unknown	65.5	86.0	85.1	90.0
Mental diagnosis:				
Depression	43.6	26.8	26.6	13.1
Bipolar disorder	7.6	5.2	3.0	3.7
Anxiety disorder	2.5	2.7	1.6	0.5
Other	2.6	2.1	2.1	1.0
No/unknown	43.7	63.2	66.8	81.7

Source: Rockett, I.R.H., Caine, E.D., Connery, H.S., et al., "Discerning suicide in drug-intoxication deaths: Paucity and primacy of suicide notes and psychiatric history," *PLOS One* 2018;13:e0190200.

association between a suicide note, a prior suicide attempt, and a suicide classification was far stronger in drug intoxication cases. I suggest that psychological/psychiatric evidence is far more important in corroborating drug intoxication suicides than gunshot/hanging suicides in the United States. The findings from this study set the scene for a discussion of our second study, which also used the restricted access data of the NVDRS, where we assessed the relative importance of psychological/psychiatric evidence and physical forensic evidence in the case ascertainment of suicides by method.

Suicide method and an evidentiary suicide note

Through confining the study population to suicides in our second study, we were freed from the small subsample size constraints related to undetermined deaths (Rockett et al., 2018b). Consequently, we could examine the respective associations between more refined suicide methods or injury mechanisms and an evidentiary suicide note. In the first study, for example, we needed to combine firearm and hanging cases because, separately, they were rare among the undetermined cases.

Stated formally, we tested two hypotheses in the second study: (1) that

Table 6.5.Adjusted odds ratios and 95% confidence intervals for suicide versus undetermined manner-of-death classification by injury mechanism/cause according to documentation of a suicide note and other selected psychological/psychiatric characteristics: 17 National Violent Death Reporting System states, 2011–13

	Drug intoxication		Gunshot/hanging	
Characteristic	Odds ratio (95% CI)	*n*	Odds ratio (95% CI)	*n*
Suicide note:				
Yes	45.43 (31.06, 66.58)	1,792	8.06 (3.94, 16.49)	7,244
No/unknown	1.00	4,813	1.00	17,604
Prior suicide attempt:				
Yes	2.64 (2.19, 3.18)	1,782	1.32 (0.79, 2.19)	3,680
No/unknown	1.00	4,823	1.00	21,168
Mental diagnosis:				
Depression	1.48 (1.17, 1.87)	2,470	1.26 (0.74, 2.15)	6,579
Bipolar disorder	1.39 (0.98, 1.97)	445	0.61 (0.26, 1.39)	753
Anxiety disorder	0.62 (0.38, 1.00)	171	2.20 (0.30, 16.41)	385
Other	1.54 (0.93, 2.55)	157	1.68 (0.40, 7.10)	517
No/unknown	1.00	3,362	1.00	16,614

Source: Rockett, I.R.H., Caine, E.D., Connery, H.S., et al., "Discerning suicide in drug-intoxication deaths: Paucity and primacy of suicide notes and psychiatric history," *PLOS One* 2018;13:e0190200.

Note: Adjusted for autopsy status, blood alcohol concentration, specification of one or more drugs, selection mode of chief medical examiner / coroner, accreditation status / type of medicolegal death investigation system, mental treatment, recent crisis, number of personal problems, physical problem, age, sex, race/ethnicity, marital status, education, and county urbanicity.

an evidentiary suicide note is more common among suicides by drug intoxication and by other poisoning, as less forensically overt methods, than among suicides by firearm and by hanging/suffocation, and (2) that performance of a forensic autopsy attenuates any observed association between overtness of method and the reported presence of a note. The logic underlying the first hypothesis was that the burden of requiring a suicide note as medicolegal evidence to corroborate suicide would be greater in more equivocal cases.

Steven Stack, a prominent Wayne State University sociologist and suicidologist, and I had previously conducted an individual-level, multivariable analysis of suicide notes that utilized NVDRS data for the period 2003–6 (Stack & Rockett, 2018). We found a higher prevalence of suicide notes among suicides by poisoning, firearm, and hanging than among those by drowning or jumping from a height. Drowning, like poisoning, is less overt than the other methods. We also found that note leaving was nonrandom across decedent age, sex, race/ethnicity, and urban residence. Unlike our American study, a study from Austria, a country with high-quality suicide data, found no difference in the prevalence of suicide notes in suicide cases by method, age, sex, family status, psychiatric care, or motive (Eisenwort et al., 2006). Moreover, there is no research showing that suicides by drug intoxication and nongas poisoning are less impulsive and more planned than suicides by the more violent and overt methods, and hence more likely to be accompanied by a suicide note.

Adopting the statistical methodology used in our first NVDRS study, my coauthors and I employed a generalized linear mixed model and retained the observation period, 2011–13 (Rockett et al., 2018b). The outcome variable was the relative odds of an evidentiary or authenticated suicide note versus no note or note status unknown. We assumed that the notes that were part of the NVDRS database were authentic, but we acknowledge that capacity to authenticate can be problematic depending on training and use of predictive statistical rules and models (Bennell et al., 2011). Suicide decedents in our study totaled 32,151. In the first study, we had provided strong evidence from comparative population and mortality profiles that our results were generalizable to the American population aged 15 years and older. Fortifying the generalizability of results from both of our NVDRS analyses, based on the 17 participant states, the distributions of suicide methods were very similar in that age group and by sex between those states and the United States as a whole (table 6.6). Similar distributions in these two populations were also evident for suicides by firearm, hanging, drug intoxication, and other poisoning for non-Hispanic Whites and the two major minorities, non-Hispanic Blacks and Hispanics. The largest difference by race/ethnicity between the NVDRS and American populations occurred with Hispanics and Blacks in the jumping/drowning and residual methods groups.

Table 6.7 presents bivariable frequency data for our study population, that is, suicide decedents, for seven demographic characteristics, seven variables representing suicide circumstances, and six variables pertaining to the medicolegal death investigation. These prevalence data provide preliminary support for our hypothesis that evidentiary suicide notes (written, typed, digital, or audio) are more common among drug intoxication (42%) and other poisoning (48%) suicides than among the more forensically overt cases of firearm (29%) and hanging/suffocation (31%) suicides. Although not subjects of our hypothesis, there were large gaps in the prevalence of recovered

Table 6.6. Percent suicide by method and selected demographic characteristics: 17 National Violent Death Reporting System states and the United States, 2011–13

Characteristic/	Firearm		Hanging/ suffocation		Drug intoxication		Other poisoning		Jumping/ drowning		Other methods[a]		n	
Method	NVDRS	US	NVDRS	US	NVDRS	US	NVDRS	US	NVDRS	US	NVDRS	US	NVDRS	US
Age (years):														
All ages	52.3	51.0	24.4	24.8	13.2	13.3	3.1	3.1	2.6	3.2	4.2	4.6	37,909	121,267
0–14	18.5	33.7	53.2	62.2	0	2.4	0	0	0	0.8	28.3	0.8	314	993
15–34	47.0	45.1	35.1	35.8	8.6	8.5	2.0	2.0	2.3	3.8	5.0	4.7	10,809	33,236
35–54	47.0	45.3	25.3	25.9	16.6	16.8	3.7	3.8	2.2	3.2	5.2	5.0	14,605	46,249
55–74	60.2	58.5	14.0	14.9	15.1	15.8	3.3	3.4	1.5	2.9	5.9	4.5	9,422	30,925
75+	76.9	75.4	7.6	9.6	5.6	7.1	0.4	2.5	0	2.8	9.5	2.6	2,741	9,844
Sex:														
Female	32.9	31.6	23.1	23.5	32.6	32.5	3.0	3.4	2.3	4.3	6.1	4.7	8,406	26,429
Male	57.8	56.4	24.8	25.2	7.7	8.0	3.1	3.0	2.3	2.9	4.3	4.5	29,503	94,838
Race/ethnicity:														
White non-Hispanic	53.9	53.6	22.6	22.2	13.8	14.1	3.2	3.2	2.4	2.7	4.1	4.2	32,443	101,011
Hispanic	36.4	35.7	41.5	41.5	8.0	9.9	0	1.7	1.0	4.4	13.1	6.7	1,627	8,125
Black non-Hispanic	49.2	47.8	26.9	28.4	7.3	9.2	1.9	2.3	0.9	3.6	13.8	8.7	2,419	6,951
Other	34.7	27.6	40.7	46.0	5.4	9.8	0	3.0	0.8	6.9	18.4	6.7	1,332	4,781

Source: Rockett, I.R.H., Caine, E.D., Stack, S., et al., "Method overtness, forensic autopsy, and the evidentiary suicide note: A multilevel National Violent Death Reporting System analysis," *PLOS One* 2018;13:e019.

Note: The data source was the Web-based Injury Statistics Query and Reporting System (WISQARS), administered by the Centers for Disease Control and Prevention.

[a] Comprises both specified and unspecified suicide methods.

Table 6.7. Prevalence of suicide notes by decedent demographics, death circumstances, and investigation system characteristics: 17 National Violent Death Reporting System states, 2011–13

Demographics	Percentage	n[a]	Circumstances
Age (years):			Past suicide attempt:
15–34	28.3	9,147	Yes
35–54	32.7	12,525	No/unknown
55–74	32.9	8,125	Mental diagnosis:
75+	28.3	2,354	Depression/dysthymia
Total	31.4	32,151	Anxiety disorder
Sex:			Bipolar disorder
Male	29.6	25,100	Other
Female	37.8	7,051	None/unknown
Race/ethnicity:			Mental health treatment:
White non-Hispanic	32.7	27,333	Yes
Hispanic	26.5	1,149	No/unknown
Black non-Hispanic	19.6	1,691	Physical health problem:
Other	26.8	1,978	Yes
Marital status:			No/unknown
Single	30.2	10,891	Personal problems:
Married	29.9	11,344	0/unknown
Widowed/divorced/separated	34.5	9,655	1
Unknown	31.8	261	2
Education (years):			3+
0–8	15.0	1,154	Recent crisis:
9–12	25.1	1,704	Yes
13+	33.1	25,216	No/unknown
Unknown	28.4	4,077	Emergency medical services:
Military veteran:			Present at scene
Yes	31.7	5,795	Absent/unknown
No/unknown	31.4	26,356	
Region of death:			
Other	34.0	18,990	
South	27.7	13,161	

suicide notes between Whites and Blacks and between the most and least educated groups. There was a higher prevalence of notes for female compared to male decedents and for decedents from non-Southern states compared to those in the South.

Percentage	n^a	Investigation	Percentage	n^a
		Chief medical examiner/		
34.9	5,858	coroner:		
30.7	26,293	Elected	27.4	11,448
		Appointed	33.6	20,703
35.0	9,313	System accreditation/type:		
38.4	539	Accredited medical	34.4	8,479
34.5	1,209	examiner		
23.2	764	Accredited coroner	36.6	1,685
29.7	20,326	Unaccredited medical	33.2	12,269
		examiner		
		Unaccredited coroner	33.2	9,718
34.2	9,850	Method:		
30.2	22,301	Drug intoxication	42.2	4,154
		Other poisoning	48.2	1,014
37.5	6,010	Firearm	28.7	16,609
30.0	26,141	Hanging	30.6	8,017
		Jumping/drowning	29.1	824
		All other	25.6	1,533
28.2	17,565	Blood alcohol concentration		
34.3	10,134	(g/dl):		
37.8	3,422	0.00	34.9	10,946
37.2	1,030	0.10–0.79	37.7	1,921
		No test/unknown	29.1	14,260
33.8	3,558	≥0.80	28.1	5,024
31.1	28,593	Other drug positive:		
		0	30.4	23,860
		1	33.7	4,914
32.6	23,377	2	35.5	2,209
28.4	8,774	3+	35.8	1,168
		Autopsy:		
		Yes	30.7	16,409
		No/unknown	32.2	15,742

[a] Total number of cases within each variable subcategory.

Source: Rockett, I.R.H., Caine, E.D., Stack, S., et al., "Method overtness, forensic autopsy, and the evidentiary suicide note: A multilevel National Violent Death Reporting System analysis," *PLOS One* 2018;13:e019.

Hypothesis testing in our second study consisted of two parts, one following a cumulative process and the other involving a stratified analysis differentiating autopsy status. The first part progressively applied four models, starting with a univariable or single-variable model limited to the predictor,

Table 6.8. Odds ratios and 95% confidence intervals for an evidentiary note by suicide method, cumulatively adjusted for investigation characteristics, death circumstances, and demographics: 17 National Violent Death Reporting System states, 2011–13

Category/variable	Model 1[a] OR (95% CI)	Model 2[b] OR (95% CI)	Model 3[c] OR (95% CI)	Model 4[d] OR (95% CI)
Suicide method:				
Drug intoxication	1.71 (1.60, 1.84)	1.80 (1.66, 1.95)	1.88 (1.73, 2.04)	1.66 (1.53, 1.81)
Other poisoning	2.22 (1.94, 2.52)	2.21 (1.94, 2.52)	2.25 (1.97, 2.57)	2.13 (1.87, 2.44)
Jumping/drowning	0.93 (0.79, 1.08)	0.91 (0.78, 1.07)	1.00 (0.86, 1.18)	0.98 (0.83, 1.15)
Hanging	1.04 (0.97, 1.10)	1.04 (0.97, 1.10)	1.05 (0.99, 1.12)	1.07 (1.00, 1.14)
Other	0.81 (0.72, 0.92)	0.81 (0.71, 0.91)	0.86 (0.76, 0.97)	0.83 (0.73, 0.94)
Firearm	1.00	1.00	1.00	1.00

[a] Unadjusted for any other study variables.

[b] Adjusted for investigation characteristics (see table 6.7).

[c] Adjusted for investigation characteristics and death circumstances (see table 6.7).

[d] Adjusted for investigation characteristics, death circumstances, and decedent demographics (see table 6.7).

Source: Rockett, I.R.H., Caine, E.D., Stack, S., et al., "Method overtness, forensic autopsy, and the evidentiary suicide note: A multilevel National Violent Death Reporting System analysis," *PLOS One* 2018;13:e019.

suicide method (drug intoxication, other poisoning, firearm, hanging, jumping/drowning, all other specified methods; table 6.8). Model 2, a multivariable model, added four death investigation variables: system type, accreditation status, alcohol toxicology, and other drug toxicology. Model 3 also encompassed death circumstances (number of personal financial, family, work, legal, or school problems, and recent crisis) and four mental and physical health variables. Model 4 added seven individual-level demographic characteristics of decedents (age, sex, race/ethnicity [White non-Hispanic, Hispanic, Black non-Hispanic, other], education, marital status, military veteran status, region of death) and two county-level or contextual demographic characteristics (urbanicity [metropolitan large, metropolitan small, metropolitan adjacent, micropolitan or adjacent, rural] and poverty prevalence).

With firearm as the reference or comparison method of suicide, the univariable statistical analysis showed that a drug intoxication suicide had 71% excess odds of being accompanied by an evidentiary suicide note and suicide by other poisoning had 122% excess odds. An empirical question is whether nondrug poisoning suicides might be more planned (vs. impulsive) than poisoning suicides by drug intoxication. Hanging, as a violent and forensically overt method of suicide, showed no significant excess odds of being accompanied by an evidentiary suicide note relative to those for firearm suicides.

These results aligned with our hypothesis. They generally remained robust through the application of model 4, under an assumption that drug intoxication suicides are not more planned and less impulsive than firearm suicides. They support an expectation that a suicide note is more pivotal in medicolegal corroboration of the former suicides relative to those by violent and forensically overt methods. We replicated the model 4 multivariable analysis in the second part of our hypothesis testing, stratifying the data by autopsy status: whether an autopsy was performed versus not performed or unknown (table 6.9). We viewed the autopsy as a surrogate for the fastidiousness of a given medicolegal death investigation, as well as inherently important, in evaluating whether the association between suicide method and presence of an evidentiary suicide note was attenuated by performance of an autopsy. However, we had no information from the NVDRS data on the extent to which medical examiner and coroner offices used virtual autopsies in lieu of physical autopsies, evidence that the digital revolution has modified the practice of forensic pathology.

Virtual autopsies use such advanced imaging technologies as multislice computerized tomography and magnetic resonance imaging, and they have the capacity to render three-dimensional volumes to create vivid images of the interior of the human body (Lathrop et al., 2023). A virtual autopsy, or virtopsy, is less invasive than a physical autopsy and does not damage bodily tissues. It may, for example, be able to detect internal bleeding and gas embolism, provide vivid pictures of skeletal and soft tissue injuries, and forestall religious objections. This technology is adequate to supplant an autopsy in determining the cause of death in many types of cases, including firearm injuries, blunt force injuries, pediatric trauma, and drug overdoses in individuals older than age 50 years.

Drug intoxication suicide cases still showed excess odds relative to firearm suicides of being accompanied by an evidentiary suicide note, as did other poisoning suicides, regardless of whether there was an autopsy. In conformance with our hypothesis, performance of an autopsy attenuated the associations. Whereas drug intoxication suicides had 86% excess odds relative to firearm suicides of being accompanied by an evidentiary suicide

Table 6.9. Odds ratios and 95% confidence intervals for an evidentiary note by suicide method, stratified by autopsy status and unstratified, adjusted for investigation characteristics, death circumstances, and demographics: 17 National Violent Death Reporting System states, 2011–13

	Autopsy				Full model (includes autopsy status)
Category/variable[a]	Yes OR (95% CI)	n[b]	No/unknown OR (95% CI)	n[b]	OR (95% CI)
Suicide method:					
Drug intoxication	1.62 (1.45, 1.82)	2,866	1.86 (1.61, 2.14)	1,288	1.70 (1.56, 1.85)
Other poisoning	2.01 (1.66, 2.43)	512	2.25 (1.86, 2.72)	502	2.12 (1.85, 2.42)
Jumping/drowning	1.04 (0.85, 1.27)	527	0.96 (0.73, 1.25)	297	0.99 (0.85, 1.17)
Hanging/suffocation	0.86 (0.73, 1.01)	3,365	0.80 (0.65, 0.97)	4,652	1.04 (0.97, 1.11)
Other	1.00 (0.91, 1.11)	939	1.07 (0.98, 1.17)	594	0.83 (0.74, 0.95)
Firearm	1.00	8,200	1.00	8,409	1.00
Autopsy:					
No/unknown					1.26 (1.18, 1.34)
Yes					1.00

[a] See table 6.7 for listing of the variables constituting the investigation characteristics, death circumstances, and decedent demographics.

[b] n = sample size.

Source: Rockett, I.R.H., Caine, E.D., Stack, S., et al., "Method overtness, forensic autopsy, and the evidentiary suicide note: A multilevel National Violent Death Reporting System analysis," *PLOS One* 2018;13:e019.

note, given no autopsy, the excess odds declined to 62% with one. Similarly, excess odds for other poisoning suicides declined from 125% to 101%. Finally, I show the results from the application of the full model, which I label model 5. In testing the suicide method hypothesis, this model comprised all model 4 variables, adjusted for autopsy status. Results for the application of models 1–4 are affirmed.

Although not part of our analytic research question(s) or formal hypothesis testing, some other interesting results emerged from the application of model 5 (data not shown). Suggesting the importance of a suicide note as corroborative evidence for a suicide determination, cases with no autopsy or with unknown autopsy status showed 26% excess odds of a suicide note being in the medicolegal record. There was no association with an evidentiary note in instances where a primary mental health diagnosis was major depression, bipolar disorder, or another specified disorder. Excess odds of a note were manifest for decedents with no measurable blood alcohol concentration or one of less than 0.80 milligrams of alcohol per deciliter of blood, or no alcohol test or unknown test status, versus those decedents with a concentration of at least 0.80 milligrams, the universal legal threshold in the United States for driving impaired by the influence of alcohol. The relationship was similar for other drugs. Excess odds were also evident where there was a record of mental health treatment, a physical health problem, or personal problems. Excess odds of a note also materialized in suicide cases where the decedent was 35 years or older; was female; was not non-Hispanic Black; was single, widowed, divorced, or separated; had more than eight years of education, or whose educational status was unknown; was a military veteran; or died outside the South or in a metropolitan area. These associations call for further research.

Affirmation of the hypothesized association between type of suicide method and record of an evidentiary suicide note rested on an assumption that the odds were higher among decedents using less forensically overt methods than among those using more overt methods because medical examiners and coroners require stronger corroborative evidence, especially a suicide note, for making a suicide determination. This rationale also applies to the alcohol and other drug test variables. English research has shown that test positivity is associated with an undetermined rather than a suicide classification (Salib, 1996), and Canadian research has shown a similar association with an accident versus suicide classification (Jarvis et al., 1991). Warranting in-depth research using psychological autopsies, a suicide note may be more pivotal for determination of non–drug intoxication suicides in cases where there is evidence of alcohol or other drug positivity than when this is absent.

The NVDRS database permitted us to examine differences in medicolegal case ascertainment by less versus more forensically overt methods, with our main interest being case ascertainment or detection of suicides by drug intoxication relative to those by firearm and hanging. The first study showed that an evidentiary suicide note is important in distinguishing suicides from undetermined deaths for suicides by all three of these leading methods, but that it is more important in drug intoxication cases (Rockett et al., 2018a). However, the other psychological/psychiatric information under scrutiny, record of a prior suicide attempt and a primary diagnosis of a mental health disorder, only comes to the fore in ascertaining drug intoxication suicides. Confining the study population to registered or known suicides afforded the second study more granularity in categorizing deaths by injury mechanism or suicide method (Rockett et al., 2018b). In this study, presence versus absence of a suicide note served as the dependent or outcome variable. The principal research issue was whether drug intoxication and other poisoning suicides are harder to detect than firearm and hanging suicides; if so, then their odds of a note, as important corroborative evidence, should be higher. This expectation was supported. However, a forensic autopsy should diminish these odds, as a proxy for the fastidiousness of a medicolegal death investigation. Although reducing the relative importance of a suicide note in substantiating drug intoxication and other poisoning suicides versus firearm and hanging suicides, performance of an autopsy did not eliminate the note effect.

Supplemented by county-level data on the sociodemographic and medicolegal context of suicide case ascertainment, the NVDRS data permitted us to control for numerous potential confounding factors in evaluating the research questions in our two multilevel, multivariable studies. However, the first study would have been strengthened if CDC had not excluded accidental deaths from their data, except for motor vehicular trauma deaths. The NVDRS data that we accessed for our two studies were a compilation of linked records and reports from multiple sources. Medical examiners and coroners, the officials responsible for ascertaining suicides, likely did not have ready access to all of this information, even if predisposed toward the value of obtaining a fuller picture to assist them with their determinations.

My concern about detecting poisoning suicides, especially suicides by drug intoxication, extends back 15 years. During this time, I became better acquainted with the strengths and weaknesses of American medicolegal death investigation systems and more appreciative of the added stresses and strains the opioid epidemic has inflicted on them—although this impact must be far from uniform across the country. I began to rethink the problem of misclassification of poisoning suicides, motivated by the reality that society was unlikely to address system deficits in the foreseeable future and my recognition that self-injury mortality (SIM) transcended known (i.e., registered) suicides. Our two NVDRS studies provide compelling evidence that decedent biographies and details on the immediate circumstances of death are critical if case ascertainment of drug intoxication suicides is to be optimal, and even if it is to match the ascertainment of suicides by the more violent and forensically overt methods of firearm (gunshot wound) and hanging.

Media dissemination

The first of our two multilevel studies (Rockett et al., 2018a) was featured in a *Reuters Health* story by Cheryl Platzman Weinstock (2018) under the headline "Drug-Overdose Suicides May Be Going Undetected." In her story, I was quoted as saying, "The opioid epidemic is killing more people every year at a higher rate. Death investigation systems are highly stressed. It's going to make it very difficult to do the kind of assessments we need to do about their intentionality. The problem with inaccurate suicide counting is that it impedes our understanding and prevention of suicide and drug deaths." Platzman Weinstock inferred from our study that there were few clues in drug cases to suggest a suicide, such as a suicide note. She highlighted marked variation in the importance of the suicide note as a pivotal piece of corroborative evidence by suicide method: "The existence of a suicide note increased the odds 45-fold that a drug overdose death would be classified as a suicide, whereas a note only raised the odds of classifying gunshot or hanging deaths as suicide by eight-fold" (Platzman Weinstock 2018).

CDC injury epidemiologist Margaret Warner commented in Platzman Weinstock's story that "the biggest story here is not that death investigations are a really important way we understand how people die. The impact of this work is that it points out the inconsistencies in how deaths are certified. . . . We want consistent investigations and comparable stats between states" (Platzman Weinstock 2018). I concur. Warner also affirmed that drug intoxication deaths are very challenging for medical examiners and coroners in assigning manner of death.

Among other study findings, detailed by Platzman Weinstock, were that gunshot and hanging deaths were 41 times more likely than drug intoxication deaths to be classified as suicide versus undetermined and that deaths accompanied by a suicide note were 34 times more likely to be classified as suicide than were cases of deaths with no note or unknown note status. She also reported on excess odds for cases with documentation of a prior suicide attempt, unipolar depression, or bipolar disorder.

The *Reuters Health* story ended with a provocative quote from Jill Harkavy-Friedman, vice president for research at the American Foundation for Sui cide Research: "I want to caution about everything being called a potential suicide because if we make it a very heterogeneous group, it stops having meaning and it's hard to understand the factors that contribute to suicide. Not every overdose is a suicide. We want to be as clear as we can when you're calling something a death by suicide" (Platzman Weinstock 2018).

Clarification is necessary. My team and I have never tried to convey to readers that all fatal drug overdoses are suicides. Yes, some unknown quantity are misclassified suicides, but our main point is that the large majority of these drug deaths lie on the upper end of the self-harm continuum, irrespective of whether the decedents intended to die. Nonetheless, Harkavy-Friedman's concern showed in stark relief that we needed to improve the translation of our research to policymakers and the public. This translation is critical when we talk about SIM, our alternative and broader conceptualization of fatal self-injury than suicide. The centerpiece of the next chapter, SIM is a departure from the conventional dichotomy where there is an initial binary choice concerning a suicide assignment, such that a given death is either a suicide or a nonsuicide. It encompasses a continuum for fatal self-injury as exists for suicidal morbidity.

Comparing national and local approaches to detecting suicides

Established and maintained by CDC's National Center for Health Statistics, the National Death Index (NDI) permits researchers and other interested parties to link their databases with death certificates of any American decedents for such purposes as assessing disease and injury burdens, informing health policy, and effectively designing and targeting interventions and prevention programming. One study compared the detection of suicides in the US Department of Defense's Suicide Data Repository, which incorporates all suicides by military veterans captured by the NDI, with that reflected in the database of root cause analyses of any inpatient suicides and suicides of outpatients occurring within seven days of discharge from the inpatient mental health unit in the Veteran Administration's health care system (Riblet et al., 2019). Implemented by multidisciplinary teams, whose activities may include reviewing medical records, visiting death scenes, and interviewing key informants in a standardized process emulating psychological autopsies, root cause analyses are conducted to identify and ameliorate systematic deficits associated with rare adverse (alarm-sounding, canaryin-a-coal-mine, sentinel) events, such as suspected suicides. While the study showed that the NDI captured many more suicides than the root cause analysis database, the former was also susceptible to suicide misclassification and did miss suicides that were identified in the latter. One can readily infer from this research that, optimally, suicide case ascertainment for the national population and subpopulations (e.g., military veterans) should emanate from a combination of national surveillance databases and local health care databases and that the data collection needs to be systematic. The authors found that more than 50% of misclassified suicides were drug overdoses. They concluded that misclassification was most problematic for nonfirearm suicides. Their findings largely affirm what we reported in 2018 from our two multilevel, multivariable NVDRS studies for a general population (Rockett et al., 2018a, 2018b).

For many years, I suspected that I would be forced to conclude that American suicide data are substantially deficient and that the situation would not improve. Optimism thankfully superseded my pessimism once I became aware of the need for the fatal SIM domain to be expanded and began to work persistently for that cause with my multidisciplinary collaborators.

7

Shifting the Suicide Paradigm Toward Self-Injury Mortality

Some troubling history

Pursuant to an earlier history involving first morphine and then heroin, the modern phase of the American opioid epidemic is rooted in unscrupulous actions by global pharmaceutical corporations (Big Pharma) and indiscriminate and prolific prescribing by manifold physicians. In time, a relatively small number of superspreaders, a term coined in the early 1970s in reference to computer simulations of influenza epidemics, generated an extraordinarily high number and proportion of opioid prescriptions. Malcolm Gladwell reported that with universal state backing universal use by physicians of triplicate prescription pads across the United States—whereby prescribers keep an original for two years, send one copy to the pharmacy filling the prescription, and share a second copy in a timely fashion with a narcotics enforcement agency—would have prevented many opioid overdoses (Gladwell, 2024).

Physicians originally may have thought that opioid painkillers—developed to control cancer pain—were nonaddictive based on reading or otherwise being cognizant of the content of a single-paragraph, five-sentence, 101-word, non-peer-reviewed research letter by Jane Porter and Hershel Jick, published in the eminent *New England Journal of Medicine* in 1980 (Porter & Jick, 1980; Zhang, 2017). Porter and Jick reported that only 0.03% of their hospital sample of 11,882 patients with no history of addiction, who had been administered at least one low-dose narcotic as part of their therapy, then manifested addiction. Major methodological flaws in this research were the small opioid doses and the absence of patient follow-up. However, the interpretation of the authors was reasonable in the time and context of the letter's publication. One could argue, then, that the opioid epidemic began as an iatrogenic problem, that is, a health care problem stemming inadvertently from medical practice. However, it evolved into a much more sinister phenomenon regarding type, scope, and lethality.

A 2017 bibliometric analysis (Leung et al., 2017) showed that the brief Porter and Jick letter became the platform and bandwagon for pharmaceutical companies to rationalize opioids as therapeutically safe for treating chronic noncancer pain,[1] consequently expanding markets and inundating them with veritable tsunamis of these pills (Jacobs, 2016; Kounang, 2017). Seventy-two percent of the 608 articles citing the letter—published in the *New England Journal of Medicine* from 1980 until March 31, 2017—employed it as evidence of the rarity of opioid addiction among recipients (Leung et al., 2017).

As the opioid epidemic burgeoned, an old, derivative, but wisdom-laden quotation from the Pulitzer Prize–winning author and "muckraker" Upton Sinclair became increasingly salient: "It's difficult to get a man to understand something if his salary depends on his not understanding it" (1935, 109). Cataloging the path of the epidemic as one dominated first by prescription opioids and then by illicit ones in the black market, a plethora of books has variously humanized implicated victims, pharmacologists, manufacturers, marketers, physicians, pharmacists, and dealers for better or worse. These books include *Dream Land: The True Tale of America's Opiate Epidemic* (Quinones, 2015), *American Pain: How a Young Felon and His Ring of Doctors Unleashed America's Deadliest Drug Epidemic* (Temple, 2016), *Fentanyl, Inc.: How Rogue Chemists Are Creating the Deadliest Wave of the Opioid Epidemic* (Westhoff, 2019), *The Least of Us: True Tales of America and Hope in the Time of Fentanyl and Meth* (Quinones, 2021), and *American Cartel: Inside Battle to Bring Down the Opioid Industry* (Higham & Horwitz, 2022). The humanization of victims, in particular, is vividly and poignantly portrayed in numerous documentaries that are easily accessible through YouTube videos.

For much of this new century, Purdue Pharma, the company owned by the Sackler family, has been the malicious and avaricious face of the pharmaceutical corporations that flooded the opioid market. However, reflected in their fines and settlements from opioid litigation, many other companies similarly reaped monumental profits from wholesale or retail sales of these highly addictive drugs (see https://nationalopioidsettlement.com/). Turning to illicit fentanyl trafficking, drug laboratories run by Mexican cartels have now largely supplanted drug factories in China as sources (Greenwood & Fashola, 2021; Stoecker et al., 2023). The death toll from the opioid epidemic is not just from overdoses. For example, aggressive marketing of OxyContin during the 1990s and early 2000s contributed to long-term mortality from communicable diseases, such as acute viral hepatitis (A, B, and C) and bacterial endocarditis, which are spread by injection drug use (Dennett & Gonsalves, 2023).

Unequal justice

In 2023, my experience as an expert witness in a fatal drug case in Boston, Massachusetts, in concert with my reading, led me to ponder massive inequalities in the criminal justice system (Institute for Research on Poverty, 2020). I had accepted the invitation from an attorney (a public defender) to serve as one because the work fell squarely into my research domain and perspective, which would obviate any self-perception that I would be functioning as a hired gun (Savitz, 2023)—an unpalatable, morally repugnant, and unacceptable role. Prisons are heavily populated by poor people who are incarcerated because they sold small quantities of opioids, marijuana, and/or other drugs, as well as being addicts themselves (Pew, 2018; Baden, 2023). Generally, modest economic returns fuel their addiction, and they frequently do not receive needed drug treatment. Captains of Big Pharma, on the other hand, marketed opioids on a gargantuan scale in the knowledge that they had strong lethal potential, and yet they experienced no prison time and retained a significant proportion of their prodigious and ill-gotten gains.[2] Their civil convictions indicated that they would qualify as serial mass murderers under a more equitable and egalitarian system of criminal justice. As a paid witness, I was reinforced in the lessons I learned from my own empirical work that death investigators are not resourced and motivated to search deeply for suicidality in fatal drug overdose cases. Here that lack of motivation was apparent even when corroborative evidence resided in hospital, law enforcement, and smartphone text records, which would have supported an assignment of suicide or undetermined as the manner of death if accessed by the medical examiner. Assignment of accident in a drug overdose death, the typical default option, is presumably far more resistant to contestation by family members in a court of law than one of suicide.

Systematizing opioid death data

Led by Kurt Nolte and funded by the Centers for Disease Control and Prevention (CDC), the American College of Medical Toxicology (ACMT) and the National Association of Medical Examiners (NAME) convened an expert panel in 2012 to address and improve the investigation, detection, analysis, classification, and certification of opioid deaths. Nolte then served as the executive vice president of NAME. Chairing the panel was Lewis Nelson, a medical toxicologist at New York University, who later also became a collaborator of mine. The panel produced a systematic review of the literature on fatal opioid analgesic poisoning, which they conducted to inform public health surveillance and enhance epidemiologic research and injury prevention (Davis et al., 2013). At the time, most opioid deaths in the United States implicated prescription pharmaceuticals, not illicit drugs. A follow-up position paper from a second ACMT and NAME panel appeared in 2020 (Davis et al., 2020). This panel, which again included Nelson, reiterated the six evidence-based recommendations from the original paper:

1. Autopsy provides the best information on a decedent's medical condition for optimal interpretation of toxicology results, circumstances surrounding death, medical history, and scene findings. The panel considers autopsy an essential component of investigating apparent overdose deaths.
2. Scene investigation includes reconciling prescription information and medication counts. Investigators should note drug paraphernalia or other evidence of using intoxicating substances.
3. Retain blood, urine, and vitreous humor whenever available. Blood from the iliofemoral vein is preferable to blood from more central sites.
4. A toxicologic panel should be comprehensive, including potent depressant, stimulant, and antidepressant medications. Detecting novel substances present in the community may require special testing.
5. When death is attributed to a drug or a combination of drugs (as cause or contributing factor), the certifier should list the drugs by generic name in the autopsy report and death certificate.
6. The best classification for manner of death in an overdose without any apparent intent of self-harm is "accident." (Davis et al., 2020, 152)

Absence or paucity of evidence

Stressing collection and reporting of detailed forensic evidence, all the previous recommendations made perfect sense to me save the final one—a recommendation with which I philosophically disagree—although I appreciate that the prevailing manner-of-death classification appears immutable for the foreseeable future. My questions and concerns with that recommendation emanate from my perspective as an epidemiologist. Elaboration of my rationale will form the essence of this chapter. As the ACMT and NAME have become more committed to the generation of data that will further the purposes of epidemiology, the basic science of public health, the panel's final recommendation highlights a critical problem that the medicolegal paradigm poses for epidemiology and suicide and other injury surveillance and prevention. In the twenty-first century, medical examiners serve not only public health but also criminal justice and public safety. Coroners, particularly those in rural offices, still tend to emphasize criminal justice. Helping to document, understand, and prevent nonhomicide deaths, like suicide, is a secondary consideration for them.

Some medical examiner offices are in health departments, whereas others have public health officials serving on their oversight boards. A great preponderance of them have some components of their statutes that focus on public health, and their staff participate in child fatality and maternal mortality reviews. Emerging and reemerging communicable (infectious and parasitic) diseases from the 1990s to the present, together with waves of heroin, cocaine, prescription opioids, and methamphetamine over the past three decades and ever-increasing gun violence, have coalesced public health and medicolegal death officials. Coroners, generally, have a quite different history from that of medical examiners. Some function in law enforcement offices. Most lack medical training and hence have little familiarity with concepts of public health and the consequence of this discipline for the community. However, it is important to note that the infrastructure funding for medical examiner and coroner offices today comes from both CDC and the National Institute of Justice.

Assigning a death as an accident is a default option for medical examiners and coroners, since it is not supported by a set of affirmative criteria. Criteria for substantiating suicide are more stringent than those for substantiating homicide, but they are affirmative for both manners of death in requiring establishment of intent. Nonetheless, establishing that a person intended to die or self-harm and administered the means represents a higher standard of proof or corroborative medical or forensic evidence for suicide than does establishing that a person died from the act of another who intended harm, but not necessarily death, or had acted with reckless disregard for the consequences (Litman, 1968). Far more frequent than homicides by drug intoxication (Muazzam et al., 2012), corresponding suicides are among the most challenging for medical examiners and coroners to detect without strong corroborative evidence (Stone et al., 2017). Our two National Violent Death Reporting System (NVDRS) studies attested to both the paucity and the primacy of this evidence in suicide cases, most notably an authenticated suicide note and documentation of psychological and psychiatric problems (Rockett et al., 2018a, 2018b). However, "absence of evidence is not evidence of absence" (Altman & Bland, 1995), a quote often attributed, but likely misattributed, to the astronomer Carl Sagan (Quote Investigator, 2019). It has been noted, too, that some medicolegal jurisdictions record nonfindings as potentially important corroborative evidence of suicide, such as incidents where a deceased person found in a hotel room had no suitcase, whereas other jurisdictions do not (Gray et al., 2014).

There can be other potent information to affirm suicide besides a note and documented mental problems. A person found in a secured residence with a contact range gunshot wound of the mouth is most likely a suicide even in the absence of a note or a compelling psychological history.[3] Similarly, someone found dead with multiple empty pill bottles for a variety of medications without abusive potential (e.g., chemotherapy agents and cardiac medications) and no evidence of a note or psychological problems is also most likely a suicide. The Cuyahoga County Medical Examiner's Office in Cleveland, Ohio, has produced an excellent field guide for conducting medicolegal death investigations, which offers additional examples of corroborative evidence for suicide specific to cases differentiated by external causes of death (e.g., drowning in tubs, pools, and bodies of water; asphyxia by chemical or gas [carbon monoxide]; illicit and prescription drug overdose/intoxication; firearm; hanging; and jumping/falling from a height; Cuyahoga County Medical Examiner's Office, 2017).

Representing a status quo that mirrors societal priorities, absence or a dearth of evidence to support a determination of a true drug suicide or other true suicide seems an inevitable by-product of deficits in expertise, infrastructure, and ancillary resources. For example, medical examiners and coroners rarely use psychological autopsies, despite their obvious utility, to resolve intentionality in equivocal manner-of-death cases (Weinberger et al., 2018). However, an innovative psychological autopsy study was conducted in recent years in Utah (Gray et al., 2014). This study involved structured interviews with the next of kin of suspected suicide decedents whose injury deaths had been investigated by the state's Office of the Medical Examiner (OME) between October 2008 and 2009. The authors stated that

> suspected suicide is determined primarily by the detective who provides a report to the OME based upon interviews and evidence gathered at the scene. A smaller number of suspected suicides are discovered by the OME during autopsy. Detectives consider suicide when the following scenarios are evident or suspected: 1. The method used is firearm, hanging, or another method common in completed suicide; 2. The decedent left a suicide note; 3. Inspection of the decedent's body demonstrates self-injury; 4. There is a known pharmacological overdose; 5. Large quantities of pills are missing from pillboxes; 6. The decedent has a history of suicide ideation or attempts; 7. There are written materials or a computer website history of topics related to suicide; or 8. A relative suspects suicide based on their knowledge of the decedent. At autopsy, a few cases are added as suspected suicides if a large concretion of pills (bezoar) is found in the decedent's stomach or intestines. (Gray et al., 2014, 335–36)

Among pertinent information collected during the interviews was whether the decedents had been experiencing acute and/or chronic pain. Although geographically limited and necessarily small, a major strength of the study was its employment of a direct approach. In reinforcing the importance of detailed decedent histories and death circumstances, to facilitate medicolegal separation of suicides from accident and undetermined deaths in equivocal cases, this research underscored the complexity confronting medical examiners and coroners in detecting suicide in most drug intoxication cases, and it added specificity to the search elements.

Prior to the Utah study, Amy Bohnert at the University of Michigan and colleagues targeted psychiatric history in a cohort study of military veterans who used Veterans Health Administration services for the period 1999–2006 to examine manner-of-death classification of drug intoxication deaths as suicide, accident, or undetermined (Bohnert et al., 2013). They associated both alcohol and other substance use disorders with an accident classification. Decedents who were assigned suicide and undetermined classifications exhibited similar psychiatric comorbidity, but undetermined cases showed higher representation of substance use disorder diagnoses. The researchers concluded that undetermined drug intoxication cases were relatively more problematic than corresponding accident cases in terms of potential suicide misclassification. However, they viewed the accident cases to be of greater absolute importance.

An Australian study of suicide underreporting, conducted in Queensland during the 1990s, reported that opioid intoxication cases were the most difficult to decipher regarding decedent intentionality owing to probable or possible decedent ambivalence toward dying (Cantor et al., 2001). Moreover, the investigators likened the opioid deaths to Russian roulette—deliberate risk-taking with the possibility of a lethal outcome. A 2019 review makes explicit the importance of better comprehending links between opioid use, drug intoxication, and suicide both to surveil and prevent suicide (Bohnert & Ilgen, 2019). Complicating and inhibiting ascertainment of drug poisoning suicides, substance addiction and dependence emulate suicide in being highly stigmatized (Tsai et al., 2019; Kheibari et al., 2021).

Alcohol

Society's drug of choice, alcohol, is cheap, intensively and extensively advertised and marketed, addictive, and easily accessible by the public. Consequently, drinking alcohol to intoxication is pervasive, frequent, and hazardous. Although alcohol misuse is a well-documented determinant of suicide, acute alcohol intoxication has not been studied in relation to suicide determination in the United States (Cherpitel et al., 2004). Nonetheless, some foreign studies have implicated blood alcohol positivity in an undetermined (intent) or accident versus suicide classification (Jarvis et al., 1991; Salib, 1996; Stanistreet et al., 2001). Two of these studies indicate that suicide detection may be impeded when (other) psychoactive substances and alcohol, while involved in a death, were not the lethal agent (Salib, 1996; Stanistreet et al., 2001). Indeed, co-occurrence of alcohol and other drugs, as well as acute alcohol intoxication, may induce misclassification of true suicides, since it is known that medicolegal authorities variably factor in substance dependence as a determinant of suicide in case ascertainment (Crepeau-Hobson, 2010). Alcohol is not even routinely labeled a drug in the scientific arena, not to mention in the everyday world. Following the money, the dominance of the alcohol beverage industry in the consumer market and the continuing separation of the National Institute on Alcohol Abuse and Alcoholism from the National Institute on Drug Abuse, the major federal agencies for funding drug-related research, reinforce this data deficit.

Death from drug self-intoxication

With the goal of prevention, epidemiology is a population-based discipline that seeks to investigate and understand disease, injury, and other related health phenomena (Rockett, 1999). By contrast, medicolegal death investigations operate at a case level, serving discrete populations, and their data from all 50 states and the District of Columbia feed into the NVDRS and the National Center for Health Statistics for epidemiologic and public health purposes. These relationships have been markedly strengthened in the twenty-first century.

The complexity of assessing suicidality in drug intoxication cases amid the opioid epidemic prompted me and my colleagues to seek to mitigate longstanding scientific tensions between the medicolegal and epidemiologic paradigms by creating two new concepts. The first was death from drug self-intoxication (DDSI; Rockett et al., 2014b). This concept became our building block to create a second novel concept, self-injury mortality (SIM; Rockett et al., 2016). I conceived SIM as an enhanced category that transcended suicide and its problematic measurement. Precursors are apparent in the work of Robert Litman and Irene Ovenstone, who allowed for gradation or a continuum of decedent intentionality in suicide determination. However, its genesis for me lay in a 2006 study by Matthew Breiding and Brian Wiersema. Major inspiration for DDSI sprang from the intellectual firepower of William Haddon, whose training comprised engineering, medicine, and public health and who revolutionized injury epidemiology, in general, and motor vehicle traffic safety, in particular (Haddon, 1968).

Breiding and Wiersema were pioneers in using NVDRS data for 2003 and 2004 to critique suicide and poisoning mortality data (Breiding & Wiersema, 2006). Seven states provided data for the system in both years, and six more provided data for 2004. In 2003, those 13 states accounted for slightly less than one-quarter of the American population, American suicides, and American homicides. However, their share of violent deaths of undetermined manner exceeded two-fifths, the category most susceptible to suicide misclassification. Three states were outliers on the high side of this measure: Massachusetts, Rhode Island, and Maryland. Their respective proportions in 2004 were 50%, 42%, and 38%. The three states collectively accounted for 65% of all undetermined deaths among the 13 participant states but just 19% of total homicides and 14% of suicides. Breiding and Wiersema also used annual-averaged data from WISQARS for the period 1999–2003 for those participant states to examine comparative age-adjusted rates and ranks for undetermined deaths. They also disaggregated poisoning deaths by manner as undetermined, suicide, and accident. Based on possible discrepant reporting in the NVDRS data, their study raised serious concerns about differential misclassification of both undetermined and suicide mortality that implicated drug types: alcohol, prescription pharmaceuticals, and street/recreational drugs. Further reference to these data indicated that medical examiners in Massachusetts, Rhode Island, and Maryland were more likely than medical examiners and coroners in the other 10 states, then participating in the NVDRS, to classify a poisoning death as undetermined when drug toxicology showed a combination of alcohol, prescription drugs, and street drugs. Issues broached in this study became a topic for deliberation by the ACMT and NAME panel in generating their two position papers, which I cited at the beginning of this chapter.

Breiding and Wiersema echoed the wisdom of Robert Litman, Irene Ovenstone, and Italian psychiatrist/suicidologist Maurizio Pompili in highlighting a "need for consideration of a wide range of the continuum of intentionality, from those who leave evidence of suicidal intent to those who may be ambivalent and less likely to leave such evidence" (2006, ii53). Besides proffering cautions about the validity of comparing poisoning deaths by manner across states, they recommended that the NVDRS expand data collection to include accidental poisoning deaths, since these deaths likely obscure misclassified suicides and other self-harm injury deaths with a lesser degree of intentionality than registered suicides (Rockett & Caine, 2015b). My later research offered reinforcement (Rockett et al., 2018a, 2018b). CDC now collects these poisoning data via NVDRS software and maintains them in a separate database called the State Unintentional Drug Overdose Reporting System (SUDORS).

SUDORS incorporates undetermined (intent) deaths, as well as unintentional/"accidental" deaths, but neither suicides nor homicides (Centers for Disease Control and Prevention, n.d.-b). Like the NVDRS, it is a rich database and collects more than 600 data elements falling within three broad categories: the death certificate, medical examiner / coroner reports, and postmortem toxicology. SUDORS similarly provides narratives on each case that offer potential for textual analysis, for example, using machine learning and various qualitative approaches, most obviously content analysis. Machine learning is an artificial intelligence technology or tool, which applies computerized algorithms and statistical models to existing data to learn new patterns and make predictions and decisions without direct human programming.

SUDORS deviates marginally from the NVDRS by not yet being universal in its coverage. At the time of writing, it represented 49 states and the District of Columbia. SUDORS data are now being shared with the NVDRS. Analysis of integrated data could yield numerous insights into overdose deaths across the injury manners of death and inform SIM and suicide accounting, trends, and distribution across the sociodemographic characteristics of the decedents.

Official American statistics and mortality data coded under the *International Classification of Diseases, Tenth Revision* or other revisions equate fatal self-directed violence to suicide only. In 2011, CDC published *Self-Directed Violence Surveillance: Uniform Definitions and Recommended Data Elements* (Crosby et al., 2011). Representing a major departure from convention, this document included a flowchart that accommodated a fatal nonsuicidal category under self-directed violence (Crosby et al., 2011, 22)—"behavior that is self-directed and deliberately results in injury or the potential for injury to oneself . . . [but where there is] no evidence, whether implicit or explicit, of suicidal intent" (Crosby et al., 2011, 21). However, CDC offered no concrete examples. The following discussion of DDSI and SIM proposes certain drug poisoning deaths that would heavily populate the category in the United States, as well as perhaps in many other countries. The CDC flowchart was much more expansive in addressing nonfatal self-directed violence. Indeed, the terms "nonsuicidal self-injury" and "deliberate (nonsuicidal) self-harm" have become well accepted in the suicide literature (Skegg, 2005; Bergen et al., 2012; Butler & Malone, 2013), although they are primarily applied to youth (Hawton et al., 2012). "Self-harm" is the preferred term in the United Kingdom, and "nonsuicidal self-injury" the preferred term in the United States (Kapur et al., 2013). Even self-harm refers to injury outcomes only and does not yet encompass any disease outcomes.

Representing nonsuicidal self-injury within morbidity opened the door to a call for corresponding representation within mortality, which was the focus of DDSI and SIM. Prompted by the thinking of Breiding and Wiersema, I began contemplating the need to expand SIM beyond registered or known suicides before becoming aware of the CDC manual and its flowchart for depicting the domain of self-directed violence or self-injury. But its existence provided helpful context, and even legitimacy, for creating a working category of nonsuicide deaths from drug self-intoxication.

In late 2013 I prepared a position paper to circulate to multidisciplinary colleagues to propose a reconceptualization of suicide and other self-injury that featured drug intoxication and other poisoning mortality. My tentative title was "Shifting the Suicide Paradigm: Problematic Measurement and Nonsuicidal Self-Injury Mortality." Thanks to the reach and potency of the internet, I was able to recruit coauthors domestically and internationally, who represented such diverse fields as epidemiology, psychiatry, emergency medicine, sociology, health economics, philosophy, medical toxicology, and forensic pathology. Some had worked with me before, but a number had not. I confess that I felt considerable intellectual vulnerability in projecting my ideas before such a distinguished group.

When I became an injury epidemiologist in the mid-1980s, I rapidly immersed myself in the CDC perspective. CDC had a talented, enthusiastic, and industrious group of people working in injury epidemiology and control, and it still does. Their first emphasis was unintentional injury. The term "accident" was anathema at CDC, and I learned from some of their people that Vernon Houk, the intimidating director of the National Center for Environmental Health and later assistant surgeon general, fined people 25 cents if they said the word in his presence, an action whose symbolic importance and source of humiliation far surpassed the tokenism of the monetary value of the fine. His objection was cemented in the notion that the word "accident" connotes fatalism, chance, or an act of God. As a counterpoint, CDC heavily promoted the slogan that "injury is no accident." Injuries are predictable and preventable, and there is no room for superstition in science. Faith is another matter. I had no trouble subscribing to the CDC approach, as reflected in the monograph I prepared for the Population Reference Bureau entitled "Injury and Violence: A Public Health Perspective" (Rockett, 1998a). Therein I reported on the seminal work of the legendary William Haddon, who adopted an environmental perspective in revolutionizing motor vehicle traffic safety and provided the inspiration and laid the foundation for the early CDC initiatives in injury epidemiology and control.

The exploding epidemics of suicide and opioid mortality in the United States, as well as my realization that mismeasurement of drug intoxication suicides was accelerating, solidified for me that fatal self-injury should encompass more than registered suicides. Moreover, as much as I had been wedded to the CDC imperative to replace accidental injury with unintentional injury, my research on suicide data quality led me to view the term "accident" through fresh eyes. During my preliminary efforts to reconceptualize SIM, I maintained a naive hope that the word could be eradicated from the language of manner-of-death categorization. Later discussions with medical examiners disabused me of that notion. The label "accident" as a formal manner of death will endure for the foreseeable future. What may not be immutable or inflexible for research and prevention purposes, however, is the classification of drug intoxication deaths as accidents. I now elaborate.

My 2013 position paper, refined and buttressed by substantial inputs from my multidisciplinary team, evolved into an article published in 2014 (Rockett et al., 2014b). In this article, entitled "Confronting Death from Drug Self-Intoxication (DDSI): Prevention Through a Better Definition," we conceived DDSI as a working concept not predicated on modification of extant manner-of-death categories. It becomes apparent that if one focuses on proximal antemortem decedent behavior related to substance acquisition and misuse rather than postmortem inference of decedent intent, most drug intoxication deaths stem from the culmination of patterned and repeated self-harming behaviors. Mechanisms are increasingly in place in states and other jurisdictions that can enable an objective categorization of DDSI that could be imposed by researchers and preventionists on drug deaths whose manner is suicide, accident, or undetermined. For example, now every American state has a functional prescription drug monitoring program that could enable discernment of prescription drug misuse through evidence of multiple prescription filing via doctor or pharmacy shopping by a decedent during the weeks, months, or even years preceding his or her death. Other evidence of self-harm, consonant with a DDSI designation, would be drug paraphernalia left by the decedent at the death scene, exemplified by syringes, tourniquets, hookahs, pipes, aerosol cans, balloons, chopped pills, and rolled bills;

drug-induced scarring in the limbs or torso discernible by autopsy or external examination; and toxicologic proof of a potentially lethal dose of illicit drugs, including cocaine, semisynthetic opioids such as heroin, and synthetic opioids such as fentanyl and the elephant tranquilizer carfentanil, which is 100 times more deadly than fentanyl. Medicolegal authorities could corroborate acute alcohol poisoning through toxicology and the presence of an empty liquor bottle near the corpse.

In our article, we allowed for drug precision in designating a death a DDSI, for example, DDSI (heroin), DDSI (oxycodone), DDSI (ethanol), DDSI (ethanol, temazepam), DDSI (heroin, fentanyl, and substance X), DDSI (not otherwise specified), and DDSI (unknown). Introduction of a checkbox on the death certificate that supported a record of DDSI would greatly facilitate surveillance, research, and prevention. Incorporation of DDSIs in the NVDRS would be an excellent addition but remains aspirational.

As we were finalizing the article, my colleagues and I wrestled with DDSI terminology. At one juncture, we appeared close to settling upon "death from deliberate self-intoxication." But seeking to mute the judgmental element in "deliberate," we substituted "drug," which refined the category by eliminating from consideration deaths attributable to the intentional or inadvertent inhalation of carbon monoxide and other toxic gases. The gases can be subsumed under the nondrug poisoning category, which also includes fumes, vapors, pesticides, detergents, and such heavy metals as lead, mercury, arsenic, and chromium. Between 2000 and 2017, nondrug deaths generally constituted 11% or less of total poisoning deaths (Centers for Disease Control and Prevention, n.d.-c). By 2017, the figure was only 7%. In some poorer countries, dominated by the Asian countries of India (Rane & Nadkarni, 2014) and China (Mew et al., 2017), poisoning by organophosphate pesticides is a prominent method of suicide. Pesticides are most readily accessible by rural populations. The finding of an acute toxic concentration in a decedent more likely invites medicolegal inference of suicide compared to a similar concentration of a psychoactive drug or drugs. Such suicides may also be more amenable to means restriction and large-scale prevention. However, marked reduction in the Chinese suicide rate in the later twentieth and early twenty-first centuries may be a product more of rapid urbanization, stimulated by the greater occupational, industrial, and economic opportunities offered by cities and towns, than of restrictions on access to highly lethal pesticides (Mew et al., 2017).

Insurance industry differentiates "accidental" drug overdoses

In 2021, I learned that the insurance industry employs a basis for paying out indemnities on an accident insurance policy that approximates our logic in viewing most drug overdose deaths as reflecting self-harm, after reading this statement prepared by Tatania Kadetskaya (2023): "A drug exclusion usually says that the policy does not cover any loss resulting from an injury sustained while voluntarily taking drugs which federal law prohibits dispensing without a prescription unless the drug is taken as prescribed or administered by a licensed physician. Often this exclusion is interpreted to mean that if a deceased insured had drugs in the system at the time of death, the death would be excluded from coverage."

Life insurance policies, as distinct from accident insurance policies, are far less restrictive when the death occurs beyond a two-year window after implementation. To the advantage of insurance companies and their shareholders, these companies tend to be far more prone than medical examiners and coroners to label a drug death as suicide, especially if reinforced by the power of a psychological autopsy. Whereas medicolegally suicide is not a residual manner-of-death category, the insurance industry treats it that way. The industry considers a drug death a suicide if the decedent had not taken the drug "accidentally," consumed too much "accidentally," was administered the incorrect drug, had taken the drug inadvertently, or died "accidentally" during surgery or another medical procedure.

Overconsumption of a prescribed drug or drugs invokes patient violation of an appropriate therapeutic range and patient noncompliance. Kadetskaya provides examples of questions that insurers should address before indemnifying or denying a death claim in that domain: "1. How old was the insured? 2. What was the insured's tolerance to the drug? 3. How long after death was the postmortem exam done? 4. Did the insured have liver failure? What are the liver function test results? What other medications was the insured taking? 5. Did he [or she] have any other illness at the time of death that could have slowed his [or her] metabolism? 6. Was the medication administered to the insured while he [or she] was unconscious?"

Ideally, although generally cost inhibitive, medical examiners and coroners or their representatives should routinely address these kinds of questions in investigating deaths by drug intoxication.

Enhanced self-injury mortality

In March 2014, with input from two colleagues, a psychiatrist and an emergency physician, I published an opinion piece entitled "Beyond Suicide: Action Needed to Improve Self-Injury Mortality Accounting" (Rockett et al., 2014a). Preceding my published work on DDSI, this opinion was written in response to the continuing rise in the suicide and accidental poisoning mortality rates and concern about suicide misclassification and the mischaracterized classification of most drug intoxication deaths as accidents, given that they normally involved repetitive self-destructive or self-harming behaviors. We expressed our concerns about related challenges affecting clinical medicine, medicolegal death investigations, and public safety. Also acknowledged was the suppressive influence on suicide certification inherent in the adverse legal, insurance, religious, and stigmatic implications of case ascertainment. The enormous potential for medical examiners and coroners to misclassify drug suicides formed the core of our argument for expanding the category of SIM. We made the point that medicolegal use of the accident and undetermined manner-of-death categories, as defaults, diminishes the likelihood that people in jails and hospital emergency departments who need drug addiction treatment would be identified and referred to treatment or other health care, or even administered a brief intervention.

The prominent early twentieth-century English epidemiologist Major (first name, not military rank) Greenwood eloquently stated, "The scientific purist who will wait for medical statistics until they are nosologically exact is no wiser than [the ancient Roman poet] Horace's rustic waiting for the river to flow away" (1948, 24). I, too, see no virtue in being a prisoner of perfection or a victim of paralysis of analysis in conducting research. Appreciating that it would be years, if ever, before a comprehensive and objective accounting of DDSI could be obtained through accessing death certificates or medical/coroner records, I decided that I wanted to operationalize nonsuicide DDSIs to compute an enhanced and working measure of SIM.

NOTES

1. Bibliometric analysis is a statistical methodology for systematically analyzing published information (from books, articles, and blogs) on a research question of interest, utilizing such accessible databases as the Web of Science Core Collection, Scopus, and Medline (see Ninkov et al., 2022).

2. A notable exception was John Kapoor, an Indian immigrant and hence a "foreigner." The founder and chief economic officer of Insys Therapeutics, he served two years of a five-and-a half-year sentence in a minimum-security prison facility for racketeering conspiracy, including wire fraud and bribing physicians to prescribe unnecessary and highly addictive and potent Subsys (fentanyl) to their patients (Hughes, 2022).

3. I am indebted to Kurt Nolte for these examples.

8

Applying, Translating, and Disseminating Self-Injury Mortality

Rationale for self-injury mortality

Colleagues and I spelled out the rationale for the concept of self-injury mortality (SIM) in a study revealing hitherto unrecognized mortality trends in racial/ethnic minorities and non-Hispanic Whites (Rockett et al., 2020b). Firstly, SIM was conceived to mitigate the downward biases in suicide measurement related to method of suicide and the demographic characteristics of the decedents, especially their sex and race/ethnicity. Secondly, SIM was bridging a gap—that psychological autopsies were unlikely to be a routine feature of the medicolegal fabric in investigating deaths when decedent intent was equivocal. Thirdly, the epidemiologic and medicolegal paradigms functioned differently regarding prioritization of surveillance, etiologic or scientific understanding, primary prevention, and therapy. Fourthly, medical examiners and coroners faced more stringent standards for assigning suicide than for assigning homicide as a manner of death, and resources for investigating suicide are not equivalent to those for homicide. Fifthly, the Great Recession of 2007/8 and the opioid and suicide epidemics have intensified the workloads of the already stressed medicolegal death investigation and emergency health care systems (compounded more recently by the COVID-19 pandemic). Sixthly, assignment of "accident" as the manner of death lacks affirmative criteria in contrast to assignment of suicide or homicide; it is a default category. Seventhly, the coding of the large preponderance of drug intoxication deaths as "accident" by nosologists is a mischaracterization, given the association between substance use disorders and suicidal ideation, suicide planning, and suicide attempts. Finally, "accident" is mandated as a manner of death by statutes across the nation, and this is unlikely to be modified in the shorter term to accommodate behaviorally based non-suicide self-injury deaths.

Self-injury mortality versus suicide and drug mortality trends

Under two alternative scenarios, I had first compared SIM to suicide and accidental and undetermined drug intoxication death rates for the period 1999–2013, as part of one of my two scheduled presentations to the 2015 CDC panel, on which I served as a "thought leader." Then, I invited Eric Caine, another "thought leader" on the panel, to collaborate with me on a follow-up article (Rockett & Caine, 2015b). The multiple-cause-of-death public use files from the National Center for Health Statistics were our data source.

Under scenario 1, SIM comprised all suicides in the national population plus 70% of the accidental drug intoxication deaths and 80% of the corresponding undetermined drug intoxication deaths in the age group 15 years and older. Under scenario 2, the proportions of accidental and undetermined drug intoxication deaths were 80% and 90%, respectively. Examination of trends revealed that the two alternative estimates of the SIM rate increased more rapidly than the suicide rate. The sharpest rate increase was for accidental drug intoxication mortality, as it escalated toward the suicide rate. Whether scenario 1 or scenario 2 prevailed, the estimated rate would have placed SIM as the eighth-leading cause of death in the United States in 2013, exceeding both influenza and pneumonia combined and kidney disease. Diabetes was the seventh-leading cause, and suicide was the 10th-leading cause. In our article, Caine and I anticipated the shift from prescription opioids to illicit opioids, like heroin and fentanyl, as the predominant lethal agents in drug intoxication deaths.

Self-injury mortality versus proximal leading causes of death

As the suicide and drug intoxication mortality rates continued to rise, I pondered whether the SIM rate was converging with the diabetes mortality rate. This led me to assemble another multidisciplinary team to examine the SIM trend in relation to suicide and three proximally ranked, top 10 causes of death: diabetes, influenza and pneumonia, and kidney disease (Rockett et al., 2016). For this study, we accessed underlying cause-of-death data from WISQARS for the period 1999–2014. In computing SIM, we combined all registered suicides, 80% of accidental drug intoxication deaths, and 90% of undetermined drug intoxication deaths in the age group 15 years and older, the SIM combination under scenario 2 in the Rockett and Caine (2015b) study. The new study showed that the SIM rate had continuously exceeded the kidney disease mortality rate, surpassed the mortality rate for influenza and pneumonia by 2006, and converged with the diabetes mortality rate in 2014 at 24 deaths per 100,000 population. The SIM rate rose 65% between 1999 and 2014. It was 1.8 times higher than the suicide rate in 2014 versus 1.4 times higher in 1999. The male-to-female ratio of the SIM to suicide mortality rate declined from 3.7 to 2.6 over the observation period.

I believe, in operationalizing SIM, that our assumption that 80% of all "accidental" drug overdose deaths in the age group 15 years and older qualify is a conservative one. In other words, the actual percentage may be higher. However, like the 90% assumption for the undetermined component, the 80% assumption theoretically could be evaluated directly in a pilot test of a self-injury checkbox on the death certificate, explained and discussed in chapter 10. In the meantime, a *Morbidity and Mortality Weekly Report* from CDC provided strong support for the validity of the 80% assumption (Kariisa et al., 2022). One of its findings was that 77% of the overdose decedents had a documented history of substance use problems. In keeping with less access to the American health care system, minorities had a lower prevalence than non-Hispanic Whites—the lowest was 71% for Asian and Pacific Islanders, followed by 74% and 75% for Blacks and Hispanics, respectively. Whites had a prevalence of 78%.

Most conventional mortality rates, like crude and cause-specific death rates, treat deaths as equivalent for accounting purposes, irrespective of age at death. Annual-averaging data for two periods, 1999–2002 and 2012–14, we cumulated deaths by age as a percentage for each of the five causes of death so that we could examine premature mortality. For the first period, 77% of SIM occurred before age 55 years, versus 11% of diabetes deaths, 6% of influenza and pneumonia deaths, and 8% of kidney disease deaths. The magnitude and variation on this measure were similar in the second period. Thus, viewing SIM from the comparative perspective of crude death rates, or age-adjusted rates, yields a very incomplete picture for public health.

The rate of potential years of life lost is one well-known measure of premature mortality, especially popular in injury prevention and public health because it better portrays the true burden of injury to society than other mortality metrics (Rockett, 1998a, 12–13). This metric accords greater weight to deaths of younger people than to those of older people. We used a life table–based measure to evaluate premature mortality among the decedents—the hypothetically "saved"—in our study and estimate years of life lost (Rockett, 1998b). For male and female decedents, SIM accounted for 32 and 37 years of life lost, respectively, in 2014 (Rockett et al., 2016). Corresponding losses were 16 and 17 years from diabetes, 15 and 17 years from influenza and pneumonia, and 15 and 16 years from kidney disease.

Of course, all studies have their research limitations. The results of the foregoing study "could have been influenced by unexamined heterogeneity in death certification stemming from variable certifier training and practice, involvement of hospitals and death investigation systems and their types and professional accreditation status, autopsy and toxicologic testing rates, diagnostic competence and coding, and/or relationships and coordination between state vital recording registrars and the National Center for Health Statistics" (Rockett et al., 2016, 1079). We also acknowledged that our conceptualization and measurement of SIM have not been validated and were imprecise, and we noted that amelioration of deficits could ensue with uniform information on alcohol and other substance use, misuse, and dependence. However, our measurement of SIM was conservative since its nonsuicide component was confined to deaths whose underlying causes were directly attributed to alcohol and other drug intoxication.

Two psychiatrists from Washington University in Saint Louis, Eugene Rubin and Charles Zorumski (2017), wrote a supportive report and commentary on the 2016 SIM study for *Psychology Today*, published on February 20, 2017. They set the scene as follows:

> Many, if not most, deaths resulting from prescription opioid and other drug overdoses are listed as "accidental" or "unintentional" on death certificates because information regarding the person's state of mind prior to the overdose is unavailable. This designation is used even when there is a history of repeated, deliberate drug use and overdose, which clearly increases the potential for death. Many in the public health field believe that this results in an underestimation of poisoning suicides. . . . Ian Rockett and colleagues . . . convincingly demonstrate an increase in self-injury mortality (SIM) over the last 15 years. . . . SIM includes deaths of those who intended to die as well as deaths by people who demonstrated self-destructive behavior for which death was a likely consequence.

Rubin and Zorumski's language was crystal clear and on point. They were translating our research and concept of SIM for a general audience as succinctly and accurately as I could have wished. They noted that "suicides often occur in the context of depression and/or substance use disorders. Deaths resulting from overdoses likely involve many causes including depression, addiction, and other psychiatric illnesses." They concluded, "The rates of death in young and middle-aged individuals from self-injury are staggering. Hopefully, research such as this will alert policymakers to invest resources to reverse this disturbing trend." This is our aim.

Self-injury mortality's clinical connection

I doubted I would live long enough to see explicit links between my research on SIM and clinical research. I nearly didn't, following a cardiac incident on a transatlantic flight outside Iceland in 2014, which necessitated bypass surgery in Toronto, Canada. In 2016, Hilary Connery reached out to me from McLean Hospital in Massachusetts via email and said she thought we would be more effective working together than separately. Her statement was both fortuitous for me and prophetic. An addiction psychiatrist, she is McLean's clinical director of the Division of Alcohol, Drugs, and Addiction. Under her leadership, we delivered a training webinar under the auspices of the American Psychiatric Association on June 21, 2016. Our webinar was entitled "Addiction, Overdose, and Suicide: Preventing Deaths from Drug Self-Intoxication (DDSI)." Since our connection, we have collaborated frequently in each other's research.

Connery is building a cohort of patients with opioid use disorders, a number of whom have manifested suicidality in overdoses, which will enable evaluation of interventions (Connery et al., 2019). Her preliminary data, based on 60 adult subjects reporting a history of opioid overdose and receiving inpatient detoxification, show that "approximately 45% reported some desire to die prior to their most recent overdose, with 20% reporting they had some intention to die" (Connery et al., 2022, 109437). It is not a giant leap to assume that the prevalence of suicidal cognition would be even higher among individuals with diagnosed or undiagnosed opioid use disorder who later died from an opioid-related overdose. The deceased may have had greater comprehension than survivors of a lethal dosage and how to avoid rescue, although the potent lethality of fentanyl and fentanyl-contaminated drugs is a complicating consideration in assessing decedent motivation in overdose cases. Fentanyl may be used in very small doses therapeutically by anesthesiologists in surgery, but prospective and potential users would be wise to adopt a zero-threshold approach and thus avoid use outside prescription in selective clinical settings.

A mass media story in *HealthDay News*, published in 2018, quoted Mark Olfson, a prominent psychiatrist from Columbia University, as saying that "broad acceptance of the self-injury concept could spur much needed reforms in clinical care, by focusing on underlying risks common to drug self-intoxication and suicide deaths. That would mean more crossover in patients' care, more substance-abuse screening among patients being treated for depression or other mental health disorders, and more attention to the overall mental health of people in treatment for drug abuse" (Norton, 2018).

Another, albeit tenuous, clinical link for SIM involves lithium, a versatile chemical element with diverse applications, including lubricants, batteries, and therapeutic use as a mood stabilizer and antidepressant, and hence as a potential suicide preventive. My Austrian colleague Nestor Kapusta invited me to participate in his correlational or ecological study of lithium in public water supplies and suicide rates (Blüml et al., 2013). The data were from Texas. An inverse correlation emerged from this descriptive study, which affirmed findings from previous foreign studies suggesting a protective effect against suicide from lithium. All results were necessarily tentative and call for more analytic and definitive research. A systematic review examined the relationship between therapeutic doses of lithium and suicide prevention in clinical trials (Riblet et al., 2022). It included a meta-analysis that provided a quantitative summary of the results of the individual trials. The association between lithium and prevention was borderline, but not statistically significant, with a probability of 5 or less in 100 that it was a chance finding. Referencing SIM, the authors of the systematic review reported a sensitivity analysis showing that the association became significant with the inclusion of a single opioid overdose case with no corroborative evidence of suicide; this case was omitted for the primary analysis.

The *Diagnostic and Statistical Manual of Mental Disorders*, substance use, and self-injury mortality

The sociologist Allan Horwitz (2021) has written an excellent history of the *Diagnostic and Statistical Manual of Mental Disorders* (*DSM*), the fourth revision of which (*DSM-IV*) was central to the estimation of met and unmet substance abuse treatment need in the Tennessee Hospital Emergency Room Drug Study. His exposition includes attention to drug dependence, addiction, and persistent misuse under *DSM-IV* and the expansion of addiction in *DSM-V* to include the nonsubstance disorder of gambling. *DSM-V* even allows for the potential of addiction to further expand to include other activities, which consumers may compulsively pursue, like surfing the internet, "sex, shopping, eating, and exercise" (Horwitz, 2021, 153). Although complicated by the incorporation of adverse social implications of substance disorders in the fourth and fifth revisions, *DSM* does view these disorders as having an organic basis or connection—as brain-related conditions or diseases. Psychoactive substances, by definition, target the brain, and it is a short step to understand that intensive and extensive use of these substances could severely impair or damage this organ.

As mainstream psychiatry evolved to view serious mental illness more organically (Lieberman, 2015), while completing a 180-degree turn from the predominance of Freudian and Jungian psychotherapy,[1] it has increasingly relied on drugs for routine treatment of this illness. Ironically, some of these drugs, such as lithium, antidepressants, and tranquilizers, can themselves impair or damage the brain (Breggin, 1991; Avorn, 2004; Sloboda, 2005; Whitaker, 2010; Harrington, 2019), as can treatments for physical injury and disease—epitomized catastrophically by opioid painkillers, both prescription and illicit. Paracelsus, an enlightened Swiss physician, alchemist, and philosopher, warned in the sixteenth century of the toxic potential of medications when taken in too strong a dose (Grandjean, 2016). Robert Whitaker's (2010) *Anatomy of an Epidemic* is replete with evidence-based examples of iatrogenesis in the treatment of mental illness. In the next chapter, I share another cautionary message, highlighting that our findings on the contextual correlates of interstate SIM and suicide rates support an inference that not all mental distress needs to be medicalized for relief.

Implied in the seismic psychiatric shift in treating serious mental illness is a transformation from the subjective to the objective, from treatment as an art to treatment informed by evidence-based, neurobiological, social, and behavioral medicine (Lieberman, 2015; Harrington, 2019). In the mix are the genesis, treatment, and management of substance use disorders. From the viewpoint of addiction psychiatry, at least, they need to be on an equal footing with other mental disorders and chronic physical illnesses, like diabetes and kidney disease, which physicians can manage and treat. This perspective is consistent with our behavioral reconceptualization of fatal self-injury, SIM, to encompass most drug deaths irrespective of decedent intentionality, in addition to registered or known suicides. Whereas the medical specialties of psychiatry and neurology share overlapping interests in the mind and the brain, psychiatrists are more concerned diagnostically with mental symptoms of an illness and neurologists with the physical symptoms.

In *American Psychosis*, Fuller Torrey (2014) documented the failure of the federal government to improve the mental health care system during the second half of the twentieth century. Deinstitutionalization exemplified this failure by magnifying the problems of homelessness among the mentally ill across the United States. In raising important questions, Torrey paid ample attention to interpersonal violence, with crime and homicide being major concerns for him. Unfortunately, he gave self-directed violence and suicide short shrift, as well as public health and drug addiction.

Self-injury mortality surpasses diabetes as a killer

Three psychiatrists, Eric Caine, Hilary Connery, and Shelly Greenfield, collaborated with me on a small time-trend study of SIM (Rockett et al., 2019). Like Connery, Greenfield is an addiction psychiatrist at McLean Hospital and affiliated with the psychiatry department at Harvard Medical School. At the time of the study, she was the president of the American Academy of Addiction Psychiatry. Published in print in 2019 (online in 2018) under the title "Mortality in the United States from Self-Injury Surpasses Diabetes: A Prevention Imperative," our study examined the likelihood that SIM had surpassed diabetes as a leading cause of death. We used the same methodology and publicly accessible query-based data source, the CDC's Wide-ranging Online Data for Epidemiologic Research database, which was used in the larger 2016 SIM study. We compared SIM and diabetes mortality rates for the period 2000–2016, distinguishing the sexes. The SIM rate exceeded the diabetes mortality rate in 2015. By 2016, the respective rates were 29 and 25 per 100,000 population. For males, the SIM excess manifested over most of the observation period, and the ratio of the SIM rate to the diabetes mortality rate rose from 1.0 to 1.5. For females, the diabetes mortality rate exceeded the SIM rate over the entire period. However, their rate ratio declined from 4.1 in 2000 to 1.4 by 2016. In this brief report, we illustrated that the presence or absence of one piece of corroborative evidence of suicide, a suicide note, could be critical to a medical examiner or coroner determining that a given death was a suicide or accident. A heuristic cartoon depicts two hypothetical cases of drug intoxication death where there was a record of comorbid depression, self-intoxication by opioids, and test positivity for alcohol (fig. 8.1). In only one of the cases was there an evidentiary suicide note—enough, we posit, to induce a suicide rather than an accident manner-of-death determination. The report reemphasized the point that the accident classification is a mischaracterization, from an epidemiologic or etiologic perspective, because of the strong likelihood of a pattern of repeated self-harm or self-injurious behavior on the part of the decedent preceding death. Both the accident and suicide cases in the cartoon would constitute SIM cases.

Research translation and dissemination

A press release prepared by the authors on a given scientific study enables them to control the narrative and avoid misinterpretation or omission of key findings, an advantage not guaranteed in reports prepared by others. An example is one issued in 2018 from McLean Hospital, an affiliate of the Department of Psychiatry at the Harvard School of Medicine (McLean Hospital, 2018), which my coauthor Hilary Connery and I had prepared on the time-trend study (Rockett et al., 2019). Besides providing details on the empirical findings of the study, this press release emphasized that SIM was conceived as a unifying concept. Quoting Connery,

> It is time to end the siloed approach to prevention. We're so entrenched in separating suicide from drug overdose or alcohol poisoning deaths that people can't wrap their heads around the idea that they are related. The mental health and social risk factors preceding suicidal behaviors and substance poisonings are largely overlapping. For example, we know from epidemiologic research and clinical studies that severe childhood trauma is highly predictive of future death by either substance-related poisoning or suicide. . . .
>
> Let's talk about preventing suicide and substance-related deaths together by aggressively screening for trauma, mental health disorders, problematic substance use, and social determinants such as poverty and then providing quality evidence-based care or amelioration for these risk factors so that self-injury behaviors are prevented. It would be much more effective and efficient to look at them together and to do prevention together, because their antecedent risk factors are so overlapping. (McLean Hospital, 2018)

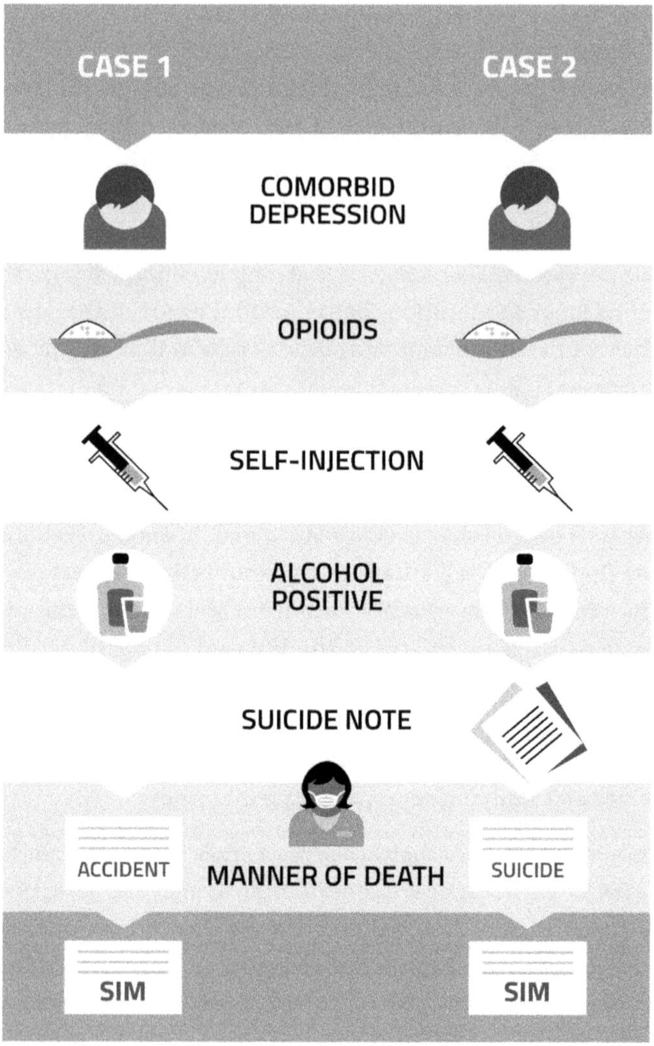

Figure 8.1. Two hypothetical cases of self-injury mortality (SIM). Source: Rockett, I.R.H., Caine, E.D., Connery, H.S., Greenfield, S.F., "Mortality in the United States from self-injury surpasses diabetes: A prevention imperative," *Injury Prevention* 2019;25:331–33.

In the McLean Hospital release, I noted that "[the United States of] America is in the midst of a persistent and major but underestimated mental health crisis. We want to unify mental health and substance use disorder experts to say we have a really serious but preventable problem of premature mortality due to self-injury, and an artificial separation of drug deaths from suicide is slowing our efforts to prevent these deaths." The press release reported that "the authors concluded that ending the SIM epidemic will require multifaceted, concerted, and sustained efforts like those that dramatically reduced mortality from cardiovascular diseases, smoking-related lung cancer, HIV, and motor vehicular traffic injury" (McLean Hospital, 2018).

Exposing minority and sex health data disparities

Our second follow-up study to the comparative 2016 study examined trends in SIM rates in the United States between 2008 and 2017 by race/ethnicity and sex (Rockett et al., 2020b). The racial/ethnic groups under scrutiny were Blacks (non-Hispanic), Hispanics, Native Americans, and Whites (non-Hispanic). With Whites serving as the comparison category, we selected the minorities according to their status as vulnerable groups, based on a long history of discrimination, segregation, and poverty. Economists Anne Case and Angus Deaton (2015), a Nobel laureate, had published a paper in 2015 showing that middle-aged Whites, especially White men, were disproportionately bearing the burden of the deaths of despair—deaths attributable to suicide, drug overdoses, and chronic alcoholism. Widely disseminated and influential, their study basically inverted an observation that colleagues and I made in our 2012 national injury mortality study (Rockett et al., 2012). In the latter study, we reported that while all major racial/ethnic groups were losing ground with respect to suicides and drug intoxication mortality—the injury deaths of despair, to adapt the terminology of Case and Deaton to these acute phenomena—Blacks and Hispanics were faring better than Whites.

Our new SIM study was motivated by a suspicion that the relative advantage held by Blacks and Hispanics over Whites, particularly that of Blacks, was eroding. While Case and Deaton included disease deaths stemming from chronic alcohol and other drug problems among their deaths of despair, they omitted analogous disease deaths like lung cancer and emphysema from tobacco smoking and anorexia from nutritional deficits. Confounding any prevention initiatives, the conditions constituting Case and Deaton's "diseases of despair" are problematic epidemiologically because they combine adverse health effects of historical disease exposures with much shorter-term injury exposure risks. Nonetheless, their work has been influential in highlighting critical health problems that have helped justify the importance of upstream approaches to address growing socioeconomic inequality and other inequities to improve public health. In his social-ecological perspective, my colleague Eric Caine (2012, 2013, 2019) has independently and forcefully argued for suicide prevention initiatives to encompass upstream modifications, such as reducing economic insecurity, strengthening economic safety nets, and restricting access to lethal means like firearms. In summary, prevention must combine biomedical micro-approaches, which treat individuals in pronounced personal distress, and macro-approaches, which address the political, social, and economic conditions that generate profound societal distress.

Our examination of the respective ratios of the minority to White suicide rates over the decade 2008–17 showed that suicide rates for Blacks and Hispanics always remained under two-fifths of the rate of Whites (Rockett et al., 2020b). By contrast, the suicide rates for Native Americans approximated parity with rates for Whites over most of the observation period, but they diverged above parity during the final three years. Corresponding ratios of SIM to suicide rates told quite a different story. Whereas Native American ratios of the two rates well exceeded parity with the White rate ratios, those for Blacks exceeded or achieved parity with the White rate ratios, and those for Hispanics approximated them or fell slightly below parity. Thus, the combination of differential misclassification of minority drug intoxication suicides and the mischaracterization of drug intoxication deaths as accidental or undetermined severely masked the true burden of SIM, beyond registered suicides alone, among the three major vulnerable minority groups vis-à-vis Whites. Attention to sex differentials in ratios of SIM to suicide rates over the observation period 2008–17 revealed profound excesses for females across all four racial/ethnic groups. Thus, just confining fatal self-injury to registered suicides distorts comparisons between females and males, as well as between the vulnerable minorities and Whites. Our results reinforce that medical examiners and coroners have greater difficulty in discerning female than male suicides owing to the excess tendency for females to use drug poisoning as a method.

More translation and dissemination

In a 2019 press release on our study from McLean Hospital, Hilary Connery placed SIM in a treatment context and reemphasized the problem with the troubling divide in the mental health domain:

> The healthcare system has a long history of separating people coming for mental health disorders care from those coming for substance use disorders care. Considering today's concurrent epidemics, this system doesn't work well at a population level because of the high rates of co-occurrence of substance use disorders and other mental health disorders. It's extremely common for a depressed person to be misusing substances but asking only for help for depression. Likewise, a person asking for help with opioid use disorder may seek medical treatment but not report suicidal thoughts and planning. In both cases, screening for suicide risk factors and overdose risk factors will improve early detection, which may then allow targeted, integrated treatments to prevent SIM deaths.
>
> [An impediment to understanding, prevention, and treatment, the] false dichotomy [between "intentional" and "unintentional" injury] leads to depictions of self-injury deaths as either intentional suicide or accidental substance poisoning. The desire to die prior to self-injury death occurs along a spectrum of low to high desire to die, which may influence risk-taking behaviors even if a person's conscious intentions are not fully suicidal. (McLean Hospital, 2019)

A story published in 2022 in *Scientific American* quoted Nora Volkow, director of the National Institute on Drug Abuse, and Kathryn Pinneri, president of the National Association of Medical Examiners (Novak, 2022). Volkow emphasized the difficulty of detecting suicide among drug intoxication cases. She also spoke about the initial protection against suicide that Blacks accrued through having less access to prescription opioid painkillers, and then their consequential loss of protection from the rapid spread of illicit fentanyl. Pinneri noted the stresses imposed on medicolegal death investigators by the opioid epidemic and the COVID-19 pandemic. She pointed out that, during the onset of COVID, Black American decedents were less likely than White American decedents to have had the external postmortem examinations that would have revealed evidence of drug involvement and other causes contributing to their deaths.

The *Scientific American* story concluded with comments from Paul Nestadt, a Johns Hopkins psychiatrist/suicidologist, who stated that clinicians in emergency departments were more attuned to assess suicidality among White men than among Black men based on differential reported risks for suicide. Nestadt's work in Baltimore County, Maryland, triggered the creation of a task force and the appointment of a suicide prevention coordinator aimed at reducing suicide among the latter demographic.

A story entitled "Overdose of Inequality," also published in *Scientific American* in 2022 (Newsome, 2022), reported that Native Americans and Blacks had fatal drug overdose rates that exceeded those of Whites and highlighted disparities between Blacks and Whites regarding drug treatment, its timeliness, and the type of medication-assisted treatment that patients receive—buprenorphine, methadone, or naltrexone. Reflected in excess drug-related arrest and incarceration rates, substance use disorders in Black populations are more heavily linked with criminal justice and less so with public health than those in White populations. Complicating access and utilization of drug treatment by Blacks, many have a strong mistrust of the health care system, which reinforces a cultural perspective that substance issues are a moral problem, not a medical one. Such mistrust was publicly validated by the scandalous revelations in the early 1970s about the Tuskegee Syphilis Study, documented in James Jones's (1981) *Bad Blood*, in which longer-term, disease-positive Black (sharecropper) participants had been denied effective antibiotic therapy by the US Public Health Service. Fear and skepticism based on inhumane treatment extend to the mental health domain (Dawes et al., 2023). For example, during the 1960s in Hattiesburg, Mississippi, a chair of a department of neurosurgery performed lobotomies on institutionalized Black children, as young as 5 years of age, as a remedial and punitive therapy for their alleged aggression or hyperactivity (Stafford et al., 2023). While general mistrust by Blacks of the health care system and related research is extremely understandable, it diminishes the likelihood that any proposed clinical suicide and overdose interventions among this population will engender an enthusiastic reception.

Translating observed data disparities

At the group level, middle-aged non-Hispanic White men, together with Native Americans, have stood out because of their high suicide rate, although all racial/ethnic groups have experienced a spike in rates during the second decade of the twenty-first century. A story in *The Atlantic* drew attention to suicide among African Americans (Yuan & Fayyad, 2018). To my knowledge, this is the first mass media story to mention health data disparities—a different concept from health disparities, even if the two are presumably interrelated. I was quoted as follows:

> We hear a lot of talk about health disparities, but what we don't hear much about at all is what I would call health data disparities. . . . If the data [are] more deficient for minorities then the gaps between whites and blacks might actually be much smaller [than reported in the vital statistics and the suicide toll much heavier]. . . . I don't know that data disparities would explain the whole gap, but I think [they are] important to consider. I think the big danger with health data disparities is that problems get more underestimated amongst the people with the more deficient data. And that has implications for targeting at-risk populations or designing interventions. It's harmful for prevention. (Yuan & Fayyad, 2018)

Austin Frakt (2020) interviewed me about the excess suicide rates for Whites relative to those of certain minorities for a story published in *The New York Times* at the end of 2020. He referenced my research on health data disparities in discussing the Black-White rate differentials. Frakt consulted many experts, and his report was balanced and, quite rightly, only attributed part of the rate gap to suicide misclassification.

Another study on minority data disparities

While noting significant improvements in drug specification, a study led by an anesthesiologist / public health researcher examined potential minority health data disparities in opioid-involved overdose deaths between 1999 and 2018 in the United States (Milam et al., 2021). Dichotomizing their observation period, the researchers reported disparities for Blacks relative to Whites in 1999–2008 but not in 2009–18. Although they did not find an association with type of medicolegal death investigation system, they concluded that inequities in resource allocation to address data specification and quality differentially impact risk of opioid-involved overdose death. Their research is a novel contribution to the literature, one that warrants in-depth research in multiple settings.

NOTE

1. Whereas psychotherapy still occupied the forefront of psychiatry in the middle of the twentieth century, the physically invasive and more controversial treatments of lobotomization and electroconvulsive therapy (still used) had traction in certain quarters (see Lieberman, 2015). Historically, lobotomies were associated with control of patients rather than cure or management of their mental illness, especially in institutions then labeled as asylums or psychiatric hospitals for the "criminally insane."

9

How Are the Nation and My State Faring?

An evolving national mental health crisis

A logical extension of the research on self-injury mortality (SIM) was to apply this concept to the American landscape over space and time in order to examine interstate SIM and suicide trends, contextual characteristics, and economic costs. For this project, I once again recruited a multidisciplinary team. Membership first included my usual blend of collaborators: social scientists, epidemiologists, psychiatrists, emergency physicians, a public health specialist, a medical toxicologist, and a medical examiner. However, I also recruited two geographers who possessed cutting-edge expertise in geographic information science.

In what morphed into a trilogy, our first study compared trends in SIM rates relative to suicide rates, nationally and across states over the period 1999–2018 (Rockett et al., 2021). Suicide has long been the conventional but heavily flawed mortal representative of imminent personal and societal distress, and I anticipated that our application of SIM would expose an unfolding national mental health crisis. Indeed, that is what the graphed and mapped data revealed, in vivid detail, as they evoked the oft-quoted adage that "a picture is worth a thousand words." Although I had included visuals in prior studies, I had never published an empirical study without at least one table. In choosing an exclusively visual approach to display the data, I was heavily influenced by the graphical depictions of Napoleon's catastrophic march to Moscow in 1812 and Hannibal's elephant-fortified war in the third century BCE against the ancient Romans by French octogenarian engineer Joseph Minard, reproduced in the scintillating work of the leading proponent of visualizing information or data, Edward Tufte (2006). Similarly in-

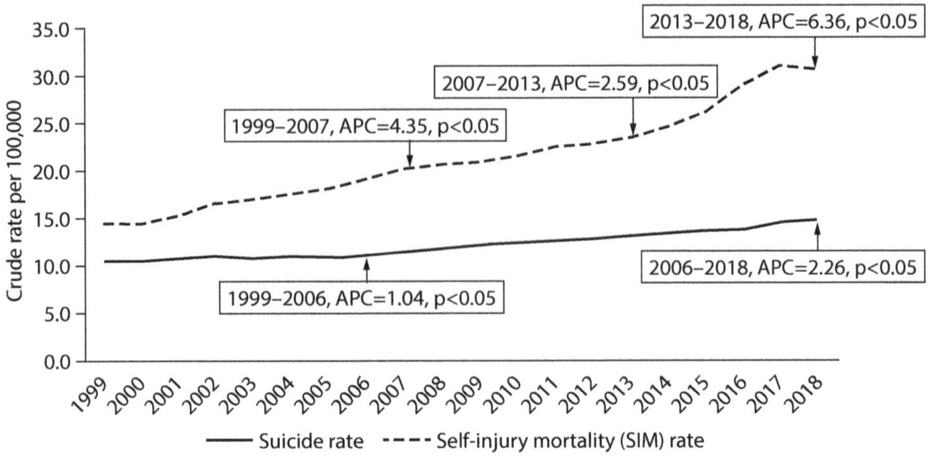

Figure 9.1. Trends and significant changes in crude suicide and self-injury mortality (SIM) rates per 100,000 population, United States, 1999–2018. Note: APC = annual percentage change based on joinpoint regression. Source: Rockett, I.R.H., Caine, E.D., Banerjee, A., et al., "Fatal self-injury in the United States, 1999–2018: Unmasking a national mental health crisis," ***EClinicalMedicine*** **2021; 32:100741.**

spirational were the ingenuity and craft of the legendary English nurse Florence Nightingale—particularly her pie or radiant chart, which she called a coxcomb (Andrews, 2022). Created by her sister, Parthenope, this chart strikingly illustrated that many more soldiers in the Crimean War succumbed to infection than to their wounds. Her military research spurred important reforms in public health and sanitation, as well as revolutionizing nursing.

Although I believe that the following images almost speak for themselves, I nonetheless offer description and a commentary. Whereas the American suicide rate increased by 41% between 1999 and 2018, the SIM rate rose more than threefold—by 128% (Rockett et al., 2021). Figure 9.1 allows for the fact that neither rate increase was linear. Use of joinpoint regression analysis revealed that there was one inflection point in the upward suicide trend and two in the corresponding SIM trend. The inflection point in the suicide rate preceded the onset of the Great Recession of 2007/8. Those for the SIM rate aligned with the Great Recession and the entry of highly lethal fentanyl and other illicit synthetic opioids, such as carfentanil. Ninety-five percent confidence intervals accompanied the point estimates. For example, the SIM rate increased by 4.4% between 1999 and 2007, with a range for the estimate of

3.3%–5.4%. In translation, we can say that we are 95% confident that the true SIM rate increase lay within this range.

Figure 9.2 displays the core of the study through a series of eight maps. The five states with the highest SIM rates in 1999/2000—Alaska, Arizona, Nevada, New Mexico, and Wyoming—became the basis for comparisons across space (states) and time, and consequently for showing the evolution of a national mental health crisis when the mortality indicator or representative of imminent personal and societal distress was SIM rather than suicide. By 2017/18, all states (and Washington, DC) except Nebraska posted SIM rates as high as that of Wyoming in 1999/2000, whose rate was the lowest for the five referent states at 21 deaths per 100,000 population; the rate for Nebraska fell just below this floor at 19 per 100,000. Also disturbing, by 2017/18 eight states in the West and West Virginia in the South registered suicide rates that entered the SIM rate range that the top five ranking states occupied in 1999/2000. Documented in the later twentieth century, a Western suicide belt is prominent across most of our observation period when we employ suicide as our mortality indicator of imminent personal and societal distress. One might, then, misleadingly infer that the poorest mental health in the United States was among populations in Western states. SIM provides a more comprehensive picture and affirms that there is a national mental health crisis.

Suggested as an effective way to display data by my emergency physician colleague Luke Larkin, two lollipop graphs provide interstate comparisons of suicide and SIM rates for four timepoints: 1999/2000, 2007/8, 2013/14, and 2017/18 (fig. 9.3). I calculated a correlational measure, Spearman's Rho, to assess the degree of congruence between the rank order of the two sets of rates at those observation points. Respective coefficients were 0.82, 0.86, 0.75, and 0.34. Thus, congruence was relatively high until 2013/14, when the precipitous decline in the correlation coefficient likely reflected the devastating impact of lethal illicit opioid use in the population. Numerous media reports indicated that medical examiner and coroner offices were being severely taxed by their added workloads. I suspect that autopsy rates and toxicologic testing became less common as a result, which would complicate detection of suicides, especially those by drug poisoning. A third lollipop graph transfers attention to the distribution across states and time of the nonsuicide component of SIM, the drug self-intoxication deaths that were either unknowable misclassified suicides or other deaths that reflected repetitive

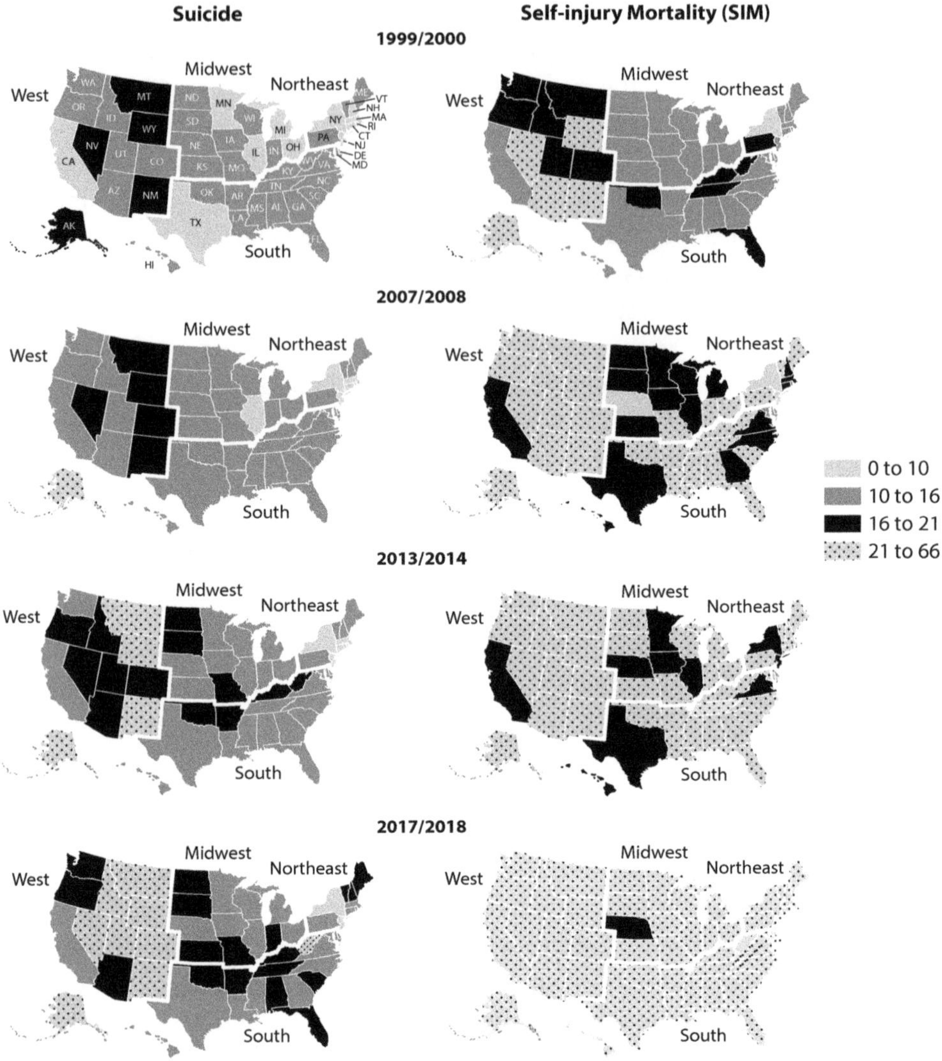

Figure 9.2. Mapped annual-averaged crude suicide and self-injury mortality (SIM) rates per 100,000 population by state and period, United States. Source: Rockett, I.R.H., Caine, E.D., Banerjee, A., et al., "Fatal self-injury in the United States, 1999–2018: Unmasking a national mental health crisis," *EClinicalMedicine* 2021; 32:100741.

self-harming behaviors (fig. 9.4). Harboring important implications for differential undercounting of suicide, due to the challenges for medical examiners and coroners to detect suicides by drugs, there was large variation in the proportion of SIM represented by these deaths. For example, in 1999/2000 the range by state extended from 9% for South Dakota to 65% for Washington, DC. In 2017/18, the same states recorded the low and the high—22% for South Dakota and 82% for DC. These results provide reason for relative confidence in the accuracy of suicide certification in South Dakota and skepticism about the DC certification. Other states appearing to have relatively high quality suicide data in the early twenty-first-century United States are North Dakota and Nebraska. On the other hand, Maryland and Massachusetts are opposites of the other two states, together with Washington, DC. Essential for effective prevention nationally, an area for future research should be a direct examination of suicide detection across states. But such research will be labor-intensive, and hence time-consuming and expensive.

Two maps enable us to look at estimated "nonsuicide" drug self-intoxication deaths both by region and by state across time, where this component of SIM qualifies as a mortality analog of "nonsuicidal self-injury" or self-harm injury morbidity and behaviorally belongs below suicide on an intentionality continuum of fatal self-injury. First, reference to a measure called the standardized mortality ratio shows us that the rate of growth is lower in the West than for the nation as a whole (fig. 9.5A). By comparison, the relative increase in these ratios tends to be higher in the Midwest and Northeast and closer to the average in the South. A smoothed map, or a "heatmap," shows that the Missouri and Lower Mississippi Rivers basically bisect the nation, with a relatively lower rate of increase in the standardized mortality rate ratios—a measure holding constant the effect of an otherwise potentially transformative variable, in this instance age—in the Western United States and a higher rate of increase in the Eastern United States (fig. 9.5B). Smoothing accommodated the fact that most American states have other states as neighbors, as many as eight each in the case of Tennessee and Missouri. Some states are even bordered by other countries, that is, Canada or Mexico. Our smoothing of the maps took account of permeability in interstate borders, although not in international ones.

If suicide detection is truly more accurate in the West than in the three other major regions of the country, it may involve two factors that, in combination, make suicide case ascertainment relatively easier for their death

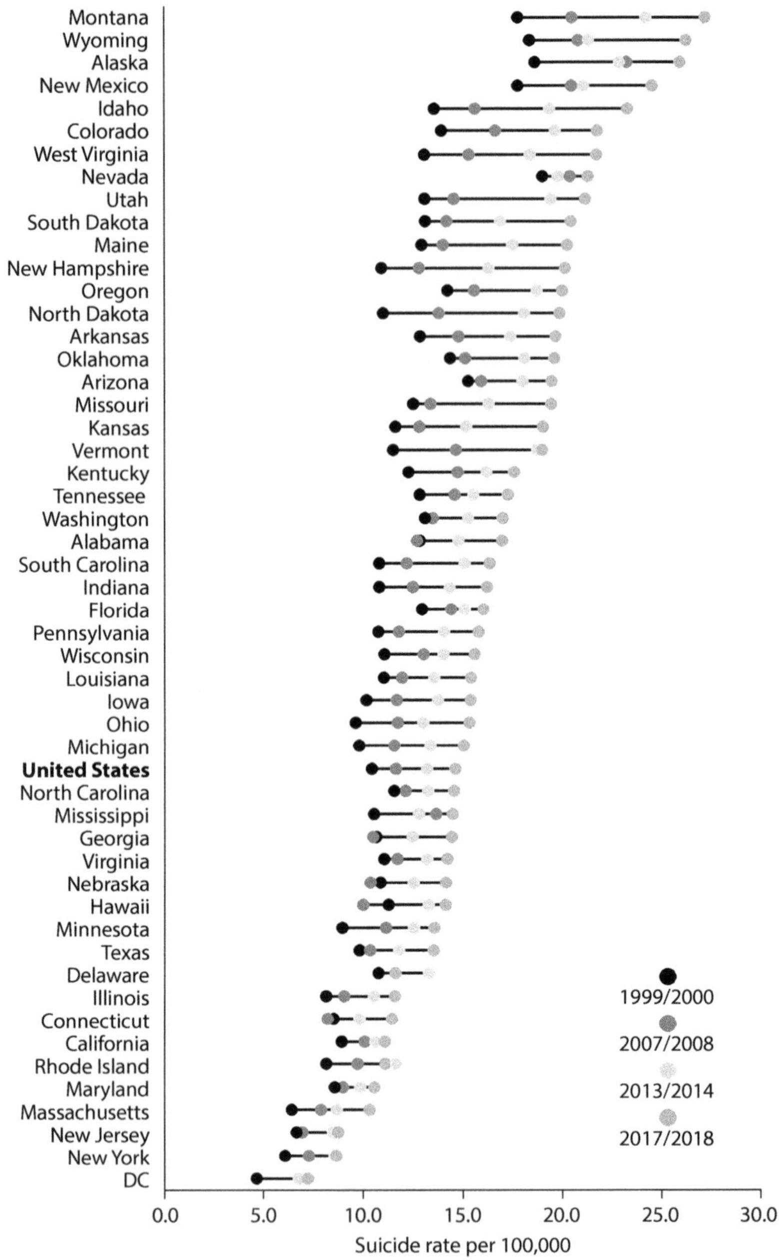

Figure 9.3. Annual-averaged crude suicide and self-injury mortality (SIM) rates by state and period, United States. Source: Rockett, I.R.H., Caine, E.D., Banerjee, A., et al., "Fatal self-injury in the United States, 1999–2018: Unmasking a national mental health crisis," *EClinicalMedicine* 2021;32:100741.

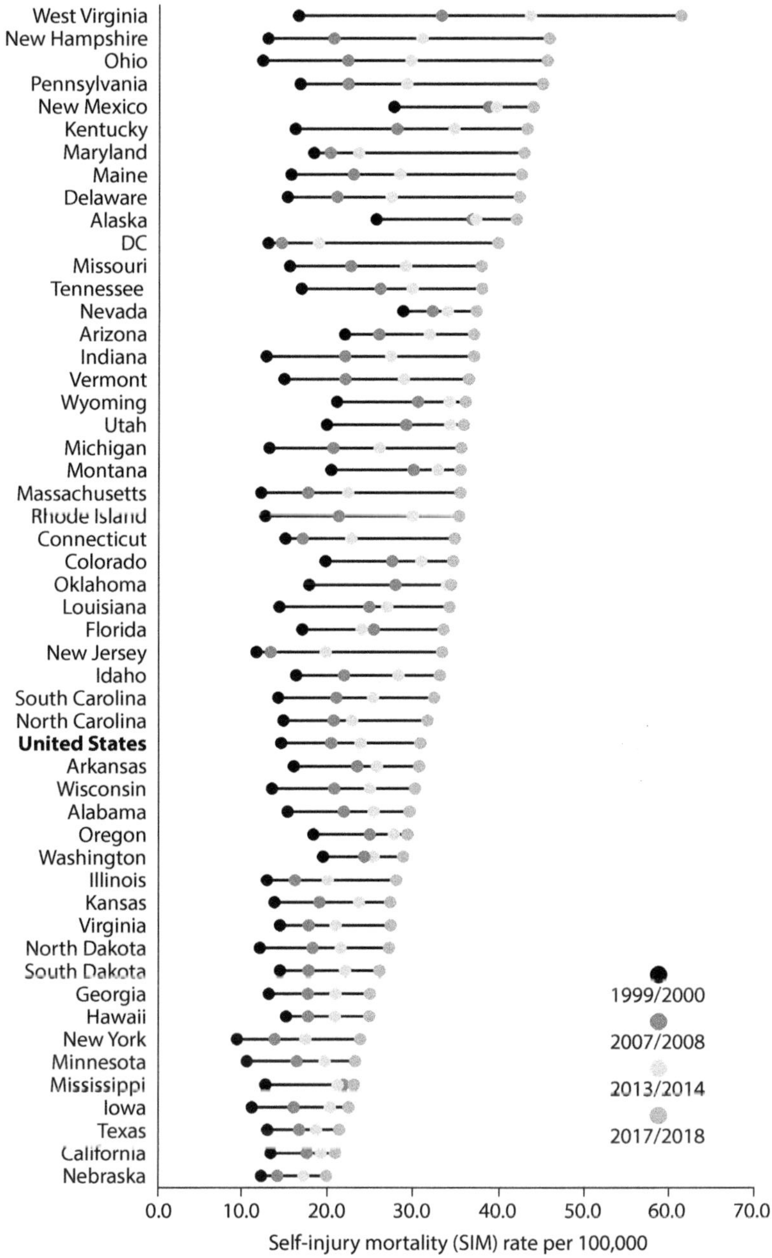
West Virginia
New Hampshire
Ohio
Pennsylvania
New Mexico
Kentucky
Maryland
Maine
Delaware
Alaska
DC
Missouri
Tennessee
Nevada
Arizona
Indiana
Vermont
Wyoming
Utah
Michigan
Montana
Massachusetts
Rhode Island
Connecticut
Colorado
Oklahoma
Louisiana
Florida
New Jersey
Idaho
South Carolina
North Carolina
United States
Arkansas
Wisconsin
Alabama
Oregon
Washington
Illinois
Kansas
Virginia
North Dakota
South Dakota
Georgia
Hawaii
New York
Minnesota
Mississippi
Iowa
Texas
California
Nebraska
1999/2000
2007/2008
2013/2014
2017/2018
0.0
10.0
20.0
30.0
40.0
50.0
60.0
70.0
Self-injury mortality (SIM) rate per 100,000

This page intentionally left blank.

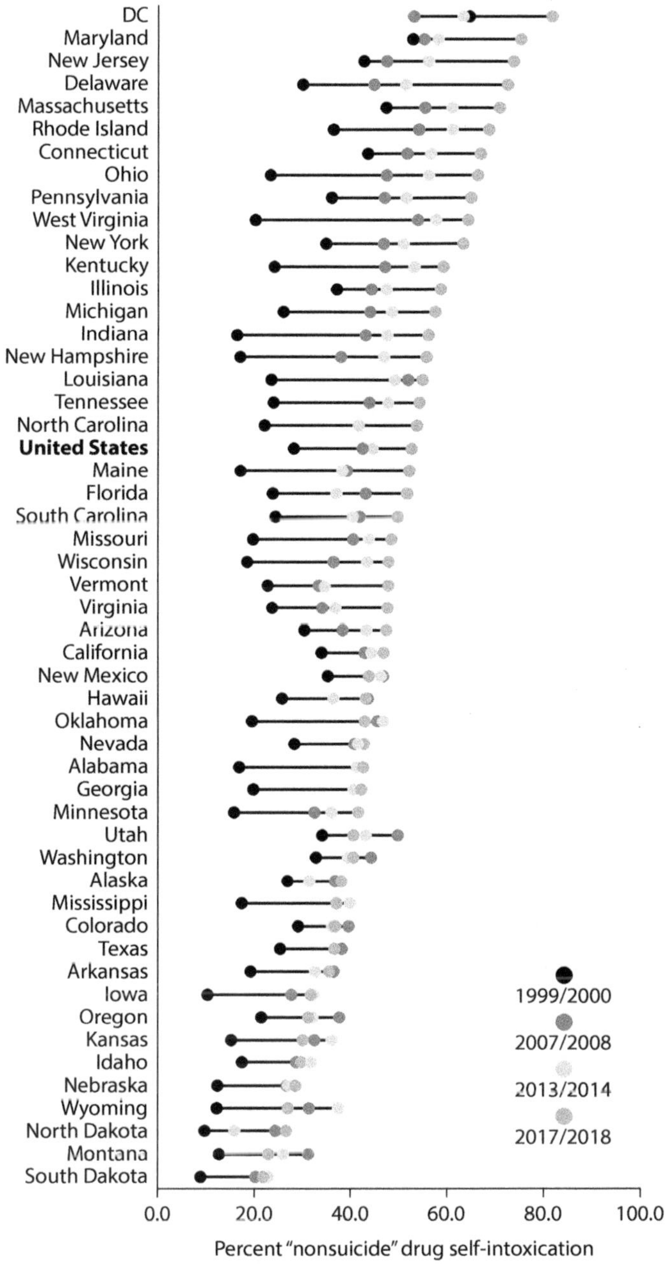

Figure 9.4. Annual-averaged percentage of "nonsuicide" drug self-intoxication deaths of self-injury mortality (SIM) by state and period, United States. Source: Rockett, I.R.H., Caine, E.D., Banerjee, A., et al., "Fatal self-injury in the United States, 1999–2018: Unmasking a national mental health crisis," ***EClinicalMedicine*** **2021;32:100741.**

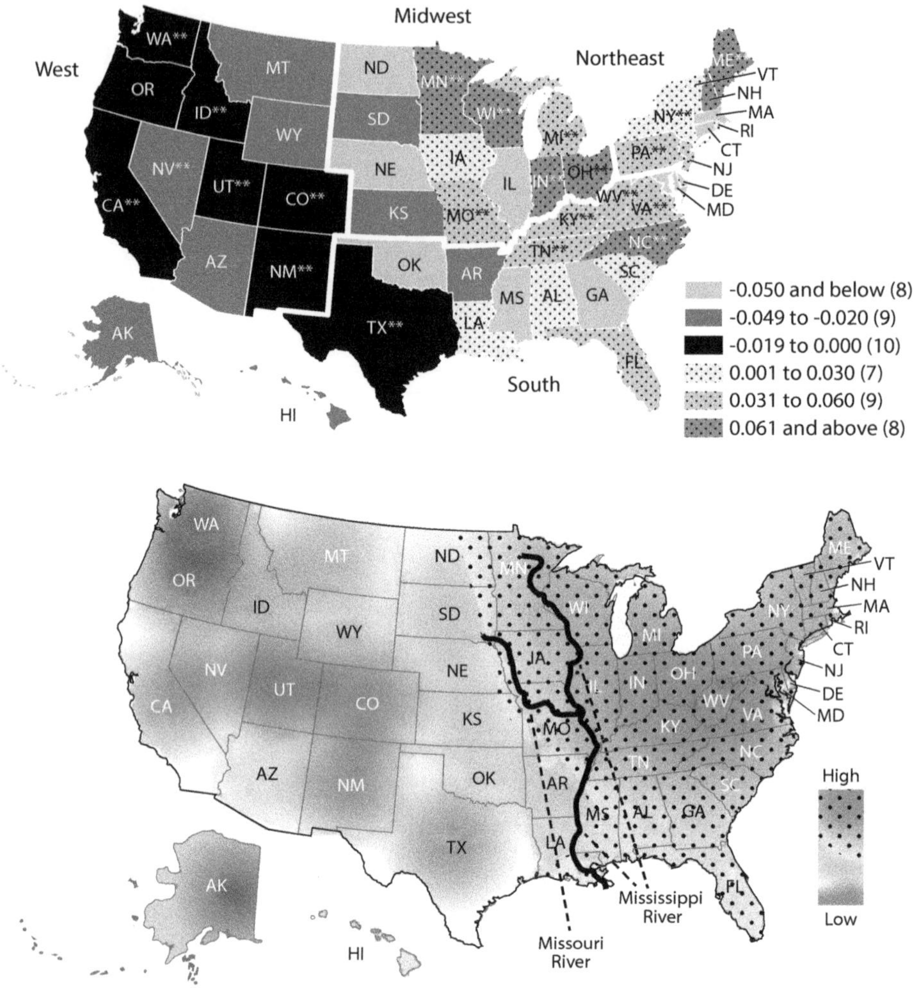

Figure 9.5. *A*, Spatiotemporal percentage change in standardized mortality ratios for "nonsuicide" drug self-intoxication by state, United States, 1999/2000–2017/18 (states with ratios statistically significantly different from the national ratio, $p \leq 0.05$, are depicted by twin asterisks). *B*, "Heatmap" of spatiotemporal change in standardized mortality ratios for "nonsuicide" drug self-intoxication, United States, 1999/2000–2017/18. Source: Rockett, I.R.H., Caine, E.D., Banerjee, A., et al., "Fatal self-injury in the United States, 1999–2018: Unmasking a national mental health crisis," *EClinicalMedicine* 2021;32:100741.

investigators. Not only had there been less penetration by the opioid epidemic in the West during the period of study, but firearm suicides were more prominent (Siegel & Rothman, 2016), as consistent with the highest prevalence of gun ownership of any region in the country (Kalesan et al., 2016). Our study of the geography of SIM versus suicide underscores a need for direct in-depth research on suicide investigation by method, resource allocation, and type of medicolegal death investigation system.

Translating the crisis

With the director of research communications at West Virginia University, Jake Stump, I prepared a press release to disseminate the findings from the previous SIM and suicide study, which in print was entitled "Fatal Self-Injury in the United States, 1999–2018: Unmasking a National Mental Health Crisis" (Rockett et al., 2021). Whereas the article itself relied heavily on visual representation of SIM and suicide rate trends by state and region, the release told the story primarily through a series of quotations from three of the authors, Hilary Connery, Eric Caine, and myself. The headline for the release was "Death by Suicide? Drug Overdoses Muddy Waters for Investigators, Amplify National Mental Health Crisis" (West Virginia University, 2021). I endeavored to set the scene by offering the following:

> Broadening the definition of SIM to encompass most drug overdose deaths, even if they don't meet the standards used by medical examiners and coroners to classify them as suicides, shows that the whole nation is afflicted by a mental health crisis. On the other hand, if we only represent SIM by registered suicides, this crisis misleadingly appears concentrated in western states.
>
> Suicides likely have been easiest to detect in the West because the leading and most highly lethal method is firearm or gunshot wound. The remainder of the country has been more severely affected by the opioid epidemic through the opening decades of the 21st century. Our previous research, which indicated there was a substantial overlap between the opioid epidemic and a more hidden suicide epidemic, led me to develop SIM in close collaboration with a very talented group of researchers and practitioners in 2015 and 2016. That the suicide epidemic was most pronounced in the west and the opioid epidemic elsewhere in the nation motivated us to look at SIM versus suicide rates across the country as a whole and time.
>
> Despite victims sharing many common risk factors, suicide and drug overdose

> deaths tend to be treated separately within the scientific literature, media, and the healthcare system, and by funding agencies and prevention programs. Among these risk factors are unemployment, family discord, unmanaged and mismanaged physical pain, and various psychiatric disorders, including alcohol, opioid, and other substance use disorders. While most people dying by overdose may not have intended to die, they were engaging in repetitive, intentional, self-injurious behaviors that they understood markedly increased their chances of a premature death. Calling these deaths "accidents" (the forensic classification most often used in the United States) or "unintentional" (the term used by the CDC) mischaracterizes what occurred, even if consistent with the classification criteria used by medical examiners and coroners. (West Virginia University, 2021)

Speaking clinically, Hilary Connery noted that "opioid and other drug-overdose deaths continue to rise in spite of medical efforts to make life-saving medications for opioid use disorder available to patients and communities. Many persons suffering drug use disorders become hopeless—they relapse frequently, continue to experience relationship losses, health consequences, and economic instability, and they frequently suffer other mental disorders, such as depression, post-traumatic stress disorder, and other anxiety disorders. We know that people with addiction have 10 times the rate of suicide compared to those without addiction" (West Virginia University, 2021).

Eric Caine underscored the major implication of the research for suicide prevention efforts, with an emphasis on "upstream" health promotion principles that well precede an individual's suicidality. He acknowledged the importance of knowing a patient's history, "long before they ever become suicidal":

> Recognizing a patient's full story with respect to risk factors, health status over the long-term, and socioeconomic history are critical in providing effective comprehensive treatment. Ultimately it is less about "classifying suicide" and more about understanding that suicide and overdose fatalities reflect common social and psychological risk factors that were present long before death. There are large groups of persons in our country who have suffered adverse early life experiences, family and social turmoil, economic hardships and life disappointments, as well as chronic ailments; many die prematurely. Our goal must be to eliminate or mitigate those circumstances. Separating these groups using misclassified or misleading postmortem labels does little to enhance prevention. We need to

focus on the lives of persons in these groups long before they get close to dying if we aspire to overcome these tragic losses of life. (West Virginia University, 2021)

Assessing potential for differential suicide misclassification by state

In our second interstate study of SIM and suicide, we first sought to shed more light on differential potential for suicide misclassification and undercounting across states and regions, during the first two decades of the twenty-first century, by graphing and mapping SIM-to-suicide rate ratios (Rockett et al., 2022). Examination of these ratios enabled us to compare the changing relative contributions of suicides and drug overdose with the overall burden of self-injury fatalities, and hence to assess the potential for differential suicide misclassification. All other things being equal, the larger the gap between the two sets of rates, the greater the potential. We employed four observation points, as we had done in the first study. In this study, however, we took advantage of the release of 2019 data from the National Center for Health Statistics to make our annual-averaged endpoint 2018/19, instead of 2017/18. To reiterate, the primary motivation for the conceptualization and operationalization of SIM was to mitigate not only downward measurement biases in suicide inherent in such demographic characteristics as sex and race/ethnicity but also a similar bias related to method or injury mechanism—most notably the less forensically overt method of drug intoxication versus the more forensically overt methods of firearm / gunshot wound and hanging/suffocation.

A lollipop graph showed that rate ratios increased across all states (fig. 9.6), reflecting growing capacity for suicide undercounting in the absence of the compensatory application of SIM. The rate gap in 2018/19 was largest for Washington, DC, Maryland, and Delaware and smallest for the Dakotas and Montana. Mapping revealed that in 1999/2000 39 states had a rate ratio below 1.50, with all four major regions represented, and that by 2018/19 the number of states had shrunk to eight, with only the West being unrepresented in the top category with ratios of 2.10 or higher (fig. 9.7). Regionally, rate gaps were narrowest in Western Mountain states, adjacent Midwestern states, and Arkansas and widest in the Northeast, the Midwest, and the geographic extremes of the South. One can infer from examination of the

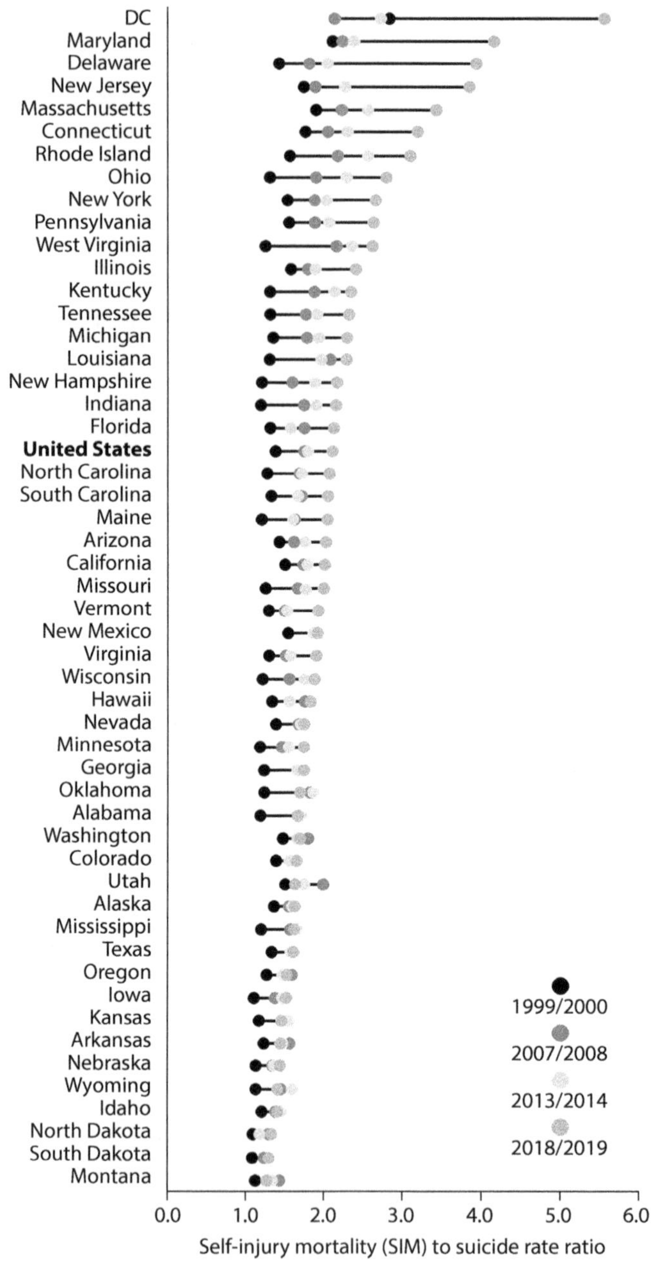

Figure 9.6. Graphed annual-averaged crude self-injury mortality (SIM) to suicide rate ratios by state and period, United States. Source: Rockett, I.R.H., Jia, H., Ali, B., et al., "Association of state social and environmental factors with rates of self-injury mortality and suicide in the United States," ***JAMA Network Open*** **2022;5(2):e2146591.**

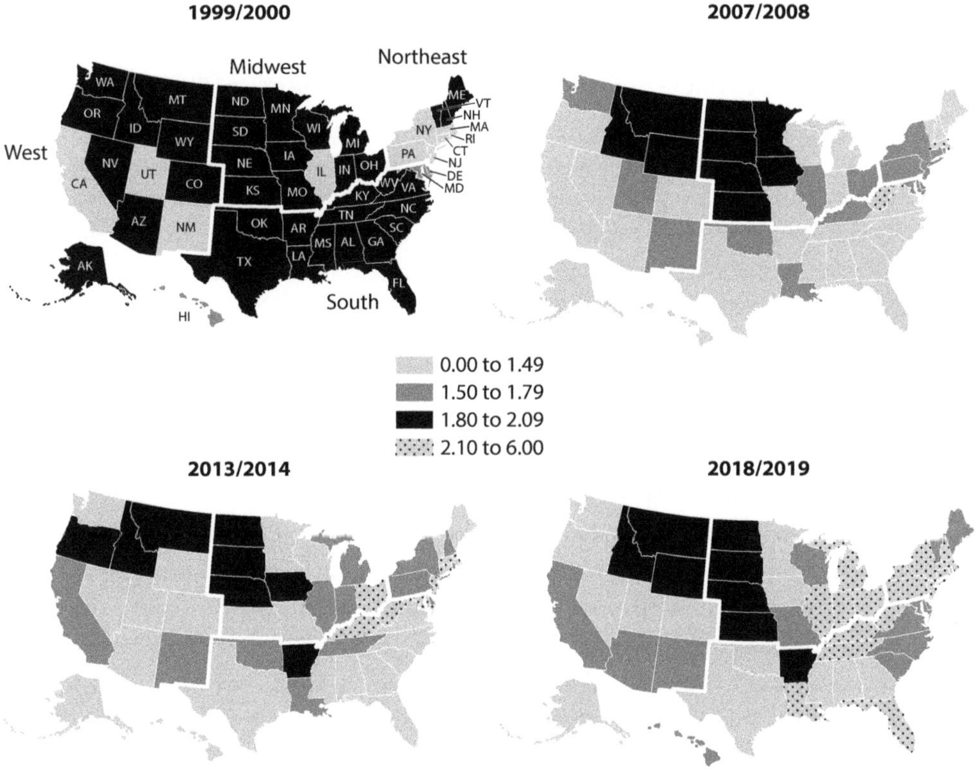

Figure 9.7. Mapped annual-averaged crude self-injury mortality to suicide rate ratios by state and period, United States. Source: Rockett, I.R.H., Jia, H., Ali, B., et al., "Association of state social and environmental factors with rates of self-injury mortality and suicide in the United States," ***JAMA Network Open*** **2022; 5(2):e2146591.**

growing gap in the SIM-to-suicide rate ratios across the nation that the reporting of American suicide rates has become increasingly unreliable in the twenty-first century.

Contextual characteristics of interstate self-injury mortality and suicide rates

The main purpose of the second study in our trilogy was to explore state-based, contextual characteristics associated with SIM and suicide rates. These characteristics broadly represented six distinct elements: social inequity and economic resources, social isolation and separation, demographics, injury mechanism, health care access, and type of medicolegal death investigation system. Incorporation of system type provided for the possibility of an artifactual component that differentiated the magnitude of SIM and suicide rates across states, after adjustment for the five substantive factors in the multivariable analysis. Our analysis utilized a statistical procedure called least absolute shrinkage and selection operator (LASSO) regression to identify the constellation of variables most strongly associated with the respective rates. A major strength of this procedure is that it can handle a relatively large number of "predictor variables," 33 in this study, some of which may highly correlate with one another, and a relatively small number of cases or observations (50 states plus Washington, DC). LASSO is predictive and exploratory but not explanatory—that is, this procedure does not enable one to infer and evaluate cause-and-effect relationships. However, application can generate testable hypotheses.

LASSO identified eight variables associated with the SIM rate: labor underutilization rate, manufacturing employment, homelessness rate, percentage nonreligious, non-Hispanic White race and ethnicity, percentage of the population prescribed opioids for 30 days or more, percentage without health insurance, and a medicolegal death investigation system that was led by a medical examiner with centralized authority. The manufacturing employment, homelessness, and health insurance variables manifested negative associations. The last two relationships appear anomalous. A plausible and testable explanation is that the homeless and uninsured were less likely than respective opposites to have interacted with the health care system and thus to have been prescribed opioids leading up to the observation point 2018/19. I hypothesize that any such associations with the SIM rate were later modified as illicit fentanyl-related drugs engulfed the country, whose use is increasingly being accompanied by use of such stimulants as methamphetamine and cocaine (Ciccarone, 2021) and tranquilizers, including the nonopioid animal sedative xylazine (US Drug Enforcement Administration, 2023); this speculation warrants in-depth research.

This study is the first where I have investigated variables associated with suicide, as distinct from the determinants of this manner-of-death classification. However, in deference to my usual focus on suicide data quality, it did not neglect the possibility of an artificial component that implicated diversity in medicolegal death investigation systems (Rockett et al., 2022). Five substantive, contextual variables were associated with the suicide rate: percentage male, military veteran, rural, firearm ownership, and pain reliever misuse. These associations are unsurprising and align with the literature. Illustrating the demographic bias in suicide measurement, the first three of the five correlates enumerated were demographic characteristics, while only non-Hispanic White race and ethnicity was associated with the SIM rate. System type showed no association with suicide, perhaps because suicide determination by medical examiners and coroners is conservative. Again, suicide is not a default manner-of-death assignment. However, the finding that a statewide centralized medical examiner system was associated with detection of more SIM cases than the other systems may reflect superior training, experience in death investigations, and capacity to conduct forensic autopsies or advanced imaging and toxicologic testing (Robinson, 2017). Pointing to geographic and rural/urban health data disparities, this is a topic calling for additional research and one that assumes even greater urgency amid the havoc the COVID-19 pandemic wrought during its onset—including the additional pressures on scarce medicolegal resources from fear of spread of the disease (Moretti et al., 2021), prior to the development and use of effective vaccines, and also of effective personal protective equipment in hospital and other medical settings. Although more people are served by centralized medical examiner systems than other death investigation system types, a greater geographic and predominantly rural area is served by decentralized county coroner systems (Hanzlick, 2014). Problematic for any initiatives to standardize medicolegal death investigations, the nation has a patchwork quilt of medicolegal death investigation systems by type (fig. 9.8).

None of our contextual variables was associated with both SIM and suicide rates; the two measures shared broader associations with demographics and injury mechanism, but not with social inequity / economic resources, social isolation, and health care access. SIM rates were positively associated with social inequity and social isolation, both upstream factors.

Mass media dissemination

Published in 2022, my coauthors and I entitled our second interstate study on SIM and suicide "Association of State Social and Environmental Factors with Rates of Self-Injury Mortality and Suicide in the United States" (Rockett et al., 2022). In an accompanying and detailed press release from West Virginia University, I explained, "A relatively new concept, SIM was conceived as a combination of all registered or known suicides and the pre-

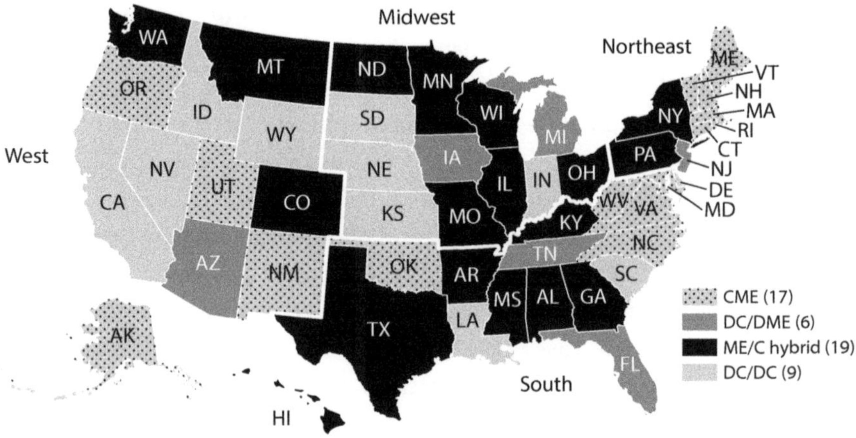

Figure 9.8. Type of medicolegal death investigation system by state and region, United States, 2018. Note: CME = centralized authority with (state) medical examiner system; DC/DME = decentralized county/district medical examiner system; ME/C hybrid = mixed medical examiner and coroner systems; DC/DC = decentralized county/district coroner system. Source: Rockett, I.R.H., Jia, H., Ali, B., et al., "Association of state social and environmental factors with rates of self-injury mortality and suicide in the United States," ***JAMA Network Open*** **2022;5(2):e2146591.**

ponderance of fatal opioid and other drug overdoses. The inclusion of overdoses in SIM recognizes these deaths reflect self-harm behaviors, emanating from drug addiction and procurement, even when the victims did not intend to die" (West Virginia University, 2022).

The news release reported on our proposition that the growing gaps between the SIM and suicide rates indicated increasing potential for suicide misclassification over time and across the nation, which stemmed from the opioid epidemic and attendant stresses and strains it imposed on medicolegal death investigation systems. I commented that the expanding rate gap "means that SIM was increasingly being represented by overdoses, a method of suicide that is very difficult for medical examiners and coroners to detect without strong corroborative evidence in the form of an authenticated suicide note, testimony by a reliable witness, and record of a previous suicide attempt or serious mental illness. Generally, such evidence is either absent or grossly deficient, and medical examiners and coroners understandably and typically use accident as their default classification for fatal overdoses, whether truly unintentional or not." The press release also included my rationale for suggesting the assumption that 80% of fatal overdoses in the age group 15 years and older are self-injury is a conservative one: "We take the view that most opioid and other drug deaths involve a pattern of self-harm, which is associated with acquiring the drugs and satisfying the motivating cravings. To meet their needs, overdose victims frequently had pharmacy shopped and doctor shopped or purchased illicit drugs on the street from dealers. It's high-risk behavior, and many people who misuse drugs are aware this is hazardous because they have known people who died as a consequence" (West Virginia University, 2022).

The West Virginia University news release noted that our study revealed that SIM rates were higher in states where labor underutilization was more common, states with populations more non-Hispanic White and nonreligious, and states where longer-term prescribing of opioids was also more common. Findings suggested an artifactual component in interstate differences in SIM rates. States whose medicolegal death investigation systems were centralized, like that of West Virginia, appeared to detect more SIM cases. An explanation may be that economies of scale allow them to conduct more toxicologic testing.

The press release further included our unanticipated findings that lower SIM rates were found in states having a higher prevalence of homelessness and larger populations lacking health insurance. Echoing a blog post by Eric Caine and myself (Rockett & Caine, 2015a), I proffered the following testable propositions in response: "Ordinarily, you'd think 'health insurance is protective,' and you would be correct. But if you're not in the healthcare system, you're not going to be prescribed opioids. Yes, now there are many illicit opioids out there, such as highly lethal fentanyl, but for a long-time opioid distribution was fundamentally a medical and pharmaceutical issue. This may also help explain why minorities had much lower overdose rates for many years. But they're catching up to non-Hispanic Whites because illicit opioids have become so common and all too readily accessible by the public." In conclusion, I noted that "drug misuse and addiction are precursors to the high-risk behaviors that always potentially, and actually often, lead to SIM. Strategies aimed at reversing the upward trend in the SIM rate must involve large-scale, diverse, and sustained interventions at the general population level, in combination with clinical and community-based interventions that target high-risk individuals among hospital emergency department patients, school and college students, and arrestees and prisoners" (West Virginia University, 2022). In a briefer story in Healio, a news source servicing medical and other health care professionals, I remarked,

> This national study breaks new ground by identifying characteristics of states that are associated with high or low rates of self-injury mortality. These characteristics represent economic inequality, social isolation, demographics, barriers to health care, means or mechanisms of injury, and system type as a surrogate for the variable quality of the medicolegal death investigations themselves.
>
> This study suggests that reversal of the rising SIM trends in the 21st century, intensified by the COVID-19 pandemic, will require upstream preventive measures that target the economy, healthcare industry, schools and colleges, the military, jails and prisons, and other major institutions, as well as the need to scale treatment interventions with high-risk patients in hospital emergency department and psychiatric care settings. (Herpen, 2022)

Local heterogeneity

Major policy formulation and implementation occur at the state level, important justification for our choice of the state as the unit of analysis in the preceding study. Yet suicides tend to be local phenomena, and future research should consider including a multilevel analysis using states, counties, and even smaller geographic units like census tracts or zip (postal) codes. A recent systematic review examined county-level predictors of drug overdose mortality in the United States and showed significant variation across some of the predictors (Cano et al., 2023). Among their research limitations, the authors reported likely geographic variation in the completeness of drug reporting on death certificates—an issue related to our finding that type of medicolegal death investigation was associated with the magnitude of reported SIM rates (Rockett et al., 2022).

National and state costs of self-injury mortality and suicide

Published in 2023 as "Escalating Costs of Self-Injury Mortality in the 21st Century United States: An Interstate Observational Study," the final study in our geographic trilogy estimated annual-averaged economic costs of SIM and suicide in terms of medical spending and losses of work productivity and quality of life in 2019 US dollars (Rockett et al., 2023). Details of the methodology and research limitations are reported in that article. The

Box 2. Valuing Lost Quality of Life

"We valued the lives lost [to suicide and SIM, respectively] with the $10.7 million average value per statistical life that the US Department of Health and Human Services uses in regulatory analysis. Value of a statistical life is the value per life saved that results from aggregating across the population the amount that people pay (or state in surveys that they are willing to pay) for small reductions in their own or an immediate family member's chance of dying. The $10.7 million value of a statistical life comes from a meta-analysis of a large literature. Subtracting lifetime work loss from [that value] yields the value of lost quality of life. Quality of life encompasses all of life's nonmonetary aspects, including a person's health, comfort, and ability to participate in and enjoy social and role functions. Dividing average lifetime quality of life loss by life expectancy yields a cost per year of quality of life lost that can be used to tailor losses by decedent age and sex. Based on previous work that suggests reduced quality of life for individuals with substance use and mood disorders (e.g., 9%–25% loss of quality of life for substance use disorders; and 15%–20% loss for people with mood disorders and suicide risk, conservatively), we valued loss of a lifetime of quality of life from each self-injury mortality (SIM) death at 80% of the loss for the average person of the same age and sex. Costs beyond the first year were discounted to present value using a widely recommended 3% annual discount rate. We inflated all costs to 2019 dollars and used two-year annual-averaged rates and costs to stabilize the data."

Source: Ted R. Miller in Rockett, I.R.H., Ali, B., Caine, E.D., et al., "Escalating costs of self-injury mortality in the 21st century United States: An interstate observational study," *BMC Public Health* 2023;23(1):3.

concepts of medical spending and work losses are rather intuitive, but future quality-of-life losses are less so. In an email communication to me on February 2, 2023, my colleague Ted Miller expressed quality-of-life costs simply as the "dollar value placed on the pain, suffering, and lost enjoyment of life of the people who died and their immediate families." He elaborated on its constituents in box 2.

In our study, costs related to the work and quality-of-life loss elements for SIM and suicide dwarfed those of medical spending, but those for lost quality of life predominated. Respective ratios of quality-of-life and work losses to medical spending in 2019 US dollars for SIM were 1,419 and 526 in 1999/2000 and 1,476 and 526 in 2018/19. Estimated annual-averaged national costs of SIM increased by 143% from $0.46 trillion in 1999/2000 to $1.12 trillion in 2019 US dollars in 2018/19, as the crude SIM rate rose by 125%—from 14.6 to 32.9 deaths per 100,000 population. Corresponding national suicide costs rose by 58%—from $318.6 billion to $502.7 billion. Respective ratios of quality-of-life and work losses to medical spending for suicide were 1,489 and 544 in 1999/2000 and 1,585 and 552 in 2018/19. National per capita costs of SIM doubled from $1,638 to $3,413 between the beginning and the end of the observation period, while the per capita costs of the suicide component increased by 35%—from $1,137 to $1,534.

Figure 9.9 depicts interstate variation in per capita SIM and suicide costs. In these lollipop graphs, states are ranked by per capita SIM and suicide costs for the annual-averaged years of 2018 and 2019. Also shown for each state are their comparative data for the years 1999/2000. First-ranked West Virginia, my home state, was a clear outlier on SIM in 2018/19, with a per capita cost of $6,534. It ranked 13th on per capita suicide cost at $2,113. Delaware ranked second on per capita SIM cost at $5,351 and 42nd on corresponding suicide cost at $1,256. Nebraska posted the lowest per capita SIM cost at $2,215 while ranking 32nd on per capita suicide cost at $1,591. The highest per capita suicide cost was posted by Alaska at $3,245, and Wyoming was second at $2,895. Washington, DC had the lowest cost at $781. Implicating drug intoxication cases, wide gaps in SIM and suicide cost rankings by state likely reflect large potential for suicide misclassification, as previously discussed.

Expressed in quintiles (five equal-sized categories depicting a range of values for a measure of interest), choropleth maps display the interperiod growth in per capita SIM and suicide costs by state and region using variable shading to differentiate gradation (fig. 9.10). States whose per capita SIM cost increase exceeded 152%, the top quintile, were concentrated in the Great Lakes, Southeast, Mideast, and New England regions. States with per capita SIM cost increases below 70%, the bottom quintile, were in the Far West, Southwest, Plains, Rocky Mountains, and Southeast. West Virginia had the largest increase at 263%, and Nevada had the smallest at 22%. Percentage per capita cost increases for SIM surpassed those for suicide. The only regions

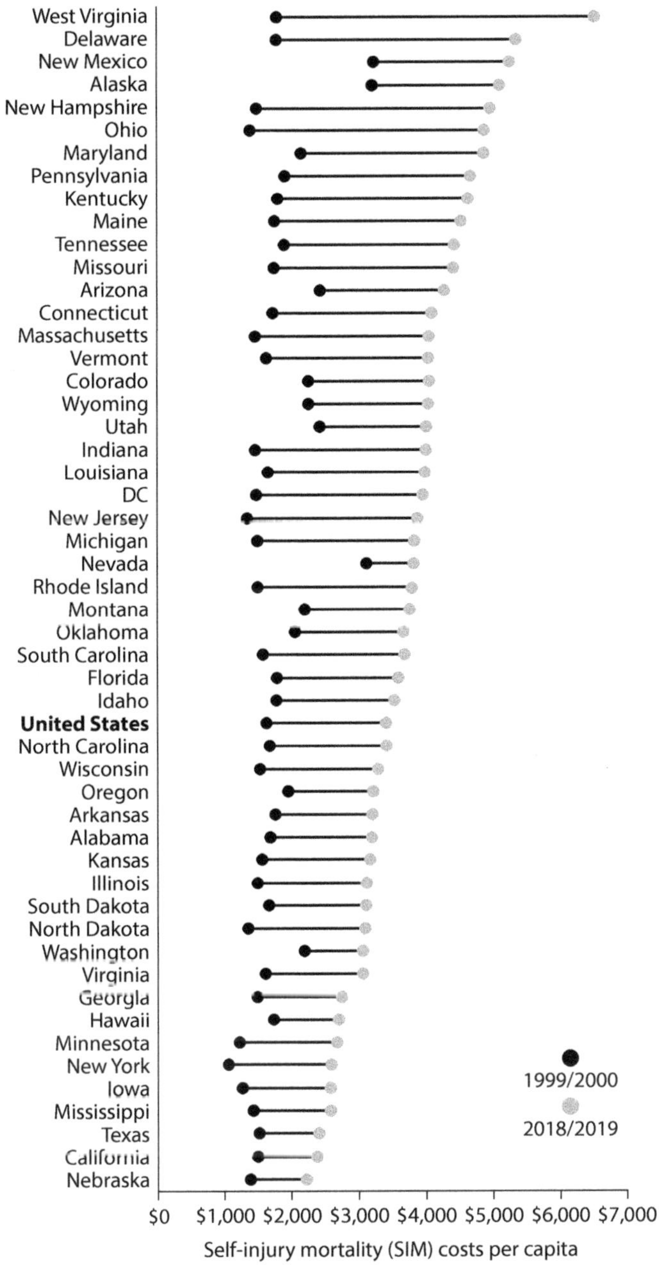

Figure 9.9. Ranked self-injury mortality (SIM) and suicide per capita costs by state, 2018/19 versus 1999/2000. Source: Rockett, I.R.H., Ali, B., Caine, E.D., et al., "Escalating costs of self-injury mortality in the 21st century United States: An interstate observational study," *BMC Public Health* 2023;23(1):28.

(continued)

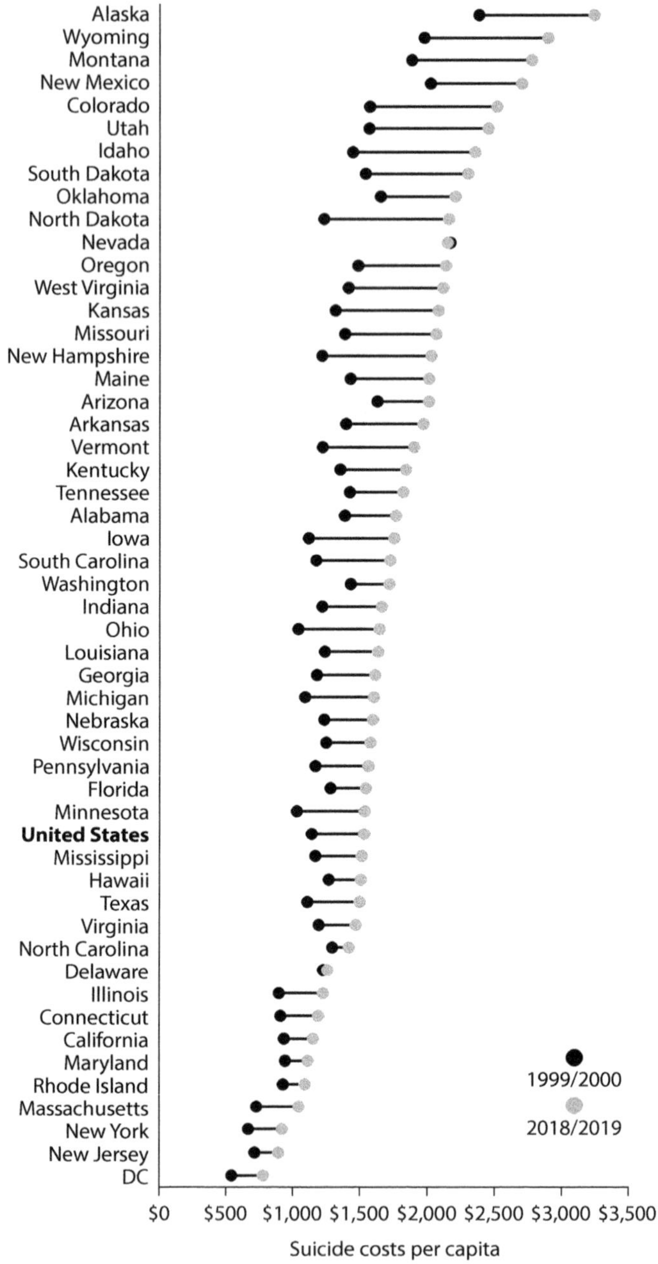

Figure 9.9. *Continued.*

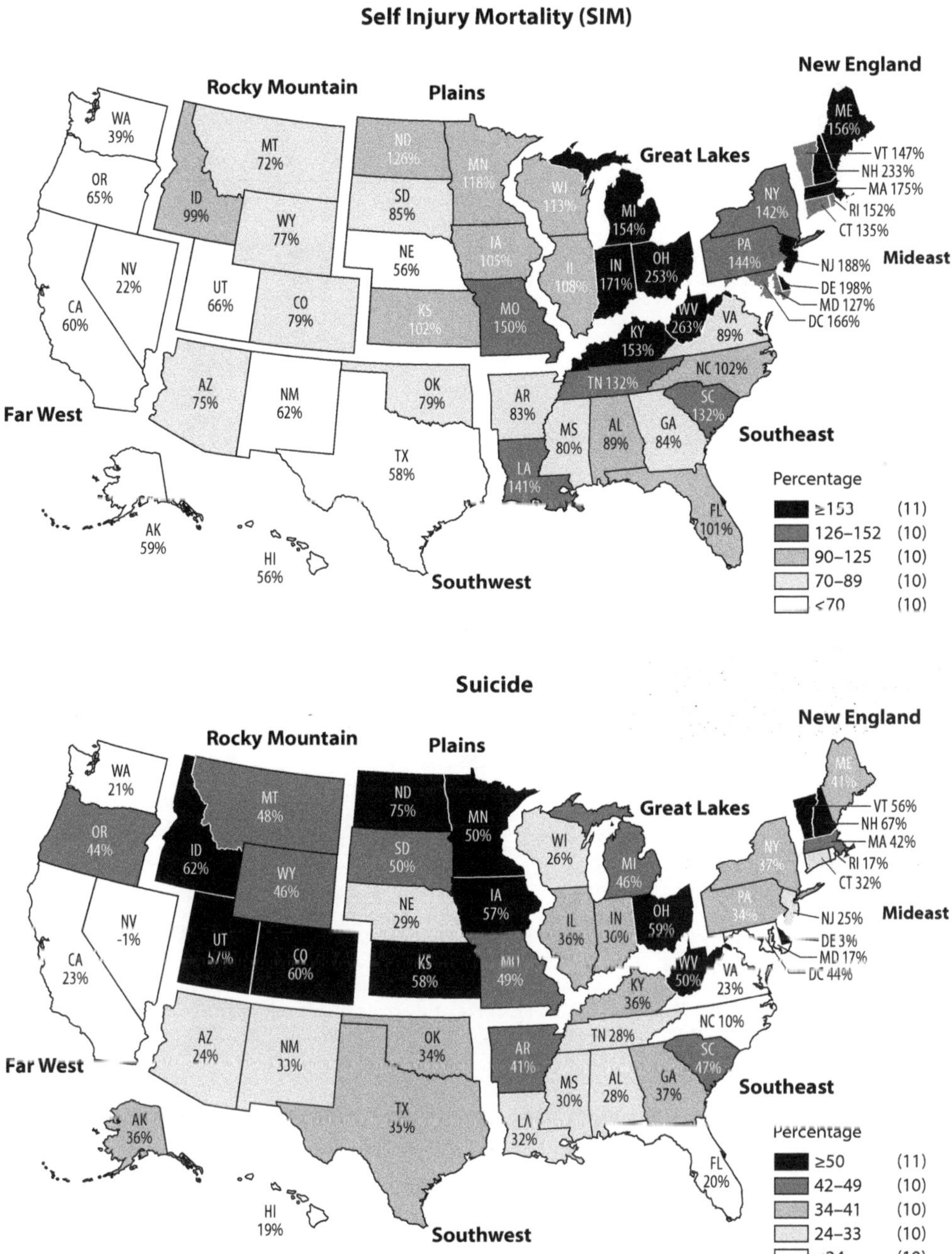

Figure 9.10. Percentage increase in self-injury mortality (SIM) and suicide costs per capita by region and state, 1999/2000–2018/19. Source: Rockett, I.R.H., Ali, B., Caine, E.D., et al., "Escalating costs of self-injury mortality in the 21st century United States: An interstate observational study," *BMC Public Health* 2023; 23(1):28.

Table 9.1. Self-injury mortality (SIM) and suicide costs per capita by state, 1999/2000 and 2018/19

	SIM cost per capita			Suicide cost per capita		
State	1999/2000 ($)	2018/2019 ($)	Change from 1999/2000 to 2018/19 (%)	1999/2000 ($)	2018/2019 ($)	Change from 1999/2000 to 2018/19 (%)
Alabama	1,689	3,186	89	1,382	1,763	28
Alaska	3,220	5,112	59	2,385	3,245	36
Arizona	2,439	4,271	75	1,621	2,008	24
Arkansas	1,752	3,203	83	1,390	1,967	41
California	1,487	2,378	60	937	1,151	23
Colorado	2,267	4,050	79	1,571	2,515	60
Connecticut	1,735	4,076	135	906	1,193	32
Delaware	1,797	5,351	198	1,224	1,256	3
DC	1,488	3,962	166	542	781	44
Florida	1,788	3,591	101	1,	1,545	20
Georgia	1,492	2,742	84	1,175	1,606	37
Hawaii	1,734	2,702	56	1,270	1,506	19
Idaho	1,780	3,537	99	1,445	2,344	62
Illinois	1,498	3,120	108	897	1,220	36
Indiana	1,477	4,006	171	1,218	1,654	36
Iowa	1,256	2,579	105	1,114	1,750	57
Kansas	1,568	3,165	102	1,315	2,084	58
Kentucky	1,831	4,635	153	1,351	1,838	36
Louisiana	1,655	3,986	141	1,235	1,630	32
Maine	1,769	4,525	156	1,427	2,009	41
Maryland	2,153	4,877	127	947	1,113	17
Massachusetts	1,471	4,050	175	730	1,039	42
Michigan	1,506	3,831	154	1,089	1,595	46
Minnesota	1,226	2,673	118	1,025	1,536	50
Mississippi	1,425	2,566	80	1,162	1,516	30
Missouri	1,765	4,414	150	1,383	2,063	49

Source: Rockett, I.R.H., Ali, B., Caine, E.D., et al., "Escalating costs of self-injury mortality in the 21st century United States: An interstate observational study," *BMC Public Health* 2023;23(1):28.

not represented in the top quintile for suicide costs, that is, states with increases of 50% or greater, were the Far West, Southwest, and Mideast. The bottom quintile comprised states whose per capita suicide cost increases were below 24%. Regional representatives were the Far West, Southeast, Mideast, and New England. North Dakota and Nevada, respectively, manifested the largest and smallest suicide cost changes by state at 75% and −1%. More detailed information on per capita costs is reported in table 9.1.

Cost estimation of SIM and suicide can inform health planning and both

Table 9.1. Continued

State	SIM cost per capita 1999/2000 ($)	SIM cost per capita 2018/2019 ($)	SIM cost per capita Change from 1999/2000 to 2018/19 (%)	Suicide cost per capita 1999/2000 ($)	Suicide cost per capita 2018/2019 ($)	Suicide cost per capita Change from 1999/2000 to 2018/19 (%)
Montana	2,189	3,773	72	1,877	2,773	48
Nebraska	1,416	2,215	56	1,233	1,591	29
Nevada	3,128	3,817	22	2,166	2,148	−1
New Hampshire	1,492	4,973	233	1,215	2,028	67
New Jersey	1,349	3,882	188	714	892	25
New Mexico	3,233	5,249	62	2,027	2,698	33
New York	1,069	2,589	142	672	917	37
North Carolina	1,680	3,400	102	1,295	1,421	10
North Dakota	1,365	3,088	126	1,229	2,154	75
Ohio	1,385	4,890	253	1,036	1,642	59
Oklahoma	2,061	3,682	79	1,644	2,204	34
Oregon	1,954	3,216	65	1,477	2,134	44
Pennsylvania	1,917	4,681	144	1,163	1,555	34
Rhode Island	1,508	3,808	153	928	1,088	17
South Carolina	1,585	3,679	132	1,171	1,726	47
South Dakota	1,681	3,105	85	1,536	2,301	50
Tennessee	1,904	4,423	132	1,421	1,818	28
Texas	1,515	2,400	58	1,105	1,495	35
Utah	2,422	4,014	66	1,558	2,453	57
Vermont	1,638	4,050	147	1,215	1,900	56
Virginia	1,617	3,047	89	1,191	1,468	23
Washington	2,192	3,053	39	1,420	1,715	21
West Virginia	1,800	6,534	263	1,408	2,113	50
Wisconsin	1,547	3,290	113	1,249	1,576	26
Wyoming	2,273	4,030	77	1,978	2,895	46
United States	1,638	3,413	108	1,137	1,534	35

clinical and public health interventions, serve as a basis for evaluating them, and ultimately undergird broad dissemination of evidence-based policies and practices. The cost study would have been infeasible without the indispensable input from two of my coauthors, Ted Miller and Bina Ali, who both work at the Pacific Institute for Research and Evaluation, a not-for-profit organization in Calverton, Maryland. They generated the cost estimates and wrote up the underlying methods. Their estimation utilized a cost-of-injury module that Miller and other colleagues had developed for the Centers for

Disease Control and Prevention's (CDC) Web-based Injury Statistics Query and Reporting System. I was most fortunate to be able to tap his expertise as a highly seasoned health economist who, along with his colleague Bruce Lawrence, represents the brainpower behind much of the scholarship and practice on injury mortality and morbidity cost estimation in the United States.

It was unanticipated that, given the annual trillion-dollar estimate for SIM costs nationally in terms of medical expenditures and losses in productivity and quality of life, the cost study attracted minimal interest in the mass media despite a press release from West Virginia University. Perhaps a deterrent to dissemination, given the gulf between the suicide and addiction research and prevention domains, was the omission of "suicide" in the article title.

Mounting bodies and diminishing autopsies

No researchers have directly studied the stresses of the opioid epidemic on suicide detection. However, with negative implications for identifying SIM cases among fatal drug overdoses, newspaper stories chronicle grave problems for medical examiners and coroners in distinguishing manners of death more generally. For example, a *Wall Street Journal* article published in May 2017 reported that some medical examiners in New England and the Rust Belt states of Pennsylvania and Ohio were neglecting the conduct of autopsies (and, I would also predict, toxicologic testing) because of these primarily fentanyl-fueled stresses and pressures (Calvert & Kamp, 2017). Referencing coverage deserts, especially in large rural areas, a February 2020 *New York* magazine article showed geographic magnification of this medicolegal crisis. The article also reported the following:

> No matter whether a state or a county runs on the medical-examiner system or the coroner system, in a vast majority of cases only a forensic pathologist can perform an autopsy of a body of a person who appears to have died of unnatural causes; coroners who aren't forensic pathologists outsource that labor. [In 2009] the National Research Council issued a warning that there were fewer than 500 forensic pathologists in the United States, a number that couldn't cover even half the annual deaths that require autopsy (for scale, there are more than 12,000 dermatologists). In the years since, the opioid epidemic has increased their caseload so drastically that the system is threatening to collapse. In the last 10 years,

> medical examiner's offices with a glut of cases have lost accreditation with the National Association of Medical Examiners, their national supervising association. The bodies in their districts are often shipped to other offices—which then become overloaded and risk losing accreditation in turn. . . . Over the past few years, news outlets reported that bodies in Cleveland, Ohio [for example] were being stacked two to a gurney and piled in refrigerator trailers to catch the morgue overflow. (Kisner, 2020)

Akin to similar resignations noted in the *New York* magazine article, *The Baltimore Sun* reported that Maryland's high-profile chief medical examiner, David Fowler, resigned in 2019 while citing his office's crushing workload amid inadequate funding and forensic resources (Baltimore Sun Editorial Board, 2019).

With this background, I was unsurprised that the COVID-19 pandemic grossly aggravated an already dire predicament, driven by the fentanyl-infused opioid epidemic, which afflicted numerous medicolegal death investigation systems across the United States (Moretti et al., 2021). Exponentiation of the woes of both coroners and medical examiners, associated with the eruption in early 2020 of this "once-in-a-century" pandemic after the Spanish Flu pandemic of 1918, was illuminated in *Kaiser Health News*:

> Funeral director Kevin Spitzer has been overwhelmed with COVID-19-related deaths in the small city of Aberdeen, South Dakota. He and his two colleagues at the Spitzer-Miller Funeral Home are working 12–15 hours a day, seven days a week, to keep up with the demand in the community of 26,000. . . . Private enterprise has created a solution for smaller communities. In Bozeman, Montana, a specialty truck company is retrofitting trailers that can be pulled by an SUV or a pickup . . . [the] Acela Truck Co. has already sold hundreds of the pull-behind refrigerated units created in response to the COVID-19 pandemic. They range from 9 to 53 feet and have racks that each hold four body trays. "We're very busy and have orders in all of the lower 48 states," said CEO David Ronsen. (Loose, 2020)

New York City was the epicenter during the onset of the pandemic, and stresses on systems were commensurate with its onslaught, as reported in a *New York Times* article:

> At the height of the outbreak in April, a New Yorker was dying almost every two minutes—more than 800 per day, or four times the city's normal death rate. And

> though the daily toll has recently slowed, hundreds of bodies are still emerging each day from private homes and hospitals.
>
> While hospitals bore the initial brunt of the crisis as sick people flooded emergency rooms, the sheer volume of human remains has pushed the system for caring for the dead to its limits, too: Hospital morgues, funeral homes, cemeteries, and crematories are all overflowing and backed up. . . . In normal times, the medical examiner's office would involve itself in a death only if it was sudden, violent, or unexpected. But during the pandemic, the office has become the official backstop for an overburdened system. (Feuer & Rashbaum, 2020)

A story out of Rhode Island in December 2022 noted that state's reliance on external forensic pathologists to meet the caseload of forensic autopsies given the shortage of permanent staff, including a chief medical examiner, against a background of the opioid epidemic and low salaries (White, 2022). Related costs more than tripled from fiscal year 2020/21 to 2021/22. This medicolegal reliance on external contractors is apparently common throughout the nation. The deputy director of the Rhode Island Department of Health stated that the main driver for external hires was the opioid epidemic and the need to prosecute drug dealers. Such situations reinforce the notion that criminal justice concerns trump those of public health in medicolegal death investigation offices. I speculate that case ascertainment of suicide deteriorates when contractors rather than permanent staff conduct autopsies of persons who died from drug intoxication, although these contractors will improve the ascertainment and specification of drug cases.

Sparking this speculation, I recall an admonition from the Medieval Italian diplomat, philosopher, and sage Niccolo Machiavelli (1532/1998). In his classic treatise *The Prince*, he cautioned the Florentine principality (city-state) against hiring mercenaries to fight its wars because he reasoned that they would not fight as tenaciously and persistently as loyal native soldiers. Mercenaries owe allegiance to others and are accessible by the highest bidder. Someone I view as a measured and insightful political scientist rather than an evil genius, Machiavelli might have derived his thinking on the malleability of mercenaries from the New Testament. In John 10 Jesus contrasted the good shepherd, who will lay down his life under threat to his flock of sheep from a wolf, with a hired hand who will flee. I hypothesize that external forensic pathologists are less fastidious than permanent internal ones in revealing suicides among drug overdose deaths.

"Mortal" psychiatric disorders obscure suicide

There is another mortality category in American vital statistics, besides undetermined (intent), accidental/unintentional drowning and poisoning, and ill-defined conditions and unknown causes, that appears highly prone to hiding suicides, together with fatal drug overdoses and hence SIM cases. Identified by Amy Bohnert and Srijan Sen, this category is mental and behavioral or psychiatric disorders, which are reported as underlying causes of death under natural causes, a disease, not injury, manner-of-death rubric. Many of the disorders in this category are anomalous because they do not implicate an injury or disease (pathobiological) mechanism essential to induce death. In an innovative study, Bohnert and Sen (2020) found that between 2010 and 2018 115,442 deaths of Americans were so classified versus 834,763 suicides and accidental/unintentional and undetermined intent drug overdoses. Annually, these "psychiatric" deaths, which predominantly implicated dependence on or "harmful use" of alcohol and to a much lesser extent that of opioids and other, multiple, or unspecified substances, ranged between 10,000 and 16,000 during the observation period. The authors excluded diagnoses for cognitive impairment or developmental childhood disorders. This decision aligns with our decision to exclude accidental and undetermined drug intoxication deaths among decedents under age 15 years in computing SIM.

Inspired and guided by the Bohnert/Sen study, Eric Caine, Cheuk Yui Yeung, and I explored changes in the crude rates of the selected mental and behavioral death rates between 2010 and 2022 in the United States (Caine et al., unpublished). Our study population was aged 15 years and older. We extracted the requisite underlying and multiple-cause-of-death data from CDC's Wide-ranging Online Data for Epidemiologic Research (WONDER) database. With deaths totaling nearly 200,000, the mental and behavioral rate virtually doubled from 4.2 to 8.2 per 100,000 population over the observation period. The rate for males was 2.6 times higher than that for females, and rates for the middle-aged and elderly populations were approximately six times higher than those for younger adults and youth. Differentiating urbanization status, rates peaked among residents of nonmetropolitan and small metro areas and were lowest in large metro centers. Other important findings were that psychoactive substance use disorders constituted 88.5% of the mental and behavioral deaths between 2020 and 2021 by underlying cause, and autopsy prevalence decreased from 33.4% to 25.7%—a 23.1% decline.

Many of the aforementioned "psychiatric" deaths would not have been evaluated by medical examiners or coroners. I predict that in-depth investigation of them from the perspective of sociodemographic characteristics, such as age, sex, race/ethnicity, educational attainment, and urbanization status or rurality, would uncover profound data disparities—a serious concern for the design and targeting of injury interventions and prevention programs. I suggest that, in due course, these deaths should be factored, along with deaths classified by nosologists under ill-defined conditions and unknown causes (Snowdon & Choi, 2020), into comparative assessments of suicide data quality. In some respects, they are reminiscent of deaths attributed to "lunacy" in Greater London in medieval times and later, which Samuel Sprott (1961) viewed as disguised or hidden suicides.

Did the suicide rate really decline in 2019 and 2020?

The knowledge I accumulated over most of this century, which informed the prior section, led me to question the validity of declines reported by CDC in the official national suicide rates (expressed as a rate adjusted for changes in age composition) in 2019 and 2020, especially that in 2020 (Ehlman et al., 2022). The two reported annual declines in the suicide rate followed a strong upward trend since 2000 (Rockett et al., 2021). The year 2020 marked the beginning of the COVID-19 pandemic, and by the end of that year one-third of the American population had contracted the disease and over 350,000 of them had died as a result (Pei et al., 2021). My untested expectation was that lockdowns, school closings, and increased social isolation and loneliness; massive business closures, employee layoffs, and economic deprivation; fear and excess domestic violence (Lu & Lin, 2021; Weinstock, 2021; Pekevski, 2022); quarantining and a dearth of personal protective equipment and quarantining; and ineffective therapy and the absence of effective vaccines would induce an increase in the true suicide rate. Moreover, I expected such pressures to further stress the medicolegal death investigation systems, in the process increasing, not depressing, the suicide rate. I conducted what I would term a preliminary examination of the question for those two years with reported suicide rate declines.

For this investigation, I compared the declines in the crude suicide rate (*International Classification of Diseases, Tenth Revision* [*ICD-10*] UO3, X60–84,

Y87.0), rather than a hypothetical age-adjusted rate, with changes in corresponding underlying cause-of-death rates for undetermined injury intent (*ICD-10* Y10–34, Y87.2), accidental/unintentional drug overdose (*ICD-10* X40–45), and psychiatric disorders (*ICD-10* F06.0–06.6, F10–19, F20–29, F30–39, F40–48, F51.0–51.9, F53–55, F59, F60–64, and F68), three categories prone to suicide misclassification. My data source was CDC WONDER. This investigation incorporated suicides and undetermined deaths at any age; both the drug and psychiatric deaths were confined to ages 15 years and older, reflecting the rarity of purposive self-harm fatalities among younger people.

Table 9.2 shows that the official suicide rate rose 2% between 2017 and 2018, declined by 2% between 2018 and 2019, and declined by 3% between 2019 and 2020, before increasing by 4% in 2021 in returning to its modal rate for the five-year observation period of 14.5 suicides per 100,000 population. Parenthetically, I note that the national suicide rate continued to rise between 2021 and 2022—by 2.1% to 14.8 per 100,000 population. The drug overdose death rate declined by 4% to 18.7 per 100,000 between 2017 and 2018, and then it rose monotonically (each year the rate was higher than in the previous year) to 30.4 in 2021—a 63% increase. Emulating this trend, the rate for the combined causes under scrutiny increased by 34%, from 40.1 deaths per 100,000 in 2018 to 53.9 in 2021. The psychiatric death rate rose monotonically from 4.8 per 100,000 in 2017 to 7.1 in 2021, a 48% increase. Varying between 1.7 and 1.9 per 100,000, the undetermined death rate remained very low throughout the observation period and contributed minimally to the magnitude of the combined rate.

While the decline in the suicide rate between 2019 and 2020 was small, at 3%, corresponding death rates for drug overdoses, psychiatric disorders, and combined causes increased by 33%, 27%, and 18%, respectively. The death rates for these three comparison categories also registered increases in 2019, but they were much smaller at 5%, 4%, and 2%. Adjusting the 2020 suicide rate, under an assumption that 6.3% of the combined excess overdose and psychiatric death rate (2020 vs. 2019) represented misclassified suicides, would negate the observed decline. Assuming 20% misclassification would yield an 8% suicide rate increase. However, indirect evidence from this investigation for suggesting that the official decline in the 2019 suicide rate was an artifact of scarce medicolegal resources is much weaker than in the case of the 2020 decline. The large decline in national life expectancy at birth between 2019 and 2020—from 78.8 to 77.0 years (Arias & Xu, 2022; Arias et

Table 9.2. Crude mortality rates and annual percentage change in suicide and other selected manner/causes, United States, 2017–21

	All suicide		Undetermined		"Accidental" drug intoxication		Psychiatric disorders		Combined causes		
Year	Rate	Change (%)	Rate	Change (%)	Rate	Change (%)	Rate	Change (%)	Rate	Change (%)	n^a
2017	14.5		1.8		19.5		4.8		40.6		132,164
2018	14.8	2.1	1.7	−5.6	18.7	−4.1	5.0	4.2	40.1	−1.2	131,325
2019	14.5	−2.0	1.7	0.0	19.6	4.8	5.2	4.0	41.0	2.2	134,576
2020	14.0	−3.4	1.8	5.9	26.1	33.1	6.6	26.9	48.5	18.3	159,758
2021	14.5	3.6	1.9	5.6	30.4	16.5	7.1	7.6	53.9	11.1	178,739

Source: Centers for Disease Control and Prevention, *Wide-ranging Online Data for Epidemiologic Research (WONDER)*, https://wonder.cdc.gov/ucd-icd10.html and https://wonder.cdc.gov/ucd-icd10-expanded.html.

Note: Rates are expressed per 100,000 population; Death rates for "accidental" drug intoxication and psychiatric disorders are confined to the population 15 years and older.

[a] n = absolute annual number of deaths.

al., 2022)—would also be consistent with a rise in the true suicide rate. On the other hand, life expectancy increased marginally between 2018 and 2019 from 78.7 to 78.8 years. CDC mainly attributed the annual decline in this measure in 2020 to drug overdoses and the onset of the COVID-19 pandemic (Arias et al., 2022). Not included in table 9.2, the SIM rate rose 2% between 2018 and 2019, by 17% during the onset of the pandemic (between 2019 and 2020), and by 11% between 2020 and 2021.

Likely fueling a spike in the SIM rate during the opening year of the pandemic were disruptions and uncertainties in the supply chains of illicit drugs. Multistate survey research revealed volatile patterns among large proportions of drug users that implicated this odious new disease threat and associated variables, such as homelessness, hunger, and transactional sex (Schneider et al., 2024). Recruited from drug treatment and harm reduction programs, sizable proportions of participants reported desiring more drugs (53%), taking higher doses (45%), and using different drugs (23%) than normal, as well as responding to different triggers (43%). Fourteen percent of study participants said they had overdosed in the month prior to the survey. The pandemic-related volatility in drug use would have increased deliberate and inadvertent participant exposure to drugs that manufacturers and dealers had contaminated with lethal fentanyl and analogs. A modest inferential leap is that this volatility would have aggravated feelings of fear, frustration, anxiety, and hopelessness among this very vulnerable population, further elevating their high risk for both suicide and a fatal overdose. Highly plausible is that people with untreated substance use disorder(s) bear a substantially higher risk than those in treatment.

A 33-country (interrupted) times series analysis, which included the United States, generated mixed findings regarding increases and declines in expected suicide numbers in the early onslaught of COVID-19—more specifically, in the first 9–15 months (Pirkis et al., 2022). The researchers reported that suicide declines were common. However, none of the other countries in their analysis have experienced an opioid epidemic on the scale of the one affecting the United States, and the study ignored the impact of the pandemic and variation in COVID-19 case fatality rates (number of deaths from COVID-19 divided by confirmed cases of COVID-19 as a percentage) and excess death rates on the medicolegal resources available to investigate suicide across their populations of interest. The latter omission is a critical research limitation. For example, in a needs assessment in Pennsylvania—a state with a hybrid medicolegal death investigation system—during the onset of COVID-19, a quantitative and qualitative survey of medical examiner and coroner offices found increased workloads and usage of personal protective equipment, such as filtering facepiece respirators, face shields, goggles, Tyvek suits, and nonabsorbent gowns, and decreased usage of surgical masks and gloves (Attwood et al., 2022). Workload included performance of autopsies, laboratory testing, field investigations, and transportation. Qualitative findings included rising staff shortages and burnout, insufficient storage for the increased number of decedents, constraints on budget and access to personal protective equipment, and inadequate emergency planning and response at the state level. Two countries that appear to have excellent suicide data, Hungary (Rockett et al., 2011) and Japan (Matsubayashi & Ueda, 2021), both reported suicide rate increases in 2020, the first year of the COVID-19 pandemic (Bálint et al., 2022; Watanabe & Tanaka, 2022).

The United States falls on the upper end of the continuum for high-income countries regarding both the case fatality rate for COVID-19, adjusted for variation in age composition, and pandemic-related excess deaths. Its percentage age-adjusted case fatality rate, as of April 6, 2021, was 0.97 (Hong et al., 2021). By comparison, for example, Austria, Belgium, Denmark, Finland, Sweden, Italy, Canada, Japan, the Netherlands, Spain, Switzerland, and New Zealand recorded appreciably lower rates. The American case fatality rate was exceeded by that of the United Kingdom but resembled Australia's. Cumulative data for the two calendar years of 2020 and 2021 showed that most American states had an excess death rate above 150 per 100,000 population, whereas most Western European countries, Japan, Canada, Australia, and New Zealand had lower rates (COVID-19 Excess Mortality Collaborators, 2022). The excess death rate is a more reliable measure than the case fatality rate, which is impacted by serious international variation in registration of both COVID-19 cases and deaths.

Preceding the pandemic, a 2019 needs assessment of American forensic laboratories and medical examiner and coroner offices from the National Institute of Justice, which was prepared for Congress, documented shortfalls in staff, training, and resourcing for the conduct of medicolegal death investigations and forensic testing (Office of Justice Programs and National Institute of Justice, 2019). As I shared previously from newspaper reports, strains were intensified by the opioid epidemic, especially its fentanyl-related component. The report from the needs assessment stated that while "medical examiners and coroners investigate deaths that are sudden, unexpected, unusual, suspicious, or violent, and deaths in which there is no attending physician," only a few involved criminality (Office of Justice Programs and National Institute of Justice, 2019, 74). Most related to disease and/or public health, and they included drug overdoses. Lying on the periphery of the criminal justice sphere, suicide, unlike overdoses, was not highlighted in the report.

Adding to the plausibility of a true rise in the American suicide rate during the onset of the COVID-19 pandemic is a 2024 report from CDC, which documented a 37.5% increase in the age-adjusted rate of deaths attributable to excessive alcohol use between 2018–19 and 2020–21—from 9.6 to 13.2 deaths per 100,000 population (Esser et al., 2024). This compared to a 6.7% increase between 2016–17 and 2018–19—from 9.0 to 9.6 per 100,000. Adjusting the death rates for age enables comparisons of rates across time in populations that have a different age composition, for example, very different proportions of young and elderly members. Reinforcing the plausibility of a true increase in the national suicide rate between 2019 and 2020, both age adjusted and crude, is the jump in the age-adjusted homicide rate following a prolonged period of relative stability (Akinyemi et al., 2024). Are we to believe that Americans responded to the pressures exerted by the advent of COVID-19 with an increased level of other-directed violence but a reduced level of self-directed violence? I don't.

Too simple?

Appealing to logic and reason, the data I share to question the national suicide rate declines in 2019 and 2020 are simple; there is no statistical analysis. In mollifying my concerns about possible criticism on that score, I take inspiration from Richard Feynman's demonstration of the loss of resilience, or fragility, of rubber O-rings in cold temperatures. In a simple but elegant experiment before the Rogers Commission, a Presidential Commission, he placed a sample in a glass of ice water to substantiate the case that the National Aeronautics and Space Administration should not have authorized the catastrophic launch of the space shuttle *Challenger* in 1986 in Florida, at a time when the anticipated ground temperature was 26 degrees Fahrenheit (Tufte, 1997).

Increased resilience under a common threat?

Digging into the plausible artifactual nature of the American suicide rate decline in 2020, in particular, I question a hypothetical argument that this decline occurred because people became more resilient with the onslaught of COVID-19, a common threat. Anecdotally, I first heard the resiliency argument in the context of an apparent decline in suicides in London during the Blitz in World War II. However, I could not imagine that suicide investigations received high priority among medicolegal authorities during this late phase of the Battle of Britain, which had mainly transitioned from a daylight to a night operation, with German aircraft and rockets inflicting relentless waves of vast death and destruction of habitat, which induced homelessness, school closings, evacuations, and family separations.

A qualitative account published in 2002 provided some pro and con circumstantial evidence that would be consonant or dissonant with a decline in London's suicide rate during the Blitz:

> Before the war psychiatrists had made dire predictions about the likely number of psychiatric casualties. These proved mistaken in the extreme. The London Emergency Region recorded an average of slightly more than two "bomb neuroses" cases during the first three months of the Blitz. . . . While chronic and incapacitating neurosis was rare, there was no way of knowing how many less serious cases went untreated since physical injury preoccupied rescue squads. . . . The strain of the raids manifested itself in a variety of less acute signs of emotional stress: anxiety attacks, extreme fatigue, eating disorders, apathy, feelings of helplessness, trembling, tics, and weeping spells. . . . A rising incidence of peptic ulcers, coronary symptoms, angina attacks, cerebral hemorrhages, miscarriages, and various menstrual disorders can also be linked to the tension under which people were living. . . . What was strikingly different in the early months of the raids . . . was that the [mass communal bomb] shelters were central to public debate about official apathy and social inequity; if anything they symbolized social division and fragmentation rather than national unity. (Field, 2002, 15, 23)

In 2021, a comparative review on the mental health outcomes of the London Blitz and COVID-19, conducted by Edgar Jones (2021), included contrary accounts of resilience / psychological robustness and excess mental trauma / "defeatism" in heavily bombed areas of London and other parts of the United Kingdom, including Scotland, Wales, and elsewhere in England. Understandably, a narrative of resilience, stoicism, and minor mental health problems possessed strong propaganda value for the British government and a besieged nation. The "myth of the Blitz," that the nation was withstanding mental trauma from the bombing, fostered the suppression of contradictory reports and follow-up research, the marginalization of mental health and minimization of psychiatry during those desperate times and beyond, and the need to create or fabricate a favorable climate for securing wartime military and economic support from the United States. Among the strongest adverse mental health effects of the onset of the COVID pandemic in the United Kingdom were on children, according to the review's author. Jones concluded his report by remarking, "Ironically, children who survived the Blitz are now among those at greatest risk of the severe physical and psychological effects of COVID-19" (2021, 714).

I did not have access to London's suicide data for the period of the Blitz, and thus I could not empirically evaluate the question of a suicide rate decline. However, logic and reason applied in consideration of the massive and relentless aerial campaign of terror by the Nazis, exceedingly scarce resources, and radically changing governmental and personal priorities lead me to hypothesize that the rate would not have declined and likely increased. Regardless, in no way do I wish to demean or diminish the extraordinary bravery and courage displayed by the citizenry of London and the United Kingdom during that harrowing period and the larger Battle of Britain. Moreover, mentally ill and/or highly desperate individuals who die by suicide are always very small minorities in the general population. Although ignoring suicide per se, historian Robert MacKay (2002) addressed the morale of the British people during World War II. His comparative account reinforced the likelihood that most of the besieged London population coped remarkably well in the Blitz, whether their true suicide rate rose, declined, or remained stable. Most importantly, Adolf Hitler's navy and army never bridged the 21 miles of the English Channel, and the United Kingdom did not surrender to Germany.

10

Into the Future

Academic transition

I have become a much more proactive researcher toward the end of my career as I strive to improve the characterization and measurement of suicide and other fatal self-injury. Facilitating my research on new populations and subpopulations, especially those in the United States, was the capacity to employ increasingly complex statistical procedures that utilized more publicly accessible and comprehensive databases. Crucial in grounding my more recent projects has been my ability online to contact and recruit outstanding collaborators, a few of whom I have still not met in person. They work in various professions and include social science and humanities scholars, medical examiners, psychiatrists, emergency physicians, health economists, and medical toxicologists. Integrating the insights from many disciplines is essential for understanding the underlying complexity of suicide as a clinical, forensic, and public health challenge for our society. My collaborations have been personally fruitful and gratifying, and I hope they have been mutually beneficial for my colleagues.

Seven years post-retirement from West Virginia University, my role as a lead investigator in research on suicide determination and data quality has likely ended. However, I look forward to continuing to assist other researchers as they pursue similar lines of inquiry and push boundaries in the name of suicide and other self-injury mortality (SIM) surveillance, scientific understanding, treatment, prevention, and public policy. Such work demands a healthy skepticism about data conceptualization, collection, and analysis and persistence in securing funding and achieving publication in higher-impact journals.

In chapter 5, I reported that the twain did meet between my previously separate lines of substance-related research in clinical settings and armchair statistical research on suicide data quality. My hospital emergency department–based studies on motor vehicular traffic trauma morbidity and mortality in the 1980s and on unmet substance abuse treatment need around the turn of the twenty-first century did inform my later research on suicide data quality—particularly that concerning the nexus between fatal drug overdoses and suicide misclassification. I inferred that suicide undercounting in the United States was becoming increasingly problematic, within the context of the opioid epidemic and high susceptibility of drug poisoning suicides to medicolegal misclassification. In turn, this realization eventually motivated me to write the position paper that resulted in two new concepts, death from drug self-intoxication (DDSI; Rockett et al., 2014b) and SIM (Rockett & Caine, 2015b). DDSI was the bridge to create SIM, which in its current incarnation is a composite of registered suicides and estimated non-suicide drug intoxication self-injury deaths. The latter include suicides attributable to drug intoxication that were missed by medical examiners and coroners or could be attributable and did not even enter their realm.

Self-injury mortality in the longer term

I envisage that augmentation of registered suicides in SIM will eventually encompass other deaths besides overdoses whose pertinence authorities could affirm on sound behavioral and other forensic evidence, most notably selected motor vehicular traffic trauma deaths. One most welcome contrarian reviewer of a rejected National Institutes of Health grant application I had submitted, which proposed a study of the Black/White suicide paradox, commented that the work would represent a paradigm shift. In drafting the article on DDSI, I feared that the concept might become submerged by potential tensions between the needs of epidemiology and those of medicolegal death investigations. Stated directly, concluding that suicide data are deficient could easily be construed as criticism of how medical examiners and coroners conduct investigations of equivocal intent cases and state and federal nosologists code and classify injury mortality data for ensuing reports. However, I eventually became sensitive to the impact of the stresses of severe underresourcing on the functioning of medicolegal death investigation systems and the government agencies charged with compiling, classifying, and reporting on the data under the constraints imposed by the mandated manner-of-death categories. These stresses coincide with low societal demands and expectations regarding accurate identification and recording of suicides.

One of my collaborators, Charles Naylor, the chief forensic pathologist for the Australian state of Queensland, eased my concerns about conflict between research needs and the needs of medical examiners and coroners. In a transpacific telephone conversation in 2014, he remarked that he understood what I was doing and that the epidemiologic and medicolegal paradigms have different functions. I then had an epiphany regarding the counterproductivity of viewing suicide epidemiology and medicolegal death investigations as competitors. DDSI is a working concept whose operationalization is not contingent on modifying the extant manner-of-death classification—a bridge too far in the foreseeable future—and, in concert with registered suicides, is a serviceable foundation on which to build an enhanced and more representative conceptualization of fatal self-injury as SIM.

The foregoing brings me to a discussion of a metaphorical iceberg, which I included in the position paper that had prompted the conceptualization of DDSI and SIM (fig. 10.1). Benefiting from the welcome assistance of Eric Caine, the published version provided scope for refinement and expansion (Rockett et al., 2016). We distinguished manifest and latent SIM, with the former representing what is visible above the surface, namely, registered suicides. The majority of SIM, the latent component, lies below the surface and theoretically includes all missed true suicides, irrespective of method, and all other deaths that would qualify as fatal self-injury according to proximal premortem behavior and other forensic evidence.

Conceptually, latent SIM represents not only misclassified suicides but also motor vehicular traffic trauma and other deaths that reflected self-injurious behavior, even where the decedents had not intended to die, or where their intent was uncertain (equivocal cases). Among the missed suicides are those misclassified under (*a*) natural causes and (*b*) ill-defined conditions and unknown causes. The literature indicates that the latter category is a leading candidate for obscuring suicides (Reseland et al., 2008; Ylijoki-Sørensen et al., 2014; Snowdon, 2023), a susceptibility that may be pronounced when there is long duration between time of death and discovery of the body, with consequential degradation of forensic evidence. This category is the vaguest of the garbage classification codes in the *International*

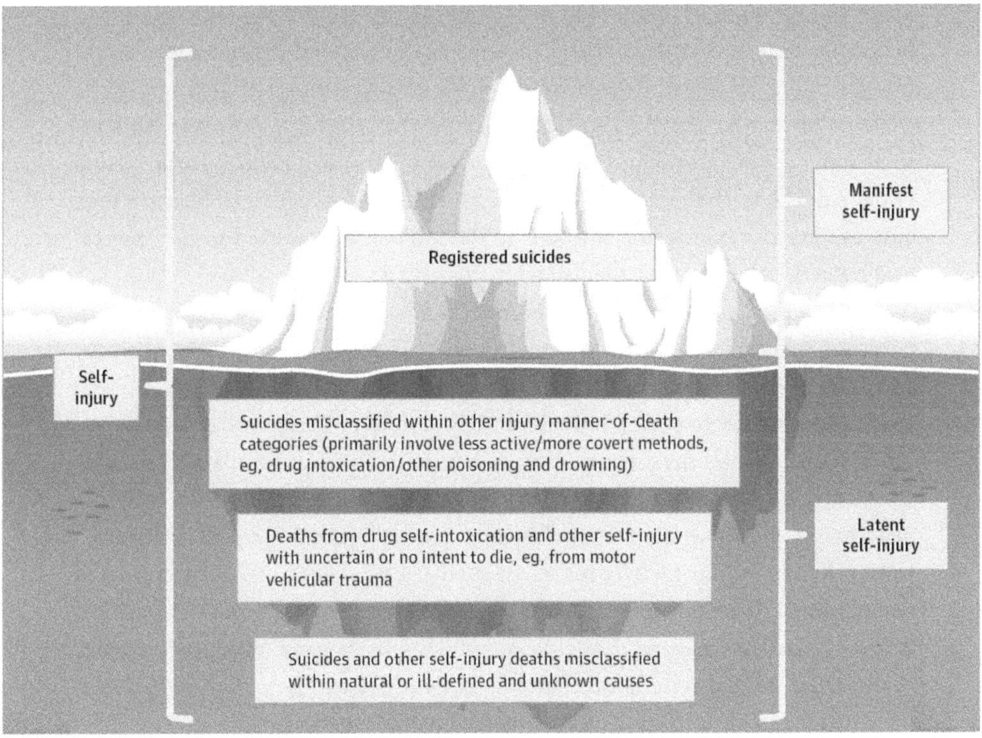

Figure 10.1. Iceberg of suicide and latent self-injury mortality (not to scale). Source: Rockett, I.R.H., Lilly, C.L., Jia, H., et al., "Self-injury mortality in the United States in the early 21st century: A comparison with proximally ranked diseases," ***JAMA Psychiatry*** **2016;73(10):1072–81.**

Classification of Diseases, Tenth Revision, mortality codes that provide little or no information on the true manner and underlying cause of death in given cases.

The natural cause or disease manner-of-death category is plausibly an immense reservoir for submerging true suicides. For example, there will be decedents, so classified, who died by suicide and whose official underlying cause of death will match their terminal diagnosis. One concern in this regard is suicides motivated by inadequate pain management for disease, especially cancer. Intensifying this problem would be the absence of an autopsy, or advanced imaging evaluation and toxicologic testing, as well as impeded access to health care. I suspect that the elderly, vulnerable minorities, and other poor people (irrespective of age) are most prone to suicide misclassification under accidents, natural causes, and ill-defined conditions and unknown causes of death. Mention of suicide misclassification also raises the issue of physician-assisted suicide or dying with dignity. However, this remains an area of ethical and moral complexity lying outside the scope of this book. Adding to the potential for the natural cause category to obscure true suicides are the increasing number of deaths being classified under mental and behavioral disorders, discussed in chapter 8.

Even when not satisfying the criteria to substantiate suicide, certain patterns of reckless drinking would qualify as SIM, beyond those directly involved in driver fatalities; think of college students who died after using a hose and funnel to pour grain alcohol directly into their stomachs. On the other hand, not all fatal drug-related "accidents" would be eligible, such as the deaths of young children from ingestion of medications that they believed were candy and patient deaths caused by lethal drug-drug interactions when compliant with prescribed medication schedules. Contemporary packaging of illicit fentanyl and analogs as multicolored tablets will predictably increase the chances that children will die from consuming these drugs under their misapprehension that they are indeed candy.

Self-injury checkbox for the death certificate

I conceived SIM to circumvent downward measurement biases in suicide and to transcend registered suicides in more expansively representing fatal self-injury, for purposes of improving injury surveillance, primary and secondary prevention, and treatment. To date, using SIM as a working category for research has been contingent on estimation through an indirect procedure. However, a direct approach is within reach and aligns with interest in the medical examiner community to bolster its relevance and ties to the public health community. With this aim in mind, I published an article with multidisciplinary colleagues in 2020 that argued for the advantages of including a checkbox for self-injury on the death certificate, distinct from the manner-of-death designation (Rockett et al., 2020a). Earlier, I had mentioned my idea of a checkbox in a telephone conversation with Robert Anderson, chief of the mortality statistics branch at the National Center for Health Statistics. He wisely counseled me that the process would need to be completed in stages, which implies the necessity of pilot testing the checkbox. Modifying a legal document of the importance of the death certificate would require acceptance and approval at many levels of government and support from various professional organizations and communities.

The 2020 position paper from the American College of Medical Toxicology and the National Association of Medical Examiners on the investigation, diagnosis, and certification of opioid and other drug intoxication deaths presented examples of medical examiner and coroner cases suggesting drug misuse (Davis et al., 2020). In turn, these examples illustrate the types of evidence that might behaviorally help induce a positive entry in a self-injury checkbox, that is, qualify as SIM whether the official manner of death is suicide, accident, or undetermined (intent):

1. Opioid medications.
2. Evidence of intravenous drug use (needles, cooker spoons, tourniquet, crushed tablets, packets of powder or crystals, other drug paraphernalia).
3. Evidence of insufflation (chopped pills or residue, chopped lines, cuts on coffee table glass, cut straws or pen tubes, rolled bills, etc.).
4. Overlapping prescriptions for the same type of prescribed controlled substances from multiple pharmacies or multiple prescribers.
5. Prescriptions in other people's names.
6. Pills not stored in prescription vials or mixed in vials.
7. Injection sites not due to resuscitation attempts.
8. Altered transdermal patches.
9. Many transdermal patches on the body or transdermal patches in unusual locations, e.g., mouth, stomach, vagina, or rectum.
10. Application of heat to increase the rate of transfer of drug from transdermal patch to decedent.
11. Presence of naloxone [as an indicator of a potential need for rescue from self-harm]. (Davis et al., 2020, 154)

These categories would be very helpful for defining and populating the nonsuicide drug self-intoxication component of SIM, and all the more so when there are two or more positives. However, in themselves they do not help medical examiners and coroners assign suicide as the manner of death. Most fatal overdoses are unwitnessed, and one can speculate that witnesses are typically drug dependent and thus unreliable. To facilitate navigation in this forest of uncertainty, the chief medical examiner of the District of Columbia, Daniel Morgan, enumerated a set of questions for follow-up with key informants after a death scene investigation, such as family members and medical personnel who had administered treatment, not only to determine whether the decedent had a history of drug misuse (abuse) or dependence but also to tap the issue of intentionality:

1. [Had] the decedent ever used illegal drugs or abused prescriptions?
   If yes, what kind? How often? When was the last use? How long has he or she been using?
   How [did] they use (route of administration, e.g., oral, inhalational, intravenous, subcutaneous, rectal)?
   [Had] he or she ever been hospitalized for an overdose? When? Where?
   [Had] he or she ever been in drug rehabilitation?
2. What precipitated initial use (it may be related to an injury)?
3. How long [had] the decedent been sober?
   Any recent life events that may have triggered relapse?
   [Had] the decedent been recently incarcerated or otherwise unable to use drugs?
4. Any indication this was an intentional overdose?
5. Who [was] the primary care physician? [Were] there any other treating physicians? (Morgan, 2017, 57)

Direct measurement of SIM would, of course, pave the way for an evaluation of the validity of my assumption in its indirect estimation that 80% of the accidental drug intoxication deaths and 90% of undetermined counterparts in the age group 15 years and older are self-injury. I hypothesize that these percentages, albeit arbitrary, are conservative. Expansion of SIM beyond a category confined to registered suicides and fatal drug overdoses would be contingent on improvements in medical, forensic, and law enforcement records and their digital linkage across data systems.

In the shorter term, a formidable barrier to the acceptance of my public health perspective on SIM among the general psychiatric and medicolegal communities in the United States is the long dominant and stigmatizing criminal justice perspective, which has prioritized punishment for drug misuse over treatment and prevention (DuFour, 2016). While there is an ongoing need for interdiction of such lethal drugs in the black market as fentanyl and other synthetic opioids, as well as the arrest and prosecution of "merchants of death," there are signs that the war on drugs is moderating with the full legalization or medical legislation of cannabis or marijuana use in many states. This change must be rapidly translated for police on the beat to avoid unnecessary confrontations and mistreatment of civilians. It will be important to combine top-down approaches with bottom-up ones in addressing the decriminalization of drug misuse (Del Pozo et al., 2021). This combination is crucial for preventing suicide and other fatal self-injury across racial/ethnic groups. Acceptance of SIM in the medicolegal and psychiatric communities would be greatly facilitated by efforts of prominent members to advance the application of their data to public health purposes.

Eventually, I hope SIM will be formally adopted by the Centers for Disease Control and Prevention (CDC) and included in mortality reports from the National Center for Health Statistics. Obviously, the inclusion of a self-injury checkbox on the death certificate would position SIM as an actionable concept. In their book *Death in Custody: How America Ignores the Truth and What We Can Do About It*, Roger Mitchell and Jay Aronson (2023) discuss several historical precedents for checkboxes, which, in adding specificity to the circumstances of given deaths, yield important public and population health benefits. The checkboxes pertain to transportation, tobacco use, and pregnancy. Mitchell and Aronson propose a new one for custodial deaths. These deaths are notoriously incomplete in their description and coverage. Misclassified deaths in prisons and jails, for example, include homicides disguised as suicides and suicides disguised as accidents. Missed deaths include decedents whom prison and jail officials had inappropriately sent to hospitals or other facilities in order to massage their data and avoid or minimize responsibility. I suspect there is considerable heterogeneity in custodial suicides, possible suicides, and other deaths across type and states, counties, and other political jurisdictions, a question requiring in depth, population-based investigations. Another outstanding research question is whether mortality misclassification varies among federal, state, and local facilities and between privately owned and publicly administered facilities.

Irrationality and suicide classification

With one exception, all key ideas I outlined in my position paper remained intact in the publication of the DDSI article (Rockett et al., 2014b). The exception? Eliciting no reaction from any of my coauthors, I had broached the notion that there is a contradiction in applying the definition of suicide, coupling decedent intention to die (or self-harm) and self-administration of the means, to deaths where people were in an irrational state of mind, whether precipitated by a substance use disorder, another mental disorder, or other factors. This contradiction reverberates through the experience of Canadian Reuters reporter Anna Mehler Paperny (2019), as a suicide survivor. A major contributor to the conundrum is that many, if not most, people classified as dying by suicide in the United States had a diagnosable psychiatric disorder. Suicide appears to defy or refute the popular notion that there is a biological imperative to survive for the continuance and maintenance of the human species—a dubious notion, however, since the longevity of females frequently far exceeds the end of their fertility.

In 2019, I enlisted Eric Caine to write an article with me critiquing the definition of suicide (Rockett & Caine, 2020). We stated that the "intention to die" criterion in the suicide definition was a cognitive phenomenon, whereas "self-administration of the means" was behavioral. To illustrate potential challenges for medical examiners and coroners—perhaps more so for elected coroners—in reconciling these cognitive and behavioral elements, we reconstructed from media reports the case of the agonizing death in 2011 of a mentally ill "(James) Bond Girl," 65-year-old English actress Angela Scoular:

> Ms. Scoular had a well-established, long-term history of active alcohol misuse, and treatment for depression and bipolar disorder. She was diagnosed with colon cancer in 2008, and while said to be cancer-free, apparently feared her cancer would return. Media reported Ms. Scoular had been arrested for "drink-driving" and crashing her vehicle just weeks prior to death, although she was freed on bail. Her physical cause of death was reported in a coroner's court as a combination of ingestion of a corrosive substance and multiple fractures from a fall down steps—the former being a drain cleaning agent containing 91% sulphuric acid. She died within two hours of drinking the liquid cleaner and pouring it over her body, with 40% burns to her throat, torso, and gastro-intestinal tract. (Rockett & Caine, 2020, 73)

Ms. Scoular had previously attempted suicide by cutting her wrists in 1992 and had a distal history of anorexia nervosa, another comorbid condition and an eating and mental health disorder associated with suicide. The English coroner ruled her death as "misadventure," that is, as an accident, because her injuries occurred "while the balance of her mind was disturbed." Thus, the coroner determined that whereas Ms. Scoular's death was self-inflicted (i.e., due to self-directed violence), it was not suicide because she lacked sufficient capacity to form intent—in contrast with the coronial decision-making in the determination of suicide in Hugo Throssell's death in Western Australia in 1933. While behaviorally Scoular's death was suicide, I am sympathetic to the coroner's position. Her overwrought husband and widower, Leslie Phillips, was a well-known character actor in English movies, and I found his performances funny. Both the determination of Scoular's manner of death and that of Throssell occurred under a shared coronial system of medicolegal death investigation. Western Australia was founded as a European political and colonial entity in 1829 under an English governor (Captain James Stirling) appointed by King George IV.

James Knoll (2008, 394–95), an American forensic psychiatrist, drew a legal distinction between sane and insane suicide in the context of insurance indemnification in differentiating a decedent who could have reasoned that his or her actions would result in death from one too impaired to comprehend the fatal consequences of these personal actions. The circumstances of Ms. Scoular's death conform to the latter situation. However, whether the English coroner had ruled the manner as accident or suicide, her death constitutes a blatant SIM case. A crucial difference, evidentiarily, between the deaths of Scoular and Throssell was that Scoular did not provide a rationale for her self-inflicted injuries in a note.

Although likely not reflecting perfect one-to-one relationships, the concepts of impulsive—what Robert Litman (1968) had termed second-degree suicide in the late 1960s—and planned suicides crudely parallel insane and sane suicides, respectively. However, there are no data systems in place in the United States that could adequately enable researchers and preventionists to distinguish planned (sane) from impulsive (insane) suicides, even including CDC's enriched, restricted access National Violent Death Reporting System (NVDRS) database, which has too much missing information. The data they need to justify a SIM designation in a suicide and an "accidental" or undetermined drug poisoning death would be attainable through the implementation of a self-injury checkbox on the death certificate. SIM could then accommodate, for example, the behavior and mortality of not only "death seekers" and "active intent" opioid and other drug overdosers but also the more ambiguous "death darers" and "passive intent" overdosers—those comprehending the hazards of their drug use and overuse but ambivalent about dying by suicide (Pergolizzi et al., 2021). People dying while engaged in Russian roulette belong in the ambiguous category.

When viewed against the backdrop of the twenty-first-century opioid epidemic, my research on suicide case ascertainment and data quality led me to infer that the suicide definition itself becomes especially problematic where a decedent's intention to die was unclear or equivocal. The distinction between the cognitive character of "intention to die" or self-harm and the behavioral character of the second pillar of the conventional suicide definition, "self-administration of the means," weighs more heavily on suicides by less forensically overt methods, such as drug intoxication and drowning, than on suicides by shooting and hanging with clear intent. Data from our two individual- and county-level, multivariable NVDRS studies indicated, generally, that medical examiners and coroners are well positioned to assign shooting and hanging deaths as suicides, based on decedent behavior and supporting physical evidence, without needing to depend on corroborative psychiatric/psychological evidence (Rockett et al., 2018a, 2018b). Australian (Elnour & Harrison, 2008) and American researchers (Conner et al., 2019) used suicide attempt data from hospital records and (completed) suicide data from the vital statistics to calculate case fatality rates for suicide methods. Both studies showed that the most lethal method was firearm (gunshot wound). Hanging emerged as the second most lethal method in the Australian study, whereas it was drowning in the American study. Drug poisoning was among the least lethal methods in both. A systematic review with meta-analysis of case fatality rates, which differentiates the sexes, largely affirms these findings (Cai et al., 2022). Also a highly lethal method, jumping from a height, together with drowning, is a method associated with equivocal decedent intent.

To reiterate, data deficits are far greater impediments for medical examiners and coroners when trying to discern true drug suicides than when trying to discern true suicides by the more forensically overt and lethal methods like hanging and shooting, as reflected in the absence of an authenticated suicide note, online or social media evidence (discussed near the end of this chapter), and/or documentation of decedent psychiatric history (Rockett et al., 2018a). They cement the need for an enhanced SIM category. However, a caveat is warranted even concerning the medicolegal determination of a potential suicide by that most forensically overt method, gunshot wound. There remains a need for a careful and comprehensive death scene investigation and follow-up with key informants, such as family members, coworkers, and physicians. Critical in assessing suicidality in a firearm case is medicolegal understanding of the lethal behavior in the context of weapon characteristics. Illustrative is a person who removed the magazine from an autoloading handgun and comprehended neither the difference between the magazine and the chamber nor the concept of the presence or absence of a magazine safety. A not uncommon situation involves individuals with this profile who waved a gun around and told their protesting friends that "it isn't loaded" before discharging it and killing either themselves or other people.

Mixed research methods

The guiding principle for my research agenda has been that high-quality suicide and other mortality data are essential for specifying risk groups, identifying risk factors, planning prevention programs, and conducting their evaluation. At a higher level of abstraction, I view accuracy as an imperative for measuring and monitoring morbidity and disability, as well as mortality, and for informing and formulating health policy. Moreover, I endorse the thrust of the following quotation from the eminent nineteenth-century British physicist and engineer Lord Kelvin: "I often say that when you can measure what you are speaking about, and express it in numbers, you know something about it; but when you cannot express it in numbers, your knowledge is of a meager and unsatisfactory kind: it may be the beginning of knowledge, but you have scarcely, in your thoughts, advanced to the stage of Science, whatever the matter may be" (1889, 73).

Although I am a quantitative researcher by training and practice, I respect the value of the purpose and procedures of qualitative research, including its capacity to pursue novel questions and generate hypotheses that are testable through rigorous quantitative research. Qualitative methods include face-to-face or virtual semistructured interviewing of key informants; focus group interviews, as well as monitoring of related interactions involving stakeholders and/or other knowledgeable or concerned parties on a common research question or issue, which are guided by an interviewer, facilitator, or moderator; content analysis of documents, often consisting of secondary data; attributional coding, which is typically based on transcripts of dialogues and extant documents and can involve translation; visual methods, such as utilization of photography and drawing; and ethnography, as an observational process aimed at describing and interpreting cultural behavior (Stier Adler & Clark, 2015; Creswell & Plano Clark, 2018). Integrating qualitative and quantitative approaches in research can be considered mixed methods (Stone et al., 2016; Ross and Kõlves, 2021) and offers great promise for capturing the big picture in addressing, understanding, and resolving data deficits, discrepancies, and disparities that plague the measurement of suicide and for refining SIM as an alternative and more comprehensive measure of fatal self-injury.

Some proposed mixed methods self-injury mortality studies

Adopting a qualitative, inductive, and exploratory perspective, a group of English social scientists wrote a book on the sociological autopsy, a contextual analog of the psychological autopsy aimed at enlightening the understanding of suicide as distinct from understanding the determination of suicide by coroners and medical examiners (Fincham et al., 2019). The core of their book was a sociological autopsy conducted on a small sample of 100 suicide cases from English coroner files. Personally, I wished that the authors had included a sample of "open" verdict cases (equivalent to undetermined intent manner-of-death cases in the United States) as a comparison group, especially since they discussed underreporting of suicides at some length. However, they concluded that underreporting was not problematic for sociological research. I object, at least in the American context, given our research findings in the twenty-first century. Moreover, research from the University of Bristol (Gunnell et al., 2013) generates cause for concern about the reliability and validity of English suicide data. This time-trend study showed a marked decline in the proportion of possible suicides among pharmaceutical drug and other poisoning cases between 1990 and 2005. In the mid-2020s, misclassification of suicides by drug intoxication may become even more problematic for coroners in England, as elements are in place for the country to experience its own opioid epidemic (Roberts & Richards, 2023).

Melanie-Angela Neuilly (2022) used mixed methods to highlight the need to examine systemic and cognitive biases in the determination of death in an article published in the *Journal of Forensic Sciences*. She had embedded herself in medicolegal offices in the United States and France, two in each country, and "propose[d] that truly understanding the sources of implicit cognitive bias in forensic pathologists and other medicolegal actors requires knowledge of legal, cultural and organizational structures that shape medicolegal systems and in turn constrain individual actors' decision-making processes" (Neuilly, 2022, 233).

While Neuilly made little mention of suicide assessment and detection per se, she commented that pertinent research, including some of my own, had identified the existence of measurement biases but largely ignored details on their sources. Indeed, I view scientific investigations of systemic and cognitive bias on the part of the diagnosticians and adjudicators of suicide determination and other contributors—particularly those of medical examiners and coroners—as important next-generation research and an extension of the ethnographic research of Maxwell Atkinson (1978) in England in the 1970s and that of Stephan Timmermans (2005) in Boston at the turn of the century. A critical issue I see in cognitive bias is the need to distinguish bias immersed in personal prejudice, such as that concerning class, sex, and race/ethnicity, from bias that is a product of differential deficits in accessible corroborative evidence, such as the availability of an authenticated suicide note, diagnosis of mental illness, knowledge of imminent distress like job loss or dissolution of marriage (official or a de facto union), and a record of any previous suicide attempts.

Small-scale studies involving focus groups of key parties could help frame questions and approaches for drilling down in both the medicolegal investigation and death certification processes. Content analysis of medicolegal records, as featured in a machine learning study of suicide classification (Rahman et al., 2021), would yield additional insights. Outstanding issues, including fiscal and social constraints on the conduct of comprehensive suicide investigations and the likely presence of racial/ethnic and sex biases in suicide case ascertainment, are predictably delicate and controversial for relevant parties. Regardless, although such research would be difficult, this need not be an insurmountable deterrent to its implementation. Other important research questions, which could be enlightened through mixed methods research, include the concealment and destruction of suicide notes, the place of gender in suicide misclassification, and the influence of familial and political pressures on medicolegal officials charged by society with investigating and determining suicide and other manners of death. Directors of funeral homes are an ignored, but potentially consequential, group for research on suicide accounting. In smaller towns, where everybody knows everybody, they likely sign knowingly, as well as unknowingly, the death certificates of many missed suicides in the natural causes bucket that were never medical examiner or coroner cases. Funeral directors in all settings would appear to be highly vulnerable to familial and political pressures, implicit and explicit, in overlooking potential suicides.

Concealment and destruction of suicide notes

In concert, our two multivariable state- and county-level studies, which utilized the restricted access data from the NVDRS, indicate the pivotal role an evidentiary suicide note plays in the medicolegal determination of suicide by drug intoxication (Rockett et al., 2018a, 2018b). Historically, Maurice Halbwachs (1978) and Gregory Zilboorg (1936) mentioned the problem of concealment of notes by survivors. Zilboorg saw this as more problematic than Halbwachs for reporting. Neither presented data. In contrast, Robert Litman and colleagues, in their 1963 psychological autopsy study of 500 equivocal suicides in Los Angeles, provided empirical evidence that it was an obstacle at a time of rampant barbiturate overdoses (Litman et al., 1963). My recent computer-based searches using Google and PubMed uncovered no contemporary scientific literature on the concealment and destruction of suicide notes.

Stephan Timmermans (2005) reported concealment of a suicide note in a drowning case study in his turn-of-the-century Boston research on suicides and other suspicious deaths. I offer weak personal but intriguing anecdotal support that concealment and destruction of suicide notes still occur. Recently, two people, without being solicited, told me in separate casual conversations that they had done so. In the first instance, a note was destroyed by a sister-in-law to hide the true manner of death of an identical twin brother of her spouse, an overdose on prescription drugs, in her conviction that it would prevent her spouse from following suit. The official manner of death was accident. The familial shroud is a potent impediment to suicide detection, and I suspect I would have acted similarly to protect a cherished one. Motive for destruction in the second instance was to shield survivors from personally damaging comments ("stinking thinking" or "stinkin thinkin") in the decedent's note. Obfuscating comprehension of the suicide, destruction of the suicide note may have mitigated guilt, shame, and helplessness among the bereaved. Receipt of life insurance payouts may also have been a motivating factor.

Gender, suicide misclassification, and self-injury mortality

Constrained by the limitations of accessible mortality databases, the inclusion of a person's sex in my research stems from the female/male distinction assigned at birth. This distinction is based on a visual anatomic examination as a proxy for biological sex. Gender is a more nuanced and complex variable than sex and blends one's social and cultural roles with one's personal identification and identity (Butler, 2024). It has also been characterized as "a [diverse] social configuration that gathers the roles, behaviors, activities, attitudes, and attributes that a given society typically associates with being masculine or feminine" (Rioux et al., 2022, 765).

Gender allows for sexual overlap, reified by transgender individuals. LGBTQIA+ is an acronym that abbreviates lesbian, gay, bisexual, transgender, queer or questioning, intersex, asexual, and other alternative groups. Targets of hateful rhetoric and actions, these groups qualify as vulnerable minorities and are associated with excess rates of suicide relative to the general population. John Blosnich, a University of Southern California epidemiologist, has written extensively on gender minorities and suicidality, focusing on the military veteran population (Blosnich et al., 2012, 2021), with its added implications for layered risk (Inoue et al., 2023). Testable within the remedial context of SIM, I hypothesize that these groups will be susceptible to excess suicide undercounting and differential misclassification by medicolegal officials, as accounting provides for both gender and sex differentiation. Referencing Blosnich, a *New York Times* article published in June 2023 signals important research being conducted in California and Utah that will advance understanding of the links between gender identity, mental health, and suicidality (Ghorayshi, 2023). The Utah study is incorporating psychological autopsies.

Race/ethnicity and social class are two other sociodemographic variables requiring more clarity and granularity with respect to the study of suicide misclassification. Racial/ethnic groups that readily spring to mind are Native Americans, Asian Americans, and Pacific Islanders, and of course no racial/ethnic groups are monolithic. Unlike in the United Kingdom, in the United States social class is not readily identifiable in official statistics. For example, Hispanics and African Americans serve as an increasingly inappropriate and inadequate surrogate for the poor. Statistical interactive terms, comprising variables combining race/ethnicity and social class or socioeconomic status, would enlighten the study of suicide misclassification and SIM.

As a word of caution, whereas ad hoc data from mixed methods and other small studies have the potential to generate more precise and accurate information than data from the large administrative databases on which I have relied for my research, they are disadvantaged in terms of capital support and underlying resources. As a necessary trade-off, ensuing results are likely to be much weaker than those from large population-based studies regarding their generalizability or external validity.

Mobile technology and death scene investigations

I see technology, buttressed by artificial intelligence and machine learning with its strong predictive capacity, as dominating future suicide detection and bolstering SIM's value as a more representative and practical alternative to suicide as a fundamental measure of mortality. I now briefly discuss the role of mobile (electronic) technology as a source of real-time data for death scene investigations and as an aid to populating a self-injury checkbox on the death certificate. As previously mentioned, I attended an in-person meeting at CDC in 2017 to discuss this technology as an aid to death scene investigators for improving the identification of suicide, particularly targeting drug intoxication cases. This meeting was part of a larger initiative (Stone et al., 2017), which also involved virtual meetings with suicidologists and death scene investigators, to facilitate the standardization, collection, accuracy, and timeliness of suicide data.

Arising from the proceedings and follow-up in a summary article (Mercado et al., 2021) was the need for a death scene investigation app using an electronic mobile device, such as a smartphone, iPad, or laptop computer. An ideal tool for conducting what is termed a social-mobile autopsy, the attributes of such a device would include being lightweight, handheld, durable, and waterproof and having long battery life, high screen resolution, a built-in camera with ≥12 megapixels, a fingerprint scanner for decedent identification, and laser capacity for distance measurement. Other important attributes would be basic smartphone features, such as an address book, note-taking and voice-recording abilities, the capacity to assign unique identifiers, and its compatibility with Windows, web-based internet browsers, and Mac software. Accessible training and adequate staff must be part of the package.

An Italian case study of a forensically overt suicide by a female, a hanging, provides a detailed application of a social-mobile autopsy to detail the circumstances of the death (Aqulia et al., 2018). In closing, the authors proposed a model for this kind of autopsy that provides the following:

1. News about the phone as it allows us to identify the type of telephone and mobile user; request the phone records with the help of a consulting

engineer; assess the geographic location where the call has been registered; search for messages, photos or videos.

2. News about [a] personal computer and other computer devices as it permits us to identify the user's email addresses, profiles and passwords through the help of a computer engineer; analyze Internet history; evaluate enrollment in dating sites; search for any documents needed for the investigation.
3. News about [a] Facebook [Meta] profile as it [gives consent to] us to investigate posts, photos, videos published in recent months; assess friends, likes, personal messages on chat, the activity log and history.
4. News about other social networks, e.g., X, Instagram, Periscope, Badoo . . . , registered with the user's account. (Aqulia et al., 2018, 82)

Centered on the Onondaga County Medical Examiner's Office in Syracuse, New York, a small qualitative study provided case examples to illustrate value in examining social network media platforms, such as Meta, LinkedIn, TikTok, X, WhatsApp, and Instagram, to inform medicolegal death investigations (Hookano et al., 2013). Benefits of this kind of examination extend from identifying a victim, establishing time of death, contacting next of kin, illuminating the circumstances and manner of death, corroborating a witness account, and discovering a suicide note. Potential pitfalls or deficits include shared use, irregular postings, masking of personal identities, deceit, postmortem removal of sensitive material, and obsolescence and evolution of social network services.

The worldwide transition to electronic communications has important implications in the search for a suicide note in medicolegal death investigations. As our two individual- and county-level, multivariable NVDRS studies strongly indicate, a suicide note is often a pivotal aid to medical examiners and coroners in ascertaining suicide as the manner of death, especially in drug cases, and a vital source of information for advancing scientific understanding and prevention. Examples of electronic counterparts to tangible notes left by decedents, which may be termed E-suicide notes, include video recordings, email messages, text messages, and postings on such online forums as X and Meta, as well as messages in files on personal computers. An Indian study used a variety of search engines, including Google, PubMed, and Scopus, to enable the authors to elaborate on the utility of the E-suicide note and to discuss some related medicolegal and judicial issues (Behera et al., 2014).

Conclusion

The big picture

The twenty-first-century United States is experiencing two injury mortality epidemics: suicide and drug overdose. While both epidemics propagate pervasive social stigma and profound personal loss, the overdose epidemic dominated the public consciousness until being temporarily overshadowed by the COVID-19 pandemic. I speculate that this is because of the role first of Big Pharma and then of foreign drug cartels and clandestine manufacturers in flooding society with highly addictive and lethal opioid painkillers. Heroin, followed by illicit fentanyl and analogs, supplanted prescription oxycodone and hydrocodone as the favored opioids when users and misusers migrated from pharmaceuticals to cheaper and more accessible alternatives, as physicians curbed their prescribing and pill mills closed under government regulations and enforcement. Although largely viewed as independent phenomena by grant-funding agencies, the suicide and overdose epidemics actually overlap. Collectively, they represent a mental health crisis that has enveloped the entire nation—not just Western regions—when suicide is the sole mortal depiction of self-injury and imminent personal and societal distress. Suicides and fatal overdoses are misconceptualized and mismeasured in medicolegal, research, treatment, and prevention settings, to the detriment of population health.

Historical antecedents

This book is a cautionary tale. It highlights the threats to population health inherent in clinicians, epidemiologists, sociologists, policymakers, administrators, planners, and preventionists uncritically accepting public health data at face value. I acknowledge some of the premier contributors to the story in the twentieth century, prior to addressing suicide undercounting in the modern era and proposing a solution to this seemingly intractable problem. The historical luminaries who deservedly occupied pride of place in my background chapters were the three principals of the Los Angeles Suicide Prevention Center—Edwin Shneidman, Robert Litman, and Norman Farberow—and their primary medicolegal collaborator, Theodore (Ted) Curphey, the chief coroner of Los Angeles County. Innovators of the first order, this multidisciplinary team conducted psychological autopsies to resolve suicide and other manners of death in equivocal barbiturate overdose cases during the third quarter of the twentieth century. Had society embraced their insights and vision, I believe we would not be in the severe accounting predicament we find ourselves in during the mid-2020s. A 2024 report of a substantial decline in overdose deaths [whites only] notwithstanding, prevention of American suicides and drug overdoses writ large remains a major public and population health problem (Nguyen et al., 2024), despite the intensive and enduring efforts of a plethora of dedicated professionals, policymakers, and community activists to reverse and end the epidemics. I suggest that this is partly a consequence of the rejection or ignorance of the research findings and didactics from the Los Angeles Suicide Prevention Center. Persistent social stigmatization commonly promotes silence among the bereaved, which, together with the siloing of the suicide and addiction domains, is a major impediment to the appropriate resourcing of medical examiners and coroners for optimizing their data collection and detecting all or most suicides and other self-injury deaths among drug and nondrug cases.

Underresourcing of emergency health care and medicolegal death investigation systems

Some of my more recent research provided specific evidence that data deficits, discrepancies, and disparities in decedent biographies and death circumstances impede the quest among medicolegal officials to detect suicides accurately, particularly in opioid and other drug cases. Previously, I shared historical data indicating that the United States was a second-tier country with respect to suicide accounting. Since then, I believe that the ravages of the opioid epidemic have eroded the American position. National reports had revealed that the emergency health care and medicolegal death investigation systems were highly stressed and underresourced, which long preceded the rapid escalation of overdose death rates in 2013/14, in the wake of the rise of fentanyl and other synthetic opioids. Onset of the COVID-19 pandemic in 2020 compounded a desperate situation.

By 2012/13, I had concluded that the plight of American suicide accounting was hopeless. A negative sparked a positive. I was empowered and assisted by talented and inspirational colleagues in creating the concept of self-injury mortality (SIM), a broader depiction of fatal self-injury than registered suicides. Behaviorally rather than cognitively based, SIM augmented these suicides with the great preponderance of overdose deaths as self-intoxication and products of high-risk behaviors. Implicated were the misuse of drugs, purchase of illicit ones in the black market, and illicit purchase of prescription drugs through doctor and pharmacy shopping. Exacerbating my growing concern with the undercounting of American suicides, I recognized that government statutes mandated suicide and other manner-of-death categories, and thus they likely will be constant for the foreseeable future. Nevertheless, I appreciated that these mandates need not hamstring us indefinitely in identifying and classifying fatal self-injury. Therefore, I posit that the incorporation of a self-injury checkbox on the death certificate, whose entries can cross the suicide, accident, and undetermined categories, would ameliorate, if not remedy, suicide's gross accounting problems for prevention and treatment. Broadening the scope of fatal self-injury, routine capture and reporting of SIM would minimize measurement biases differentially associated with the suicide methods used by the decedents, their psychological and psychiatric histories, and such sociodemographic characteristics as age, sex, race/ethnicity, and education.

Standardizing death scene investigations and utilizing mobile technology

There is an imperative to standardize death scene investigations through the creation of common protocols and adoption of mobile technology, which emanates from within and across heterogeneity in medical examiner and coroner systems and law enforcement offices. However, inertia and costs could prove formidable barriers to timely implementation. As a counterpoint, I contend that our astronomical estimated annual costs of SIM and suicide, encompassed by the Centers for Disease Control and Prevention's (CDC) $2.12 trillion estimate for total injury mortality—all in 2019

US dollars (Peterson et al., 2021)—make development, adoption, and universal implementation both commonsense and a bargain. Essential to the calculus, we cannot prevent what we cannot identify and measure.

Even if infrastructure and resources should prove too meager over the shorter term for mobile technology to improve suicide detection nationally, in a systematic and standardized way, more attainable is its application to portray death scenes in mortality reporting and populate a self-injury checkbox on the death certificate. This technology would be particularly helpful to medical examiners and coroners in identifying SIM in alcohol, opioid, and other drug intoxication cases, disaggregated by the three nonhomicide injury manners of death: suicide, accident, and undetermined. My fervent wish is that a multitude of young researchers and preventionists, in concert with health care professionals, forensic pathologists, health planners, and policymakers, will absorb the importance of comprehensively characterizing self-harm in the enablement and assurance of the ongoing capture of high-quality background, morbidity, disability, and mortality data for public health databases. A relevant initiative is already underway in the United Kingdom and on the European continent, which are anticipating their own opioid epidemics.

CDC is modernizing its medicolegal and public health data systems that generate the information central to suicide measurement. Modernization has expedited the finalization and release of mortality data for research and other public health use, through the Wide-ranging Online Data for Epidemiologic Research database, Web-based Injury Statistics Query and Reporting System, National Violent Death Reporting System, and State Unintentional Drug Overdose Reporting System, from a lag exceeding two years to closer to one. CDC's goal "is to move from siloed and brittle public health data systems to a connected, resilient, adaptable, and sustainable 'response ready' data ecosystem that can help us solve problems before they happen and reduce the harm caused by the problems that do happen" (Centers for Disease Control and Prevention, 2023, 3). It would be helpful in identifying high-risk groups and designing effective interventions and prevention and treatment programs if SIM were part of the equation. Merging NVDRS and SUDORS, in lieu of just sharing data between the two systems, would mean that drug addiction and suicide fall unambiguously under the umbrella of mental health.

Status of suicide underreporting

Ingvild Tøllefsen, a Norwegian medical researcher, led a global systematic review of the reliability of suicide statistics for the period 1963–2009, based on 31 studies with wide representation but highly variable quality, which indicated that underreporting of suicide was the norm (Tøllefsen et al., 2012). Sixteen of the selected studies provided estimates of over 10% underreporting, and 12 provided estimates exceeding 30%. To date, no one has provided a systematic, evidence-based estimate of underreporting of the American suicide rate. But I predict that underreporting now surpasses 30%. The numerator in the American rate of 15.0 per 100,000 in 2022 was 49,954 suicides. Assuming 10% undercount, the true suicide toll would be 54,949. Corrected at 30%, the toll would rise to 64,940. By comparison, estimated SIM cases would be 134,131, if that measure represented fatal self-injury rather than suicide alone. All aforementioned groups overrepresent the younger population, a prime demographic for targeting public health initiatives.

Which mortality categories are most susceptible to obscuring American suicides? Not fatal police shootings (victim-precipitated homicides), drownings, or single-occupant, single-vehicle crashes. Not the undetermined manner-of-death category, even though this is the category most prone to suicide misclassification, relatively speaking. My own research and review of that of others lead me to hypothesize that the largest repositories of hidden suicides are accidental/unintentional drug poisonings, mental and behavioral disorders, and ill-defined conditions and unknown causes. States can utilize ill-defined conditions and unknown causes as a holding category for fatal drug overdose cases, pending their manner-of-death assignment by medical examiners and coroners. Warranting an answer, empirical questions include the extent to which states do this and the proportion of these cases whose manner of death remains unresolved at the time of submission of the mortality data to the National Center for Health Statistics. Medicolegal investigations of equivocal intent cases—plausibly numerous among fatal overdoses—are resource poor. Psychological autopsies are not integral to the tool kit of medical examiner and coroner offices (Weinberger et al., 2018), and few professionals are trained to administer them (Calkins, 2019). Moreover, there is still no kindred agency to the police to facilitate and reinforce suicide and possible suicide investigations, unlike police involvement in homicide counterparts, and I don't hear a public outcry for better suicide data. This is unsurprising given the stigma and painful legacy of suicides and fatal drug overdoses.

Final thoughts

A New Zealand research team asked whether suicide is a "mental health, public health, or societal problem" (Goel et al., 2023). Obviously, the answer runs the gamut. Measurement and domain are central to the challenges posed by prevention. With suicide measurement, the United States gets what it pays for (or does not pay for), at the expense of public health data, clinical medicine, the forensic sciences, and consequently prevention and population health. Suicide detection, particularly suicide by drug self-intoxication, retains its precarious position (Moretti et al., 2021)—one consonant with my central hypothesis that American suicide data are seriously deficient. However, this situation is amenable to marked amelioration with concerted efforts by coalitions of the willing at national, state, and local levels, which include such entities as the bereaved, medicolegal and public health officials, psychiatrists, emergency physicians, hospitals, health administrators, planners, policymakers, pharmaceutical companies, nosologists, and research grant agencies. Yet fatal self-injury transcends suicide. Reflection on this observation induced me and my colleagues to propose SIM as a pragmatic and more representative measure or indicator of fatal self-injury than registered or known suicides alone.

My perception from perusing the literature and attending numerous conferences in North America and overseas is that suicidologists, generally, have minimal interest in expanding their domain to embrace the study of drug addiction and other substance issues. By the same token, the leaders of the substance misuse domain often appear indifferent about accommodating or reluctant to accommodate suicidality. The tendency of American public and private grant agencies to view suicides and fatal drug overdoses (the injury deaths of despair) as distinct phenomena and to fund research and prevention initiatives unevenly makes no sense for clinical medicine, public health, and medicolegal death investigations. Suicide, lethal drug overdose, and other fatal self-injury will be misunderstood and resistant to prevention for as long as they are misconceptualized and mismeasured by researchers, grant-funding agencies, policymakers, and preventionists, and consequently in the scientific literature and mass media stories and reports. The enormous, but largely latent, ocean of personal pain engendered by these losses merits a paradigm shift and amelioration, with initiatives by stakeholders to destigmatize mental illness, drug addiction, suicide, and other self-harm. In stark contrast to vaccination for COVID-19 mortality, there is no magic or silver bullet for markedly reversing the toll from the "injury deaths of despair."

The bottom line in my multidisciplinary research agenda is that epidemiology, demography, the forensic sciences (e.g., subspecialties of pathology, biology, toxicology, and chemistry), the humanities (e.g., literature, philosophy, and history), the social sciences (e.g., anthropology, economics, psychology, and sociology), clinical medicine, and public health principles can jointly enhance mental health and hence population health. Effective mental health treatment (including drug treatment) and prevention of suicide and other fatal self-injury demand high public confidence in the reliability and validity of the biographical, circumstantial, morbidity, disability, and mortality data that inform them.

Acknowledgments

Contributors to the development of my research career, and hence this book, are legion. I am indebted to all and remember many with great fondness and respect. Eric Caine has been a steadfast friend, colleague, and ally in the trenches since we began our collaboration in 2013. His wisdom and vast knowledge and experience have been essential in helping me reconceptualize fatal self-injury, beyond registered suicides alone, and in implementing this novel measure and translating and disseminating it to professional and lay audiences. Bina Ali, Aniruddha (Rudy) Banerjee, Joey Dacanay, James Holt, Haomiao Jia, Ted Miller, Crystal Rhodes, and Steven Stack were vital to the preparation and production of the tables, graphs, and/or maps, and Jessica White to the overall preparation of the manuscript. A number of them also contributed to various aspects of the underlying research, along with James Frost, Gerry Hobbs, Nestor Kapusta, Krista Lilly, and Shuhui Wang. Julian Rockett enriched my sensitivity to the desperation afflicting high-risk groups for suicide and overdose, as I conducted my investigations and reading that informed this book—far removed from the personal tragedies underlying my subject matter.

I am most appreciative of Franklin White for drawing from his wealth of international experience in community medicine and public health in graciously reviewing preliminary drafts of most chapters, as well as for recommending a glossary. I also deeply appreciate Kurt Nolte for reviewing the first full draft, correcting various errors in substance and interpretation, providing extensive edits to my glossary, and enhancing the underlying research, as did his medical examiner colleague Randy Hanzlick before him. Robert (Bob) Anderson, chief of the Statistical Analysis and Surveillance Branch at the National Center for Health Statistics (NCHS), made important contributions to the glossary and has always responded generously to the numerous questions I have raised with him over decades. Reviewing a full draft, William (Bill) Mosher offered me pearls of wisdom derived from his long career in designing, leading, and analyzing large fertility surveys at the NCHS. For example, he convinced me of the need for an executive summary and wisely counseled me against misusing the benefits of 20-20 hindsight in critiquing the seminal research of French sociologist Émile Durkheim. Hilary Connery brought her formidable clinical expertise and sensitivity to the forefront in reviewing the introduction and the first five chapters and has contributed substantially to the core research that informs the remainder of the book. All my research colleagues helped me clarify my intended audiences and minimize the abstruse.

I thank Alan (Lanny) Berman, Silvia Canetto, Roger Clark, Steven Stack, and Donley Studlar for their constructive comments on various sections of the manuscript. Roger has been an enthusiastic and sustained supporter of my research on suicide data quality. Rod McClure, former editor in chief of *Injury Prevention*, has also been a strong supporter of my research. I am indebted to Gordon Gee for encouraging me to translate my research for a wider audience than researchers and other professionals inhabiting the fields of suicidology, the forensic sciences, and drug addiction. Robin Coleman, Marlee Brooks, Edith Saint Preux, and Kris Lykke at Johns Hopkins University Press, together with the Faculty Advisory Board and the anonymous reviewers of my proposal and full manuscript, provided invaluable guidance and advice as I approached and entered the publication phases of the project. Robin was fully supportive of the project from our first contact, and Marlee and Edith were unfailingly conscientious in preparing me for the submission and review of my files for copyediting and proofing, as well as expeditious and thorough in responding to my queries. Jeremy Horsefield admirably and meticulously took on the onerous task of copyediting and Kathy Patterson that of indexing.

Finally, I would like to thank my wife, Sandra Putnam. A superb researcher and astute observer, she has been the major influence on the direction my suicide research has followed in the new millennium. Her corpus of work on alcohol and other substance misuse and prevention, primarily conducted for federal and state health agencies, triggered the mindset that enabled me to recognize that suicide and drug poisoning mortality are truly overlapping phenomena.

Mortality-Related Glossary

autopsy (postmortem examination): a systematic examination of a decedent to characterize the condition of the body and determine the cause of death. Autopsies start with a review of the circumstances of death and can also include a variety of laboratory testing (e.g., microbiologic, histologic, toxicologic, and radiologic).

consent autopsy: An autopsy performed with the consent of the decedent's next of kin in the interests of family members. These autopsies are generally performed by pathologists in a hospital setting on decedents who have succumbed to a natural disease. Pathologists performing these autopsies without medicolegal authority can only certify a natural manner of death.

demography: The study of size, composition, trends, and change of human and nonhuman populations. There are three components of change: fertility, mortality, and migration.

differential suicide misclassification: A measurement bias that occurs from limited investigative information where true suicides are misallocated to alternative manner-of-death categories, such as accident, undetermined, or natural causes (disease), or where true nonsuicides are misallocated to the suicide category. In democratic high-income countries, such as the United States, suicide case ascertainment is conservative, and thus the misclassification of true nonsuicides as false suicides is assumed by researchers to be exceedingly rare. Some total institutions, particularly prisons, may be a possible exception with misclassification of true homicides as false suicides.

disease: Abnormalities of the body's anatomical structure or physiological functioning from a wide variety of potential causes (e.g., genetic, communicable, toxic, metabolic, environmental, nutritional, neoplastic, degenerative).

epidemiology: The study of the distribution and determinants of disease, injury, and other health-related phenomena in populations—primarily human, but also animal populations. Epidemiology's domain extends from the macro level to the micro level, that is, from the societal to the molecular or intracellular level.

forensic: Derived from the Latin *forensis* meaning "public or open court." Pertaining to courts of law with subject matter open to public discussion and debate.

forensic (or medicolegal) autopsy: An autopsy performed in the public interest with statutory authorization. Next-of-kin consent is not required. Medicolegal autopsies are usually conducted by a forensic pathologist in a medicolegal setting. In addition to determining the cause of death, they can determine unnatural (homicide, suicide, accident, undetermined) manners of death.

forensic pathology: A subspecialty of pathology concerned with the investigation and physical examination, which is conducted on behalf of the public, of decedents who died suddenly, unexpectedly, or under suspicious, violent, unnatural, or unattended circumstances. Forensic pathology is a platform that supports public safety, public health, and the criminal justice system.

forensic toxicology: A subspecialty of forensic science concerned with the laboratory analysis of specimens (typically blood, urine, vitreous fluid, and solid organs) from individuals living or dead to detect and quantify drugs and other toxic substances on behalf of the public. Forensic toxicology is a platform that supports public safety, public health, and the criminal justice system. Medicolegal death investigative agencies have access to in-house, public, or private toxicologic laboratories.

injury: Disruption of the body's tissues, organs, or physiological processes by external agents such as guns, knives, blunt impacts, asphyxiating processes, fire, environmental conditions (extreme heat/cold), toxic agents including drugs, electric current, and radiation.

International Statistical Classification of Diseases and Related Health Problems (ICD): Under the auspices of the World Health Organization (WHO), ICD is a global system of standardized classification and coding of causes of death and illness, which are associated with disease, injury, and other health-related phenomena, used mainly for the preparation of death certificates; reporting and monitoring trends; and informing the targeting, design, implementation, and evaluation of interventions and prevention programming. Authorized by the WHO and maintained by the National Center for Health Statistics, a modified and expanded version with provision for detailed morbidity diagnoses has been adapted in the United

States to clinical settings (ICD-CM) to ground and guide health services research and service planning, in order to enhance health care quality and safety and to facilitate health care billing and reimbursement. The 11th revision of the ICD is in its implementation phase worldwide (*ICD-11*).

manner of death: Refers to the circumstances under which a death occurred and is divided into natural deaths (due to intrinsic disease processes) and unnatural deaths due to injuries from external agents (e.g., guns, knives, motor vehicles, drugs). Albeit rarely, natural deaths encompass one anomalous category, mental and behavioral disorders, which sometimes does not reflect the presence of a clear lethal disease mechanism. Only medical examiners and coroners can certify unnatural deaths, which are separated into homicide, suicide, and accident based on differing indications of intent. A homicide "occurs when death results from . . . an injury or poisoning or from . . . a volitional act committed by another person to cause fear, harm or death." A suicide "results from an injury or poisoning [due to an] an intentional self-inflicted act committed to do self-harm or cause the death of one's self." Accidents have "little or no evidence that the injury or poisoning occurred with intent to harm or cause death . . . the fatal outcome was unintentional." There is a residual category, "could not be determined" or "undetermined," which is "used when the information pointing to one manner of death is no more compelling than one or more other competing manners of death when all available information is considered" (Department of Health and Human Services et al., 2003, 29).

mechanism of injury death: The cascading anatomic and physiologic changes that occur between time of injury and time of death. Lethal mechanisms can be brief (e.g., hemopneumothorax in someone shot in the chest) or may last decades (e.g., urosepsis due to quadriplegia in a person who sustained a gunshot wound of the spine many years earlier).

psychological autopsy: A retrospective investigation of a decedent's intent and state of mind with respect to his/her premorbid behavior proximal to time of death. It combines an intensive review of medical examiner / coroner, laboratory, medical, law enforcement, and other first responder records with information acquired through semistructured, postmortem interviews with family members, health care providers, friends, and workplace acquaintances of the deceased as appropriate. Regardless of whether the manner of death is uncertain (equivocal), unexplained, or contested, the use of a psychological autopsy is usually reserved for those cases where one possible manner of death is suicide or accident.

self-injury mortality (SIM): Conceptually, SIM transcends registered suicides as the representative of fatal self-injury by embracing other deaths where the repetitive patterns of self-harming behavior of the decedent, like misuse of alcohol, opioids, stimulants, sedatives, and other drugs, and/or high speed and other negligent forms of driving, resulted in death. As of 2024, the nonsuicide component of SIM is confined to researcher-estimated deaths attributable to drug self-intoxication. Direct measurement would be facilitated by the addition of a self-injury checkbox to the death certificate, whose domain would traverse three manners of death: suicide, accident, and undetermined.

significant contributing causes of death: Concurrent diseases, injuries, impairments, or other health-related conditions that, while not directly leading to the death, contributed to the mechanism of death (i.e., comorbidities). For example, an elderly person with emphysema falls, breaks a femur, develops pneumonia, and dies. The immediate cause of death would be "bronchopneumonia," the underlying cause of death would be "fracture of femur," and a significant contributory condition would be "emphysema."

underlying (or principal) cause of death: The injury or disease that initiated the fatal sequence of events (e.g., gunshot wound of head, COVID-19 pneumonia). Immediate and intermediate causes of death are recorded sequentially on the death certificate above the underlying cause of death, for example, pulmonary embolus (immediate cause), due to deep venous thromboses of the lower extremities (intermediate cause), due to fracture of femur (underlying cause). In the case of an injury death, the circumstances of the injury are recorded on a death certificate in a box labeled "how injury occurred" (e.g., fell down stairs). Cause-of-death statements are the medical opinions of the certifier.

undetermined (cause or manner): A category typically utilized by medical examiners and coroners when they cannot determine the cause of death (e.g., skeletonized remains) or when they cannot distinguish among two or more of the injury manner-of-death categories as the appropriate assignment for a given death. Some types of injury deaths can be challenging for medical examiners or coroners to assign a manner of death because of limited investigative information, including information about decedent intent or the involvement or intent of others. Epitomizing these deaths are drug overdoses (e.g., where there is equal evidence for suicidal intent and recreational drug use), unwitnessed drownings, and falling from a height. Determination of manner could be facilitated by the implementation of a psychological autopsy in some of these cases.

References

Abe, K., Mertz, K.J., Powell, K.J., & Hanzlick, R.L. (2006). "Characteristics of Black and White suicide decedents in Fulton County, Georgia, 1988–2002." *American Journal of Public Health* 96(10):1794–98.

Acinas, M.P., Robles, J.I., & Peláez-Fernández, M.A. (2015). "Suicide note and the psychological autopsy: Associated behavioral aspects." *Actas Españolas de Psiquiatría* 43(3): 69–79.

Adcock, J.M., & Chancellor, A.S. (2016). *Death investigations* (2nd ed.). CreateSpace.

Akinyemi, O., Ogundare, T., Wedeslase, T., Hartmann, B., Odusanya, E., Williams, M., et al. (2024). "Trends in suicides and homicides in 21st century America." *Cureus* 16(5):e61010.

Altman, D.G., & Bland, J.M. (1995). "Absence of evidence is not evidence of absence." *British Medical Journal* 311(7003):485.

American Psychiatric Association. (1994). *Diagnostic and statistical manual of mental disorder* (4th ed.). Washington, DC: American Psychiatric Association.

Andersson, A.L., & Svensson, K. (2015). "Fatalities in road traffic: A result of accidents or suicide." *Journal of Local and Global Health Science* 27.

Andrews, R.J. (ed.). (2022). *Florence Nightingale mortality and health diagrams*. San Francisco: Visionary Press.

Appleby, L., Turnbull, P., Kapur, N., Gunnell, D., & Hawton, K. (2019). "New standard of proof for suicide at inquests in England and Wales." *British Medical Journal* 366:14745.

Aqulia, I., Sacco, M.A., Gratteri, S., Sirianni, M., De Fazio, P., & Ricci, P. (2018). "The 'social-mobile autopsy': The evolution of psychological autopsy with new technologies in forensic investigations in suicide." *Legal Medicine* 32:79–82.

Arias, E., & Xu, J. (2022). "U.S state life tables, 2019." *National Vital Statistics Reports* 70(19):1–57.

Arias, E., Xu, J., Tejada-Vera, B., Murphy, S.L., & Bastian, B. (2022). "U.S. state life tables, 2020." *National Vital Statistics Reports* 71(2):1–17.

Arsenault-Lapierre, G., Kim, C., & Turecki, G.. (2004). "Psychiatric diagnoses in 3275 suicides: A meta-analysis." *BMC Psychiatry* 4(1):37.

Atkinson, J.M. (1978). *Discovering suicide: Studies in the social organization of sudden death*. London: MacMillan Press.

Attwood, W.R., Quinn, T., Chiu, S.K., Li, J.F., & Steege, A.L. (2022). "Reducing occupational exposure to SARS-CoV-2: A survey of changes in caseload and controls among medical examiner and coroners' offices in Pennsylvania during 2020." *Journal of Occupational and Environmental Hygiene* 19(5):256–65.

Avorn, J. (2004). *Powerful medicines: The benefits, risks, and costs of prescription drugs*. New York: Alfred A Knopf.

Baden, M.M. (2023). *American autopsy*. Dallas: BenBella.

Bakst, S.S., Braun, T., Zucker, I., Amitai, Z., & Shohat, T. (2016). "The accuracy of suicide statistics: Are true suicide deaths misclassified?" *Social Psychiatry and Psychiatric Epidemiology* 51(1):115–23.

Bálint, L., Osváth, P., Németh, A., Kapitány, B., Rihmer, Z., & Döme, P. (2022). "Suicide mortality in Hungary during the COVID-19 pandemic." *Orvosi Hetilap* 163(48):1895–901.

Baltimore Sun Editorial Board. (2019). "Maryland medical examiner's resignation underscores resource limitations amid opioid crisis." *Baltimore Sun*, December 10. https://www.baltimoresun.com/2019/12/10/maryland-medical-examiners-resignation-underscores-resource-limitations-amid-opioid-crisis/.

Barell, V. (1995). "Injury data definitions: The need for standards." In *Proceedings of the International Collaborative Effort on Injury Statistics*, 16-1–16-14. Hyattsville, MD: US Department of Health and Human Services.

Barker, J. (2023). "The death of Stalin's son." *History Today* 73(4). https://www.historytoday.com/archive/history-matters/death-stalins-son.

Barraclough, B.M. (1973). "Differences between national suicide rates." *British Journal of Psychiatry* 122:95–96.

Barth, A., Sögner, L., Gnambs, T., Kundi, M., Reiner, A., & Winker, R. (2011). "Socioeconomic factors and suicide: An analysis of 18 industrialized countries for the years 1983 through 2007." *Journal of Occupational and Environmental Medicine* 53(3):313–17.

Behera, C., Karthik, K., Dogra, T.D., Lalwani, S., Millo, T., & Singh, S.R. (2014). "E-suicide note: A newer trend and its medico-legal implications in India." *Medico-Legal Journal* 82(2):80–82.

Bennell, C., Jones, N.J., & Taylor, A. (2011). "Determining the authenticity of suicide notes: Can training improve human judgment?" *Criminal Justice and Behavior* 38(7):669–89.

Bergen, H., Hawton, K., Waters, K., Ness, J., Cooper, J., Steeg, S., et al. (2012). "Premature death after self-harm: A multicentre cohort study." *Lancet* 380(9853):1568–74.

Berman, A.L., & Pompili, M. (eds.). (2011). *Medical conditions associated with suicide risk*. Washington, DC: American Association of Suicidology.

Best, J. (2004). *More damned lies and statistics: How numbers confuse public issues*. Berkeley: University of California Press.

Blosnich, J.R., Bossarte, R.M., & Silenzio, V.M.B. (2012). "Suicidal ideation among sexual minority veterans: Results from the 2005–2010 Massachusetts Behavioral Risk Factor Surveillance Survey." *American Journal of Public Health* 102(suppl. 1):S44–47.

Blosnich, J.R., Boyer, T.L., Brown, G.R., Kauth, M.R., & Shipherd, J.C. (2021). "Differences in methods of suicide death among transgender and nontransgender patients in the Veterans Health Administration, 1999–2016." *Medical Care* 59:531–35.

Blüml, V., Regier, M.D., Hlavin, G., Rockett, I.R.H., König, F., Vyssoki, B., et al. (2013). "Lithium in the public water supply and suicide mortality in Texas." *Journal of Psychiatric Research* 47(3):407–11

Bohnert, A.S.B., & Ilgen, M.A. (2019). "Understanding links among opioid use, overdose, and suicide." *New England Journal of Medicine* 380(1):71–79.

Bohnert, A.S.B., McCarthy, J.F., Ignacio, R.V., Ilgen, M.A., Eisenberg, A., & Blow, F.C.

(2013). “Misclassification of suicide deaths: Examining the psychiatric history of overdose decedents.” *Injury Prevention* 19(5):326–30.

Bohnert, A.S.B., & Sen, S. (2020). “Deaths attributed to psychiatric disorders in the United States, 2010–2018.” *American Journal of Public Health* 110(12):1825–27.

Botello, T., Noguchi, T., Sathyavagiswaran, L., Weinberger, L.E., & Gross, B.H. (2013). “Evolution of the psychological autopsy: Fifty years of experience at the Los Angeles County Chief Medical Examiner-Coroner’s Office.” *Journal of Forensic Sciences* 58(4): 924–26.

Breggin, P. (1991). *Toxic psychiatry*. New York: St. Martin’s Press.

Breiding, M.J., & Wiersema, B. (2006). “Variability of undetermined manner of death in the US.” *Injury Prevention* 12(suppl. 2):ii49–54.

Brossard, B., & Chandler, A. (2022). *Explaining mental illness: Sociological perspectives*. Bristol: Bristol University Press.

Bugeja, L., Ibrahim, J.E., Ferrah, N., Murphy, B., Willoughby, N., & Ranson, D. (2016). “The utility of medico-legal databases for public health research: A systematic review of peer-reviewed publications using the National Coronial Information System.” *Health Research Policy and Systems* 14(28).

Burr, V. (1995). *Social constructionism*. London: Routledge.

Butler, A.M., & Malone, K. (2013). “Attempted suicide v. non-suicidal self-injury: Behaviour, syndrome or diagnosis?” *British Journal of Psychiatry* 202(5):324–25.

Butler, J. (2024). *Who’s afraid of gender?* New York: Farrar, Strauss & Giroux.

Cai, Z., Junus, A., Chang, Q., & Yip, P.S.F. (2022). “The lethality of suicide methods: A systematic review and meta-analysis.” *Journal of Affective Disorders* 300:121–29.

Caine, E.D. (2012). “Suicide prevention is a winnable battle.” *American Journal of Public Health* 102(suppl. 1):S1–6.

Caine, E.D. (2013). “Forging an agenda for suicide prevention in the United States.” *American Journal of Public Health* 103(5):822–29.

Caine, E.D. (2019). “Building the foundation for comprehensive suicide prevention—based on intention and planning in a social-ecological context.” *Epidemiology and Psychiatric Sciences* 29:e69.

Caine, E.D., Yeung, C.Y., & Rockett, I.R.H. (Unpublished). “Deaths attributed to mental and behavioral disorders in the United States: Rising rates from 2010–2022.”

Calkins, C.G. (2019). “The psychological autopsy: What, who and why.” *Forensic Mental Health Practitioner* 2(1):1–10.

Calvert, C., & Kamp, J. (2017). “Medical examiners skip some autopsies, as opioid crisis mounts.” *Wall Street Journal*, May 3. https://www.wsj.com/articles/opioid-crisis-strains-medical-examiners-1493812801.

Canetto, S. (2008). “Women and suicidal behavior: A cultural analysis.” *American Journal of Orthopsychiatry* 78(2):259–66.

Canetto, S., Tatum, P.T., & Slater, M.D. (2017). “Suicide stories in the US media: Rare and focused on the young.” In *Media and suicide: International perspectives on research, theory, and policy*, T. Niederkrotenthaler, Steven Stack (eds.), 27–39. New York: Routledge.

Canetto, S.S, Antonelli, P., Ciccotti, A., Dettore, D., & Lamis, D.A. (2021). “Suicidal as normal—a lesbian, gay, and bisexual youth script?” *Crisis* 42(4):292–300.

Cano, M., Oh, S., Osborn, P., Olowolaju, S.A., Sanchez, A., Kim, Y., et al. (2023). "County-level predictors of US drug overdose mortality: A systematic review." *Drug and Alcohol Dependence* 242:109714.

Cantor, C., McTaggart, T., & De Leo, D. (2001). "Misclassification of suicide: The contribution of opiates." *Psychopathology* 34(3):140–46.

Cantor, C.H., & Dunne, M.P. (1990). "Australian suicide data and the use of 'undetermined' death category (1968–1985)." *Australian and New Zealand Journal of Psychiatry* 24(3): 381–84.

Case, A., & Deaton, A. (2015). "Rising morbidity and mortality in midlife among white non-Hispanic Americans in the 21st century." *Proceedings of the National Academy of Sciences USA* 112(49):15708–83.

Cato, J.E., & Canetto, S.S. (2003). "Young adults' reactions to gay and lesbian peers who became suicidal following 'coming out' to their parents." *Suicide and Life-Threatening Behavior* 33(2):201–10.

Cavanagh, J.T.O., Carson, A.J., Sharpe, M., & Lawrie, S.M. (2003). "Psychological autopsy studies of suicide: A systematic review." *Psychological Medicine* 33(3):395–405.

Centers for Disease Control and Prevention. (2023). *Data modernization plan user guide*. https://www.cdc.gov/csels/dmi-support/docs/DMI_Plan_User_Guide.pdf.

Centers for Disease Control and Prevention. (n.d.-a) *Coroner and medical examiner laws*. U.S. Department of Health and Human Services. https://www.cdc.gov/phlp/php/coroner/index.html.

Centers for Disease Control and Prevention. (n.d.-b). *State Unintentional Drug Overdose Reporting System (SUDORS)*. U.S. Department of Health and Human Services. https://www.cdc.gov/nchs/comec/sudors.htm.

Centers for Disease Control and Prevention. (n.d.-c). *Web-Based Injury Statistics Query and Reporting System (WISQARS)*. U.S. Department of Health and Human Services. https://wisqars.cdc.gov/.

Centers for Disease Control and Prevention. (n.d.-d). *Wide-Ranging Online Data for Epidemiologic Research (WONDER)*. U.S. Department of Health and Human Services. https://wonder.cdc.gov/.

Cherpitel, C., Borges, G.L., & Wilcox, H.C. (2004). "Acute alcohol use and suicidal behavior: A review of the literature." *Alcoholism: Clinical and Experimental Research* 28(suppl. 5):S18–28.

Chikazawa, K. (1974). "Statistical observation of suicide by the aged: Its relationship with the welfare problem (in Japanese)." *Kango Gijustsu* 20:54.

Chiswick, B.R., Lee, Y.L., & Miller, P.W. (2002). *The determinants of the geographic concentration among immigrants: Application to Australia*. Bonn: Institute for the Study of Labor.

Choi, N.G., Marti, C.N., DiNitto, D.M., & Choi, B.Y. (2020). "Suicides and deaths of undetermined intent by poisoning: Reexamination of classification differences by race/ethnicity and state." *Archives of Suicide Research* 24(suppl. 2):S264–81.

Ciccarone, D. (2021). "The rise of illicit fentanyls, stimulants and the fourth wave of the opioid overdose crisis." *Current Opinion in Psychiatry* 34(4):344–50.

Claassen, C.A., Yip, P.S., Corcoran, P., Bossarte, R.M., Lawrence, B.A., & Currier, G.W.

(2010). "National suicide rates a century after Durkheim: Do we know enough to estimate error?" *Suicide and Life-Threatening Behavior* 40(3):193–223.

Committee on Identifying the Needs of the Forensic Sciences Community, National Research Council. (2009). *Strengthening forensic science in the United States: A path forward*. Washington, DC: National Academies Press.

Conner, A., Azrael, D., & Miller, M. (2019). "Suicide case-fatality rates in the United States, 2007 to 2014: A nationwide population-based study." *Annals of Internal Medicine* 171(12):885–95.

Connery, H.S., Taghian, N., Kim, J., Griffin, M., Rockett, I.R.H., Weiss, R.D., et al. (2019). "Suicidal motivations reported by opioid overdose survivors: A cross-sectional study of adults with opioid use disorder." *Drug and Alcohol Dependence* 205:107612.

Connery, H.S., Weiss, R.D., Griffin, M.L., Trinh, C.D., Kim, J., Rockett, I.R.H., et al. (2022). "Suicidal motivations among opioid overdose survivors: Replication and extension." *Drug and Alcohol Dependence* 235:109437.

COVID-19 Excess Mortality Collaborators (2022). "Estimating excess mortality due to the COVID-19 pandemic: A systematic analysis of COVID-19-related mortality, 2020–21." *Lancet* 399(10334):1513–36.

Crepeau-Hobson, F. (2010). "The psychological autopsy and determination of child suicides: A survey of medical examiners." *Archives of Suicide Research* 14(1):24–34.

Creswell, J.W., & Plano Clark, V.L. (2018). *Designing and conducting mixed methods research* (3rd ed.). Los Angeles: Sage.

Crosby, A.E., Ertl, A., Lyons, B.H., Ivey-Stephenson, A.Z., & Jack, S. (2021). "Circumstances associated with suicides among females—16 states, United States, 2005–2016." *Medical Care* 59:S92–99.

Crosby, A.E., Ortega, L., & Melanson, C. (2011). *Self-directed violence surveillance: Uniform definitions and recommended data elements, version 1.0*. Atlanta, GA: Centers for Disease Control and Prevention, National Center for Injury Prevention and Control.

Curphey, T.J. (1965). "The role of the social scientist in the medicolegal certification of death from suicide." In *The cry for help*, N.L. Farberow, E.S. Shneidman (eds.), 110–17. New York: McGraw-Hill.

Curphey, T.J. (1967). "Role of the forensic pathologist in the medicolegal certification of modes of death." *Journal of Forensic Sciences* 13(2):163–76.

Curtin, S.C., Tolson, G., Arias, E., & Anderson, R.N. (2019). *Funeral director's handbook: Death registration and fetal death reporting*. Hyattsville, MD: National Center for Health Statistics.

Cuyahoga County Medical Examiner's Office. (2017). *Medicolegal death investigation: A step-by-step field guide*.

Davis, G.G., Cadwallader, A.B., Fligner, C.L., Gilson, T.P., Hall, E.R., Harshbarger, K.E., et al. (2020). "Position paper: Recommendations for the investigation, diagnosis, and certification of deaths related to opioid and other drugs." *American Journal of Forensic Medicine and Pathology* 41(3):152–59.

Davis, G.G., Nelson, L.S., Aiken, S.S., Druid, H., Gill, J.R., Goldberger, B.A., et al. (2013). "National Association of Medical Examiners position paper: Recommendations for the investigation, diagnosis, and certification of deaths related to opioid drugs." *Academic Forensic Pathology* 3(1):77–83.

Davis, J.H., & Spelman, J.W. (1968). "The role of the medical examiner or coroner." In *Suicidal behaviors*, H.L.P. Resnik (ed.), 453–514. Boston, MA: Little, Brown.

Dawes, D.E., Holden, K.B., & Williams, D.R. (eds.). (2023). *Health equity: African Americans and public health*. Washington, DC: American Public Health Association.

De Leo, D., Burgis, S., Bertolote, J.M., Kerkhof, A.J.F.M., & Bille-Brahe, U. (2006). "Definitions of suicidal behavior: Lessons learned from the WHO/EURO Multicenter Study." *Crisis* 27(1):4–15.

De Leo, D., Dudley, M.J., Aebersold, C.J., Mendoza, J.A., Barnes, M.A., Harrison, J.E., et al. (2010). "Achieving standardised reporting of suicide in Australia: Rationale and program for change." *Medical Journal of Australia* 192(8):452–56.

Del Pozo, B., Beletsky, L., Goulka, J., & Kleinig, J. (2021). "Beyond decriminalization: Ending the war on drugs requires recasting police discretion through the lens of a public health ethic." *American Journal of Bioethics* 21(4):41–44.

Denham, A., Vasu, T., Avendano, P., Boslett, A., Mendoza, M., & Hill, E.L. (2022). "Coroner county systems are associated with a higher likelihood of unclassified drug overdoses compared to medical examiner county systems." *American Journal of Drug and Alcohol Abuse* 48(5):606–17.

Dennett, J.M., & Gonsalves, G.S. (2023). "Early OxyContin marketing linked to long-term spread of infectious diseases associated with injection drug use." *Health Affairs* 42(8):1081–90.

Department of Health and Human Services. (2004). "Instructions for completing the cause-of-death section of the death certificate for injury and poisoning." https://www.cdc.gov/nchs/data/dvs/red_form.pdf.

Department of Health and Human Services, Centers for Disease Control and Prevention, and National Center for Health Statistics. (2003). *Medical examiners' and coroners' handbook on death registration and fetal death reporting 2003 revision*. Hyattsville, MD: US Department of Health and Human Services.

Dhossche, D.M. (2003). "Toxicology of suicide: Touchstone for suicide prevention?" *Medical Science Monitor* 9(4):SR9–19.

Donaldson, A.E., Larsen, G.Y., Fullerton-Gleason, L., & Olson, L.M. (2006). "Classifying undetermined poisoning deaths." *Injury Prevention* 12(5):338–43.

D'Onofrio, G. (2003). "Treatment for alcohol and other drug problems: Closing the gap." *Annals of Emergency Medicine* 41(6):814–17.

Douglas, J.D. (1967). *The social meanings of suicide*. Princeton, NJ: Princeton University Press.

Drewe, R. (2000). *The shark net*. Melbourne: Penguin Australia.

DuFour, S.N. (2016). "Perpetuating the cycle: Opioid addiction and the criminal justice system." *Inquiries* 8(7):1–2.

Durkheim, E. (transl. J.A Spaulding & G. Simpson). (1897/1951). *Suicide: A study in sociology*. New York: Free Press.

Egger, M., Davey Smith, G., & Altman, D.G. (eds.). (2001). *Systematic reviews in health care: Meta-analysis in context* (2nd ed.). London: BMJ.

Ehlman, D.C., Yard, E., Stone, D.M., Jones, C.M., & Mack, K.A. (2022). "Changes in suicide rates—United States, 2019 and 2020." *MMWR Morbidity and Mortality Weekly Report* 71:305–12.

Eisenwort, B., Berzlanovich, A., Willinger, U., & Eisenwort, G. (2006). "Suicide notes and their importance to suicide research: The representativeness of suicide note writers (in German)." *Nervenarzt* 77(11):1355–56, 1358–1360, 1362.

Elnour, A.A., & Harrison, J. (2008). "Lethality and suicide methods." *Injury Prevention* 14(1):39–45.

Eskin, M., Kujan, O., Voracek, M., Shaheen, A., Carta, M.G., Sun, J.M., et al. (2016). "Cross-national comparisons of attitudes toward suicide and suicidal persons in university students from 12 countries." *Scandinavian Journal of Psychology* 57(6):554–63.

Esser, M.B., Sherk, A., Liu, Y., & Naimi, T.S. (2024). "Deaths from excessive alcohol use—United States, 2016–2021." *MMWR Morbidity and Mortality Weekly Report* 73(8): 154–57.

Evans, A., & Abrahamson, K. (2020). "The influence of stigma on suicide bereavement: A systematic review." *Journal of Psychosocial Nursing and Mental Health Services* 58(4): 21–27.

Feuer, A., & Rashbaum, W.K. (2020). "We ran out of space: Bodies pile up as N.Y. struggles to bury its dead." *New York Times*, November 18. https://www.nytimes.com/2020/04/30/nyregion/coronavirus-nyc-funeral-home-morgue-bodies.html.

Field, G. (2002). "Nights underground in darkest London: The Blitz, 1940–1941." *International Labor and Working-Class History* Fall:11–49.

Fincham, B., Langer, S., Scourfield, J., & Shiner, M. (2011). *Understanding suicide: A sociological autopsy*. London: Palgrave MacMillan.

Frakt, A. (2020). "What can be learned from differing rates of suicide among groups." *New York Times*, December 30. https://www.nytimes.com/2020/12/30/upshot/suicide-demographic-differences.html.

GBD 2017 SDG Collaborators. (2018). "Measuring progress from 1990 to 2017 and projecting attainment to 2030 of the health-related sustainable development goals for 195 countries and territories: A systematic analysis for the Global Burden of Disease Study 2017." *Lancet* 392:2091–2138.

Ghorayshi, A. (2023). "No one knows how many L.G.B.T.Q. Americans die by suicide." *New York Times*, June 1. https://www.nytimes.com/2023/06/01/health/lgbtq-suicide-data.html.

Gjertsen, F., Bruzzone, S., & Griffiths, C.E. (2019). "Burden of suicide presented as one of the leading causes of death: Uncover facts or misrepresent statistics?" *Journal of Global Health* 9(1):010401.

Gladwell, M. (2024). *Revenge of the tipping point: Overstories, superspreaders, and the rise of social engineering*. New York: Little, Brown.

Goel, D., Dennis, B., & McKenzie, S.K. (2023). "Is suicide a mental health, public health or societal problem?" *Current Opinion in Psychiatry* 36(5):352–59.

Goldsmith, S.K., Pellmar, T.C., Kleinman, A.M., & Bunney, W.E.E. (2002). *Reducing suicide: A national imperative*. Washington, DC: National Academies Press.

Goodin, J., & Hanzlick, R. (1995). "Mind your manners part II: General results from the

National Association of Medical Examiners manner of death questionnaire." *American Journal of Forensic Medicine and Pathology* 18(3):224–27.

Grandjean, P. (2016). "Paracelsus revisited: The dose concept in a complex world." *Basic and Clinical Pharmacology and Toxicology* 119(2):126–32.

Gray, D., Coon, H., McGlade, E., Callor, W., & Byrd, J. (2014). "Comparative analysis of suicide, accidental, and undetermined cause of death classification." *Suicide and Life-Threatening Behavior* 44(3):304–16.

Greenwood, L., & Fashola, K. (2021). *Illicit fentanyl from China: An evolving global operation*. U.S.-China Economic and Security Review Commission. https://www.uscc.gov/sites/default/files/2021-08/Illicit_Fentanyl_from_China-An_Evolving_Global_Operation.pdf.

Greenwood, M. (1948). *Medical statistics from Graunt to Farr*. Cambridge: Cambridge University Press.

Gunnell, D., Bennewith, O., Simkin, S., Cooper, J., Klineberg, E., Rodway, C., et al. (2013). "Time trends in coroners' use of different verdicts for possible suicides and their impact on officially reported incidence of suicide in England: 1990–2005." *Psychological Medicine* 43:1415–22.

Haddon, W., Jr. (1968). "The changing approach to the epidemiology, prevention, and amelioration of trauma: The transition to approaches etiologically rather than descriptively based." *American Journal of Public Health Nations Health* 58(8):1431–38.

Halbwachs, M. (transl. H. Goldblatt) (1978). *The causes of suicide*. London: Routledge & Kegan Paul.

Hamilton, J. (2012). *The price of valour*. Sydney: Pan Macmillan Australia.

Hanschmidt, F., Lehnig, F., Reidel-Heller, S.G., & Kersting, A. (2016). "The stigma of suicide survivorship and related consequences: A systematic review." *PLOS One* 11(9):e0162688.

Hanzlick, R. (2006). "Medical examiners, coroners, and public health: A review and update." *Archives of Pathology and Laboratory Medicine* 130(9):1274–82.

Hanzlick, R. (2007). *Death investigation: Systems and procedures*. Boca Raton, FL: CRC Press.

Hanzlick, R.L. (2014). "A perspective on medicolegal death investigation in the United States: 2013." *Academic Forensic Pathology* 4(1):2–9.

Hanzlick, R.L., & Combs, D. (1998). "Medical examiner and coroner systems: History and trends." *JAMA* 279(11):870–74.

Hanzlick, R.L., & Parrish, G. (1996). "The use of medical examiner/coroner data in public health surveillance and epidemiologic research." *Annual Review of Public Health* 17:383–409.

Harrington, A. (2019). *Mind fixers: Psychiatry's troubled search for the biology of mental illness*. New York: W. W. Norton.

Harris, E.C., & Barraclough, B. (1997). "Suicide as an outcome for mental disorders: A meta-analysis." *British Journal of Psychiatry* 170:205–28.

Hasnain, A. (2022). "Suicide is not a crime—countries must stop treating it as one." *Al Jazeera Newsletter*, October 10. https://www.aljazeera.com/opinions/2022/10/10/suicide-is-not-a-crime-countries-must-stop-treating-it-as.

Hawton, K., Bergen, H., Kapur, N., Cooper, J., Steeg, S., Ness, J., et al. (2012). "Repetition of self-harm and suicide following self-harm in children and adolescents: Findings from the Multicentre Study of Self-Harm in England." *Journal of Child Psychology and Psychiatry* 53(12):1212–19.

Health Resources and Services Administration, Bureau of Health Workforce, National Center for Health, and Workforce Analysis. (2015). *The county Area Health Resources File (AHRF) 2014–2015 release*. Rockville, MD: US Department of Health and Human Services, Health Resources and Services Administration.

Henry, A.F., & Short, J.F., Jr. (1954). *Suicide and homicide: Some economic, sociological and psychological aspects of aggression*. New York: Free Press.

Herpen, R. (2022). "Social, environmental factors key to assessing rates of self-injury mortality and suicide." *Healio News*, February 11. https://www.healio.com/news/psychiatry/20220211/social-environmental-factors-key-to-assessing-rates-of-self injury-mortality-and-suicide.

Higham, S., & Horwitz, S. (2022). *American cartel: Inside the battle to bring down the opioid industry*. New York: Twelve.

Hjelmeland, H., Dieserud, G., Dyregrov, K., Knizek, B.L., & Leenaars, A.A. (2012). "Psychological autopsy studies as diagnostic tools: Are they methodologically flawed?" *Death Studies* 36(7):605–26.

Hobby, N. (2022). *The red witch: A biography of Katharine Susannah Prichard*. Melbourne: Miegunyah Press.

Hong, D., Lee, S., Choi, Y.-J., Moon, S., Jang, Y., Cho, Y.-M., et al. (2021). "The age-standardized incidence, mortality, and case fatality rates of COVID-19 in 79 countries: A cross-sectional comparison and their correlations with associated factors." *Epidemiology and Health* 43:e2021061.

Hookano, R., Knight, L.D., Brunelli, R.A., & Stoppacher, R. (2013). "Applications of social network media in medicolegal death investigation." *Journal of Forensic Sciences* 58(6):1628–32.

Horwitz, A.V. (2021). *DSM: A history of psychiatry's bible*. Baltimore: Johns Hopkins University Press.

Hoyert, D.L. (2011). "The changing profile of autopsied deaths in the United States, 1972–2007." *NCHS Data Brief* 67:1–8.

Hughes, E. (2022). *The hard sell: Crime and punishment at an opioid startup*. New York: Doubleday.

Huguet, N., Kaplan, M.S., & McFarland, B.H. (2012). "Rates and correlates of undetermined deaths among African Americans: Results from the National Violent Death Reporting System." *Suicide and Life-Threatening Behavior* 42(2):185–96.

Humphry, D. (2010). *Final exit: The practicalities of self-deliverance and assisted suicide for the dying* (rev. 3rd ed.). New York: Delta Trade Paperbacks.

Inoue, C., Shawler, E., Jordan, C.H., Moore, M.J., & Jackson, C.A. (2023). *Veteran and military mental health issues*. St. Petersburg, FL: StatPearls.

Institute for Research on Poverty. (2020). *Connections among poverty, incarceration, and inequality*. Madison: University of Wisconsin–Madison.

Institute of Medicine. (2006a). *Emergency medical services at the crossroads*. Washington, DC: National Academies Press.

Institute of Medicine. (2006b). *Hospital-based emergency care: At the breaking point*. Washington, DC: National Academies Press.

International Association of Coroners & Medical Examiners. (n.d.). "Accreditation." http://www.theiacme.com/accreditation.

Jacobs, H. (2016). "This one-paragraph letter may have launched the opioid epidemic." *Business Insider*, May 26. https://www.businessinsider.in/This-one-paragraph-letter-may-have-launched-the-opioid-epidemic/articleshow/52455353.cms.

Jarvis, G.K., Boldt, M., & Butt, J. (1991). "Medical examiners and manner of death." *Suicide and Life-Threatening Behavior* 21(2):115–13.

Jentzen, J.M. (2009). *Death investigation in America: Coroners, medical examiners, and the pursuit of medical certainty*. Cambridge, MA: Harvard University Press.

Jobes, D.A., Berman, A.L., & Josselson, A.R. (1986). "The impact of psychological autopsies on medical examiners' determination of manner of death." *Journal of Forensic Sciences* 31(1):177–89.

Jobes, D.A., Berman, A.L., & Josselson, A.R. (1987). "Improving the validity and reliability of medical-legal certifications of suicide." *Suicide and Life-Threatening Behavior* 17(4): 310–25.

Johnson, S. (2023). "It's a huge sign of progress: The battle to decriminalise suicide." *Guardian*, July 20. https://www.theguardian.com/global-development/2023/jul/20/its-a-huge-sign-of-progress-the-battle-to-decriminalise-suicide.

Jones, E. (2021). "COVID-19 and the Blitz compared: Mental health outcomes in the UK." *Lancet Psychiatry* 8:708–16.

Jones, J.H. (1981). *Bad blood: The Tuskegee syphilis experiment*. New York: Free Press.

Jougla, E., Pequignot, J., Chappert, J., Rossollin, F., Le Toullec, A., & Pavillon, G. (2002). "Quality of suicide mortality data (in French)." *Revue d Epidemiologie et de Sante Publique* 51:49–62.

Kadetskaya, T. (2023). "Does life insurance cover accidental drug overdose?" https://life-insurance-lawyer.com/accidental-death-claim-denied-due-to-drug-exclusion/.

Kalesan, B., Villarreal, M.D., Keyes, K.M., & Galea, S. (2016). "Gun ownership and social gun culture." *Injury Prevention* 22(3):216–20.

Kapur, N., Cooper, J., O'Connor, R.C., & Hawton, K. (2013). "Non-suicidal self-injury v. attempted suicide: New diagnosis or false dichotomy?" *British Journal of Psychiatry* 202(5):326–28.

Kapusta, N.D., Tran, U.S., Rockett, I.R.H., De Leo, D., Naylor, C.P.E., Niederkrotenthaler, T., et al. (2011). "Declining autopsy rates and suicide misclassification: A cross-national analysis of 35 countries." *Archives of General Psychiatry* 68(10):1050–57.

Karch, DL, Dahlberg, L.L., & Patel, M. (2010). "Surveillance for violent deaths—National Violent Death Reporting System, 16 states, 2007." *MMWR Morbidity and Mortality Weekly Reports* 59:1–50.

Kariisa, M., Davis, N.L., Kumar, S., Seth, P., Mattson, C.L., Chowdhury, F., et al. (2022). "Vital signs: Drug overdose deaths, by selected sociodemographic and social determinants of health characteristics—25 states and the District of Columbia, 2019–2020." *MMWR Morbidity and Mortality Weekly Report* 71(29):940–47.

Khan, K.S., Kunz, R., Kleijnen, J., & Antes, G. (2003). *Systematic reviews to support evidence-*

based medicine: How to review and apply findings of healthcare research. London: Royal Society of London Press.

Kheibari, A., Cerel, J., & Victor, G. (2021). "Comparing attitudes toward stigmatized deaths: Suicide and opioid overdose deaths." *International Journal of Mental Health and Addiction* 20:2291–305.

Kisner, J. (2020). "Piled bodies, overflowing morgues: Inside America's autopsy crisis." *New York Times Magazine*, February 26. https://www.nytimes.com/2020/02/25/magazine/piled-bodies-overflowing-morgues-inside-americas-autopsy-crisis.html.

Kleinig, J. (2012). "Active drug users as social change agents: Some ethical dimensions." *Substance Use and Misuse* 47(5):596–98.

Klugman, J., Condran, G., & Wray, M. (2013). "The role of medicolegal systems in producing geographic variation in suicide rates." *Social Science Quarterly* 94(2):462–89.

Knoll, J.L. (2008). "The psychological autopsy, part 1: Applications and methods." *Law and Psychiatry* 14(6):393–97.

Knox, K.L., Conwell, Y., & Caine, E.D. (2004). "If suicide is a public health problem, what are we doing to prevent it?" *American Journal of Public Health* 94:37–45.

Kochanek, K.D., Murphy, S.L., Xu, J., & Arias, E. (2019). "Deaths: Final data for 2017." *National Vital Statistics Report* 689(9):1–62.

Koehler, S.A., & Wecht, C.H. (2006). *Postmortem: Establishing the cause of death*. Buffalo, NY: Firefly Books.

Kounang, N. (2017). "One short letter's huge impact on the opioid epidemic." *CNN Health*, June 1. https://www.cnn.com/2017/06/01/health/opioid-epidemic-1980-letter-origins-study/index.html.

Krieger, N. (2000). "Refiguring 'race': Epidemiology, racialized biology, and biological expressions of race relations." *International Journal of Health Services* 30(1):211–16.

Kushner, H.I. (1991). *American suicide: A psychocultural exploration*. New Brunswick, NJ: Rutgers University Press.

Larsen, S.T., & Lynnerup, N. (2011). "Medico-legal autopsies in Denmark." *Danish Medical Bulletin* 58(3):1–4.

Lathrop, S.L., Wiest, P.W., & Andrews, S.W. (2023). "Can computed tomography replace or supplement autopsy?" *Journal of Forensic Sciences* 68(2):524–35.

Leung, P.T.M., Macdonald, E.M., Stanbrook, M.B., Dhalla, I.A., & Juurlink, D.N. (2017). "A 1980 letter on the risk of opioid addiction." *New England Journal of Medicine* 376(22): 2194–95.

Levine, R.S., Foster, J.E., Fullilove, R.E., Fullilove, M.T., Briggs, N.C., Hull, P.C., et al. (2001). "Black-white inequalities in mortality and life expectancy, 1933–1999: Implications for Healthy People 2010." *Public Health Reports* 116:474–83.

Lieberman, J.A. (2015). *Shrinks: The untold story of psychiatry*. New York: Little, Brown.

Lim, J.S., Buckley, N.A., Cairns, R., Schumann, J., & Chitty, K.M. (2023). "Substances detected during coroner postmortem toxicology analyses in poisoning- and non-poisoning-related suicides." *JAMA Psychiatry* 80(11):1121–30.

Litman, R.E. (1968). "Psychological-psychiatric aspects in certifying modes of death." *Journal of Forensic Sciences* 13(1):46–54.

Litman, R.E. (1989). "500 psychological autopsies." *Journal of Forensic Sciences* 34(3):638–46.

Litman, R.E., Curphey, T., Shneidman, E.S., Farberow, N.L., & Tobachnick, N. (1963). "Investigations of equivocal suicides." *Journal of the American Medical Association* 184:924–29.

Logan, J.E., Karch, D.L., & Crosby, A.E. (2009). "Reducing 'unknown' data in violent death surveillance: A study of death certificates, coroner/medical examiner and police reports from the National Violent Death Reporting System, 2003–2004." *Homicide Studies* 13(4):385–97.

Loose, C. (2020). "Funeral homes, morgues grapple with surge in US Covid-19 deaths." *CNN Health*, December 15. https://www.cnn.com/2020/12/15/health/funeral-homes-morgues-covid-deaths-wellness-partner/index.html#:~:text=Funeral%20homes%2C%20morgues%20grapple%20with%20surge%20in%20US%20Covid%2D19%20deaths,-By%20Cindy%20Loose&text=Acela%20Truck%20Co.%20has%20already,to%20the%20Covid%2D19%20pandemic.&text=Funeral%20director%20Kevin%20Spitzer%20has,city%20of%20Aberdeen%2C%20South%20Dakota.

Lord Kelvin. (1889). "Lecture to the Institution of Civil Engineers." *Popular Lectures and Addresses* 1:73.

Love, D.K. (2023). *Edmond Halley: The many discoveries of the most curious Astronomer Royal.* Essex, CT: Prometheus Books.

Lu, X., & Lin, Z. (2021). "COVID-19, economic impact, mental health, and coping behaviors: A conceptual framework and future research directions." *Frontiers in Psychology* 12:759974.

Lunetta, P., Lounamaa, A., & Sihvonen, S. (2007). "Surveillance of injury-related deaths: Medicolegal autopsy rates and trends in Finland." *Injury Prevention* 13(4):282–84.

Machiavelli, N. (transl. R. Goodwin). (1532/1998). *The Prince* (2nd ed.). Chicago: University of Chicago Press.

MacKay, R. (2002). *Half the battle: Civilian morale in Britain during the Second World War.* Manchester: Manchester University Press.

Mansfield, D. (2003). "Study: ERs miss drug-abuse cases." *Knoxville News Sentinel*, June 7.

Massey, D. (1995). "The new immigration and ethnicity in the United States." *Population and Development Review* 21(3):631–52.

Matsubayashi, T., & Ueda, M. (2021). "Is suicide underreported? Evidence from Japan." *Social Psychiatry and Psychiatric Epidemiology* 57:1571–78.

McLean Hospital. (2018). "Researchers call for a unified approach to preventing suicides and other self-injury deaths." Mass General Brigham, August 27. https://www.mcleanhospital.org/news/researchers-call-unified-approach-preventing-suicides-and-other-self-injury-deaths.

McLean Hospital. (2019). "Investigating the full spectrum of suicide: New self-injury mortality study allows closer look at trends in suicide and drug overdose deaths." Mass General Brigham, October 12. https://www.mcleanhospital.org/news/investigating-full-spectrum-suicide.

Mercado, M.C., Stone, D.M., Kokubun, C.W., Trudeau, A.R.T., Gaylor, E., Holland, K.M., et al. (2021). "Inconsistencies in overdose suicide death investigation practice and potential remedies using technology: A Centers for Disease Control and Prevention consultation meeting summary." *Academic Forensic Pathology* 11(2):83–93.

Mergl, R., Koburger, N., Heinrichs, K., Székely, A., Tóth, M.D., Coyne, J., et al. (2015). "What are reasons for the large gender differences in the lethality of suicidal acts? An epidemiological analysis in four European countries." *PLOS One* 10(7):e0129062.

Mew, E.J., Padmanathan, P., Konradsen, F., Eddleston, M., Chang, S.-S., Phillips, M.R., et al. (2017). "The global burden of fatal self-poisoning with pesticides 2006–15: Systematic review." *Journal of Affective Disorders* 219:93–104.

Meyers, M.A. (2007). *Happy accidents: Serendipity in modern medical breakthroughs*. New York: Arcade.

Milam, A.J., Furr-Holden, D., Wang, L., & Simon, K.M. (2021). "Health data disparities in opioid-involved overdose deaths from 1999 to 2018 in the United States." *American Journal of Public Health* 111(9):1627–35.

Miller, T.R., Swedler, D.I., Lawrence, B.A., Ali, B., Rockett, I.R.H., Carlson, N.N., et al. (2020). "Incidence and lethality of suicidal overdoses by drug class." *JAMA Network Open* 3(3):e200607.

Mishara, B.L., & Weisstub, D.N. (2016). "The legal status of suicide: A global review." *International Journal of Law and Psychiatry* 44:54–74.

Mitchell, R.A., Jr., & Aronson, J.D. (2023). *Death in custody: How America ignores the truth and what we can do about it*. Baltimore: Johns Hopkins University Press.

Mohandie, K., Meloy, J.R., & Collins, P.I. (2009). "Suicide by cop among officer-involved shooting cases." *Journal of Forensic Sciences* 54(2):456–62.

Mohler, B., & Earls, F. (2001). "Trends in adolescent suicide: Misclassification bias?" *American Journal of Public Health* 90(1):150–53.

Moretti, M., Malhotra, A., Visonà, S.D., Finley, S.J., Osculati, A.M.M., & Javan, G.T. (2021). "The roles of medical examiners in the COVID-19 era: A comparison between the United States and Italy." *Forensic Science, Medicine and Pathology* 17:262–70.

Morgan, D. (2017). "Opioid drug death investigations." *Academic Forensic Pathology* 7(1): 50–59.

Morselli, H. (1882). *Suicide: An essay in comparative moral statistics*. New York: D. Appleton.

Moynihan, D.P. (1965). *The Negro family: The case for national action*. Washington, DC: US Department of Labor.

Muazzam, S., Swahn, M.H., Alamgir, H., & Nasrullah, M. (2012). "Differences in poisoning mortality in the United States, 2003–2007: Epidemiology of poisoning deaths classified as unintentional, suicide or homicide." *Western Journal of Emergency Medicine* 13(3):230–38.

Myrdal, G. (1969). *An American dilemma: The Negro problem and modern democracy*. New York: Harper & Row.

National Association of Medical Examiners. (n.d.). https://netforum.avectra.com/eweb/DynamicPage.aspx?Site=NAME&WebCode=OrgSearch.

National Center for Health Statistics. (2019). *A reference guide for completing the death certificate for drug toxicity deaths*. Hyattsville, MD: National Center for Health Statistics.

National Center for Health Statistics. (2023). *Physician's handbook on medical certification of death*. Hyattsville, MD: National Center for Health Statistics.

National Commission on Forensic Science, National Institute of Standards and Technology. (2015). *Accreditation of medicolegal death investigation offices*. January 30. https://

www.justice.gov/sites/default/files/ncfs/pages/attachments/2015/02/25/mdi_accreditation_final_as_amended_1_30_15.pdf.

Neuilly, M.A. (2022). "Sources of bias in death determination: A research note articulating the need to include systemic sources of biases along with cognitive ones as impacting mortality data." *Journal of Forensic Sciences* 67(5):2032–39.

Newsome, M. (2022). "Overdose of inequality." *Scientific American* 327(6):60–68.

Nguyen, A., Wang, J., Holland, K.M., Ehlman, D.C., Welder, L.E., Miller, K.D., et al. (2024). "Trends in drug overdose deaths by intent and drug categories, United States, 1999–2022." *American Journal of Public Health* 114(10):1081–85.

Niederkrotenthaler, T., Stack, S., Till, B., Sinyor, M., Pirkis, J., Garcia, ID., et al. (2019). "Association of increased youth suicides in the United States with the release of *13 Reasons Why*." *JAMA Psychiatry* 76(9):933–40.

Ninkov, A., Frank, J.R., & Maggio, L.A. (2022). "Bibliometrics: Methods for studying academic publishing." *Perspectives in Medical Education* 11(3):173–76.

Norton, A. (2018). "U.S. deaths from suicide, drugs surpass diabetes." *HealthDay News*, August 27.

Novak, S. (2022). "Suicides among Black people may be vastly undercounted." *Scientific American*, June 6. https://www.scientificamerican.com/article/suicides-among-black-people-may-be-vastly-undercounted/.

Obenson, K. (2013). "Suicide versus self-inflicted: Is it time to change manner of death classification?" *Forensic Science, Medicine and Pathology* 9:576–77.

O'Carroll, P.W. (1989). "A consideration of the validity and reliability of suicide mortality data." *Suicide and Life-Threatening Behavior* 19:1–16.

Office of Justice Programs and National Institute of Justice. (2019). *Report to Congress: Needs assessment of forensic laboratories and medical examiner/coroner offices*. US Department of Justice. NCJ 253626. Washington, DC: National Institute of Justice.

Ojima, T., Nakamura, Y., & Detels, R. (2004). "Comparative study about methods of suicide between Japan and the United States." *Journal of Epidemiology* 14:187–92.

Our World in Data. (n.d.). "Share of deaths registered with an ill-defined cause of death, 2021." https://ourworldindata.org/grapher/deaths-registered-with-an-ill-defined-cause-of-death.

Ovenstone, I.M.K. (1973). "Spectrum of suicidal behaviors in Edinburgh." *British Journal of Social and Preventive Medicine* 27:27–35.

Palmer, B.S., Bennewith, O., Simkin, S., Cooper, J., Hawton, K., Kapur, N., et al. (2015). "Factors influencing coroners' verdicts: An analysis of verdicts given in 12 coroners' districts to researcher-defined suicides in England in 2005." *Journal of Public Health (Oxford)* 37(1):157–65.

Paperny, A.M. (2019). *Hello I want to die please fix me: Depression in the first person*. New York: Experiment.

Pei, S., Yamana, T.K., Kandula, S., Galanti, M., & Shaman, J. (2021). "Burden and characteristics of COVID-19 in the United States during 2020." *Nature* 598(7880):338–41.

Pekevski, J. (2022). "Preparing for the likely rise in suicides due to COVID-19: A review of the literature." *Journal of Emergency Management* 20(9):79–90.

Pergolizzi, J., Breve, F., Magnusson, P., Nalamasu, R., LeQuang, J.A.K., & Varrassi, G.

(2021). "Suicide by opioid: Exploring the intentionality of the act." *Cureus* 13(9): e18084.

Pescosolido, B.A., & Mendelsohn, R. (1986). "Social causation or social construction of suicide? An investigation into the social organization of official rates." *American Sociological Review* 51(1):80–100.

Peterson, C., Luo, F., & Florence, C. (2021). "State-level economic costs of fatal injuries—United States, 2019." *MMWR Morbidity and Mortality Weekly Report* 70(48):1660–63.

Petticrew, M., & Roberts, H. (2006). *Systematic reviews in the social sciences: A practical guide*. Malden, MA: Blackwell.

Pew. (2018). *More imprisonment does not reduce state drug problems*. https://www.pewtrusts.org/en/research-and-analysis/issue-briefs/2018/03/more-imprisonment-does-not-reduce-state-drug-problems.

Phillips, D.P., & Ruth, T.E. (1993). "Adequacy of official suicide statistics for scientific research and public policy." *Suicide and Life-Threatening Behavior* 23:307–31.

Pirkis, J., Gunnell, D., Shin, S., Del Pozo-Banas, M., Arya, V., Aguila, P.A., et al. (2022). "Suicide numbers during the first 9–15 months of the COVID-19 pandemic compared with pre-existing trends: An interrupted time series analysis in 33 countries." *EClinicalMedicine* 51:101573.

Platt, S., Backett, S., & Kreitman, N. (1988). "Social construction or causal ascription: Distinguishing suicide from undetermined deaths." *Social Psychiatry and Psychiatric Epidemiology* 23(4):217–21.

Platzman Weinstock, C. (2018). "Drug-overdose suicides may be going undetected." *Reuters Health*, January 11. https://www.reuters.com/article/business/healthcare-pharmaceuticals/drug-overdose-suicides-may-be-going-undetected-idUSKBN1F0317/.

Pompili, M., Serafini, G., Innamorati, M., Montebovi, F., Palermo, M., Campi, S., et al. (2012). "Car accidents as a method of suicide: A comprehensive overview." *Forensic Science International* 223(1–3):1–9.

Popper, K. (2002). *The logic of scientific discovery* (2nd ed.). Abingdon-on-Thames: Routledge.

Porter, J., & Jick, H. (1980). "Addiction rare in patients treated with narcotics." *New England Journal of Medicine* 302(2):123.

Powder, J. (2023). "Just before it happened: Using psychological autopsies to prevent suicide." *Hopkins Bloomberg Public Health Magazine*, Fall/Winter, https://magazine.publichealth.jhu.edu/2023/looking-for-why.

Prior, L. (1985). "Making sense of mortality." *Sociology of Health and Illness* 7(2):167–90.

Pritchard, C., & Amanullah, S. (2007). "An analysis of suicide and undetermined deaths in 17 predominantly Islamic countries contrasted with the UK." *Psychological Medicine* 37(3):421–30.

Pritchard, C., & Hansen, L. (2015). "Examining undetermined and accidental deaths as source of 'under-reported suicide' by age and sex in twenty Western countries." *Community Mental Health Journal* 51(3):365–76.

Pritt, B.S., Hardin, N.J., Richmond, J.A., & Shapiro, S.L. (2005). "Death certification errors at an academic institution." *Archives of Pathology and Laboratory Medicine* 129(11):1476–79.

Purnell, T.S., Calhoun, E.A., Golden, S.H., Halladay, J.R., Krok-Schoen, J.L., Applehans, B.M., et al. (2016). "Achieving health equity: Closing the gaps in health care disparities, interventions, and research." *Health Affairs* 35(8):1410–15.

Quinney, R. (1965). "Suicide, homicide, and economic development." *Social Forces* 43(3): 41–46.

Quinones, S. (2015). *Dream land: The true tale of America's opiate epidemic.* New York: Bloomsbury Press.

Quinones, S. (2021). *The least of us: True tales of America and hope in the time of fentanyl and meth.* New York: Bloomsbury.

Quote Investigator. (2019). *Absence of evidence is not evidence of absence. Carl Sagan? Martin Rees? William Wright? William Housman? W. J. Sollas? Dugald Bell? Anonymous?* https://quoteinvestigator.com/2019/09/17/absence/#google_vignette.

Rahman, N., Mozur, R., McHugh, R.K., Rockett, I.R.H., Chow, C.M., & Vaughan, G. (2021). "Using natural language processing to improve suicide classification requires consideration of race." *Suicide and Life-Threatening Behavior* 52(4):782–91.

Randall, B. (1997). *Death investigation: The basics.* Tucson, AZ: Galen Press.

Rane, A., & Nadkarni, A. (2014). "Suicide in India: A systematic review." *Shanghai Archives of Psychiatry* 26(2):69–80.

Ray, W.A., Hall, K., & Meador, K.G. (2007). "Racial differences in antidepressant treatment preceding suicide in a Medicaid population." *Psychiatric Services* 58(10): 1317–23.

Reseland, S., Le Noury, J., Aldred, G., & Healy, D. (2008). "National suicide rates 1961–2003: Further analysis of Nordic data for suicide, autopsies and ill-defined death rates." *Psychotherapy and Psychosomatics* 77(2):78–82.

Riblet, N.B., Shiner, B., Watts, B.V., &. Britton, P. (2019). "Comparison of national and local approaches to detecting suicides in healthcare settings." *Military Medicine* 184(9–10):e555–60.

Riblet, N.B., Shiner, B., Young-Xu, Y., & Watts, B.V. (2022). "Lithium in the prevention of suicide in adults: Systematic review and meta-analysis of clinical trials." *British Journal of Psychiatry Open* 8:e199.

Rioux, C., Paré, A., London-Nadeau, K., Juster, R.P., Weedon, S., Levasseur-Puhach, S., et al. (2022). "Sex and gender terminology: A glossary for gender-inclusive epidemiology." *Journal of Epidemiology and Community Health* 76(8):764–68.

Ritchie, H. (2019). "Does the news reflect what we die from?" World Economic Forum, June 18. https://www.weforum.org/agenda/2019/06/does-the-news-reflect-what-we-die-from/.

Roberts, A.-O., & Richards, G.C. (2023). "Is England facing an opioid epidemic?" *British Journal of Pain* 17(3):320–324.

Robins, L.N., & Kulbok, P.A. (1986). "Methodological strategies in suicide." *Annals of the New York Academy of Sciences* 487:1–15.

Robinson, R. (2017). "County coroners and their role in the heart of the opioid epidemic." *Academic Forensic Pathology* 7(4):667–704.

Rockett, H. (1933). "A case of haemolytic streptococcal meningitis, with recovery." *British Journal of Childhood Diseases* 30:196–99.

Rockett, I.R.H. (1998a). "Injury and violence: A public health perspective." *Population Bulletin* 53(4):1–40.

Rockett, I.R.H. (1998b). "Injury elimination and survival: A cross-national study." *Public Health* 112:27–30.

Rockett, I.R.H. (1999). "Population and health: An introduction to epidemiology" (2nd ed.). *Population Bulletin* 54(4):1–44.

Rockett, I.R.H. (2010). "Counting suicides and making suicide count as a public health problem." *Crisis* 31(5):227–30.

Rockett, I.R.H. (2017). "The gender suicide gap and differential misclassification: A research autobiography." *International Review of Modern Sociology* 43(1):5–32.

Rockett, I.R.H., Ali, B., Caine, E.D., Shepard, D.S., Banerjee, A., Nolte, K.B., et al. (2023). "Escalating costs of self-injury mortality in the 21st century United States: An interstate observational study." *BMC Public Health* 23(1):285.

Rockett, I.R.H., & Caine, E.D. (2015a). "Not so new." *BMJ*. http://www.bmj.com/content/351/bmj.h6180/rapid-responses.

Rockett, I.R.H., & Caine, E.D. (2015b). "Self-injury is the eighth leading cause of death in the United States: It is time to pay attention." *JAMA Psychiatry* 72(11):1069–70.

Rockett, I.R.H., & Caine, E.D. (2020). "Reconciling suicides with 'accidental' drug-intoxication deaths: A behaviorally based definition of self-injury mortality." *American Journal of Public Health* 110(1):73–74.

Rockett, I.R.H., Caine, E.D., Banerjee, A., Ali, B., Miller, T., Connery, H.S., et al. (2021). "Fatal self-injury in the United States, 1999–2018: Unmasking a national mental health crisis." *EClinicalMedicine* 32:100741.

Rockett, I.R.H., Caine, E.D., Connery, H.S., D'Onofrio, G., Gunnell, D.J., Miller, T.R., et al. (2018a). "Discerning suicide in drug intoxication deaths: Paucity and primacy of suicide notes and psychiatric history." *PLOS One* 13(1):e0190200.

Rockett, I.R.H., Caine, E.D., Connery, H.S., & Greenfield, S.F. (2019). "Mortality in the United States from self-injury surpasses diabetes: A prevention imperative." *Injury Prevention* 25(4):331–33

Rockett, I.R.H., Caine, E.D., Connery, H.S., & Nolte, K.B. (2020a) "Overcoming the limitations of 'accident' as a manner of death for drug overdose mortality: Case for a death certificate checkbox." *Injury Prevention* 27(4):375–78.

Rockett, I.R.H., Caine, E.D., Connery, H.S., Nolte, K.B., Nestadt, P.S., Nelson, L.S., et al. (2020b). "Unrecognised self-injury mortality (SIM) trends among racial/ethnic minorities and women in the USA." *Injury Prevention* 26(5):439447.

Rockett, I.R.H, Caine, E.D., Stack, S., Connery, H.S, Nolte, K.B., Lilly, C.L., et al. (2018b). "Method overtness, forensic autopsy, and the evidentiary suicide note: A multilevel National Violent Death Reporting System analysis." *PLOS One* 13(5):e0197805.

Rockett, I.R.H., Hobbs, G.R., De Leo, D., Stack, S., Frost, J.L., Ducatman, A.M., et al. (2010a). "Suicide and unintentional poisoning mortality trends in the United States, 1987–2006: Two unrelated phenomena?" *BMC Public Health* 10:705.

Rockett, I.R.H, Hobbs, G.R., Wu, D., Jia, H., Nolte, K.B., Smith, G.S., et al. (2015). "Variable classification of drug-intoxication suicides across US states: A partial artifact of forensics?" *PLOS One* 10(8):e0135296.

Rockett, I.R.H., Jia, H., Ali, B., Banerjee, A., Connery, H.S., Nolte, K.B., et al. (2022). "Association of state social and environmental factors with rates of self-injury mortality and suicide in the United States." *JAMA Network Open* 15(2):e2146591.

Rockett, I.R.H., & Kapusta, N.D. (2015). "Measuring suicide." In *An invitation to social research: How it's done*, E. Stier Adler, R.D. Clark (eds.), 141–46. Stamford, CT: Cengage Learning.

Rockett, I.R.H., Kapusta, N.D., & Bhandari, R. (2011). "Suicide misclassification in an international context: Revisitation and update." *Suicidology Online* 2:48–61.

Rockett, I.R.H., Kapusta, N.D., & Coben, J.H. (2014a). "Beyond suicide: Action needed to improve self-injury mortality accounting." *JAMA Psychiatry* 71(3):231–32.

Rockett, I.R.H., Lian, Y., Stack, S., Ducatman, A.M., & Wang, S. (2009). "Discrepant comorbidity between minority and white suicides: A national multiple cause-of-death analysis." *BMC Psychiatry* 9.

Rockett, I.R.H., Lilly, C.L., Jia, H., Larkin, G.L., Miller, T.R., Nelson, L.S., et al. (2016). "Self-injury mortality in the United States in the early 21st century: A comparison with proximally ranked diseases." *JAMA Psychiatry* 73(10):1072–81.

Rockett, I.R.H., Putnam, S.L., Jia, H., Chang, C., & Smith, G.S. (2005). "Unmet substance abuse treatment need, health services utilization, and cost: A population-based emergency department study." *Annals of Emergency Medicine* 45(2):118–27.

Rockett, I.R.H., Putnam, S.L., Jia, H., & Smith, G.S. (2003). "Assessing substance abuse treatment need: A statewide hospital emergency department study." *Annals of Emergency Medicine* 41(6):802–13.

Rockett, I.R.H., Putnam, S.L., Jia, H., & Smith, G.S. (2006a). "Declared and undeclared substance use among emergency department patients: A population-based study." *Addiction* 101(5):706–12.

Rockett, I.R.H., Regier, M.D., Kapusta, N.D., Coben, J.H., Miller, T.R., Hanzlick, R.L., et al. (2012). "Leading causes of unintentional and intentional injury mortality: United States, 2000–2009." *American Journal of Public Health* 102(11):e84–92.

Rockett, I.R.H., Samora, J.B., & Coben, J.H. (2006b). "The black-white suicide paradox: Possible effects of misclassification." *Social Science and Medicine* 63(8):2165–75.

Rockett, I.R.H., & Smith, G.S. (1987). "Injuries in relation to chronic disease: An international view of premature mortality." *American Journal of Public Health* 77(10): 1345–46.

Rockett, I.R.H., & Smith, G.S. (1989). "Homicide, suicide, motor vehicle crash and fall mortality: United States' experience in comparative perspective." *American Journal of Public Health* 79(10):1396–400.

Rockett, I.R.H., & Smith, G.S. (1993). "Covert suicide among elderly Japanese females: Questioning unintentional drownings." *Social Science and Medicine* 36(11):1467–72.

Rockett, I.R.H., & Smith, G.S. (1995). "Suicide misclassification in an international context." In *Proceedings of the International Collaborative Effort on Injury Statistics*, 26-1–26-18. Hyattsville, MD: US Department of Health and Human Services.

Rockett, I.R.H., Smith, G.S, Caine, E.D., Kapusta, N.D., Hanzlick, R.L., Larkin, G.L., et al. (2014b). "Confronting death from drug self-intoxication (DDSI): Prevention through a better definition." *American Journal of Public Health* 104(12):e49–55.

Rockett, I.R.H., & Thomas, B.M. (1999). "Reliability and sensitivity of suicide certification in higher income countries." *Suicide and Life-Threatening Behavior* 29(2): 141–49.

Rockett, I.R.H., Wang, S., Lian, Y., &. Stack, S. (2007). "Suicide-associated comorbidity among US males and females: A multiple cause-of-death analysis." *Injury Prevention* 13(5):311–15.

Rockett, I.R.H., Wang, S., Stack, S., De Leo, D., Frost, J.L., Ducatman, A.M., et al. (2010b). "Race/ethnicity and potential suicide misclassification: Window on a minority suicide paradox." *BMC Psychiatry* 10:35.

Rosenberg, M.L., Davidson, L.E., Smith, J.C., Berman, A.L., Buzbee, H., Gantner, G., et al. (1988). "Operational criteria for the determination of suicide." *Journal of Forensic Sciences* 33(6):1445–46.

Rosenberg, M.L., & Fenley, M.A. (eds.). (1991). *Violence in America: A public health approach*. New York: Oxford University Press.

Ross, O., & Kreitman, N. (1975). "A further investigation of differences in the suicide rates of England and Wales and of Scotland." *British Journal of Psychiatry* 127:575–82.

Ross, V., & Kõlves, K. (2021). "Mixed methods in suicide research." In *Advancing suicide research*, K. Kõlves, M. Sisask, P. Värnik, A. Värnik, D. De Leo (eds.), 151–59. Göttingen: Hogrefe.

Routley, V., Staines, C., Brennan, C., Haworth, N., & Ozanne-Smith, J. (2003). *Suicide and natural deaths in road traffic—review*. Clayton: Monash University Accident Research Center.

Rubin, E., & Zorumski, C. (2017). "Self-injury mortality: A deadly crisis." *Psychology Today*, February 20. https://www.psychologytoday.com/us/blog/demystifying-psychiatry/201702/self-injury-mortality-deadly-crisis.

Ruiz, L., Posey, B.M., Neuilly, M.A., Stohr, M.K., & Hemmens, C. (2018). "Certifying death in the United States." *Journal of Forensic Sciences* 63(4):1138–45.

Ruzicka, L.T., Choi, C.Y., & Sadkowsky, K. (2005). "Medical disorders of suicides in Australia: Analysis using a multiple cause-of-death approach." *Social Science and Medicine* 61(2):333–41.

Sainsbury, P., & Jenkins, J.S. (1982). "The accuracy of officially reported suicide statistics for purposes of epidemiological research." *Journal of Epidemiology and Community Health* 36:43–48.

Salib, M. (1996). "Predictors of coroner's verdict: A logistic regression model." *Medicine, Science and the Law* 36(3):237–41.

Savitz, D. (2023). "Epidemiology and the law: Reflections on serving as an expert witness." *EpiMonitor*. https://www.epimonitor.net/Epidemiology-and-the-Law.htm.

Schneider, K.E., Martin, E.M., Allen, S.T., Morris, M., Honey, K., Saloner, B., et al. (2024). "Volatile drug use and overdose during the first year of the COVID-19 pandemic in the United States." *International Journal of Drug Policy* 126:104371.

Senate Community Affairs Committee Secretariat. (2010). *The hidden toll: Suicide in Australia*. Canberra: Senate Printing Unit.

Shah, A. (2008). "A cross-national study of the relationship between elderly suicide rates and urbanization." *Suicide and Life-Threatening Behavior* 38(6):714–19.

Shi, L., & Stevens, G.D. (2021). *Vulnerable populations in the United States* (3rd ed.). Hoboken, NJ: John Wiley & Sons.

Shneidman, E.S. (1969). "Suicide, lethality, and the psychological autopsy." *International Journal of Psychiatry in Clinical Practice* 6(2):225–50.

Shojania, K.G., Burton, E.C., McDonald, K.M., & Goldman, L. (2003). "Changes in rates of autopsy-detected diagnostic errors over time: A systematic review." *Journal of the American Medical Association* 289(21):2849–56.

Siegel, M., & Rothman, E.F. (2016). "Firearm ownership and suicide rates among US men and women, 1981–2013." *American Journal of Public Health* 106(7):1316–22.

Sinclair, U. (1935). *I, candidate for governor, and how I got licked*. New York: Farrar & Rinehart.

Skegg, K. (2005). "Self-harm." *Lancet* 366(9495):1471–83.

Skinner, R., McFaull, S., Rhodes, A.E., Bowes, M., & Rockett, I.R.H. (2016). "Suicide in Canada: Is poisoning misclassification an issue?" *Canadian Journal of Psychiatry* 61(7):405–12.

Sloboda, Z. (2005). *Epidemiology of drug abuse*. New York: Springer.

Snowdon, J. (2023). "Hidden suicides: Their misclassification as accidental, 'undetermined' or unknown cause deaths." *Journal of Suicidology* 18(2):529–39.

Snowdon, J., & Choi, N. (2022). "Unanticipated changes in drug overdose death rates in Canada during the opioid crisis." *International Journal of Mental Health and Addiction* 22:1394–412.

Snowdon, J., & Choi, N.G. (2020). "Undercounting of suicides: Where suicide data lie hidden." *Global Public Health* 15(12):1894–901.

Sorenson, S.B., Shen, H., & Kraus, J.F. (1997). "Undetermined manner of death: A comparison with unintentional injury, suicide, and homicide death." *Evaluation Review* 21(1):43–57.

Speechley, M., & Stavraky, K.M. (1991). "The adequacy of suicide statistics for use in epidemiology and public health." *Canadian Journal of Public Health* 82:38–42.

Spiegelhalter, D. (2019). *The art of statistics: How to learn from data*. New York: Basic Books.

Sprott, S.E. (1961). *The English debate on suicide from Donne to Hume*. La Salle, IL: Open Court.

Stack, S. (1983). "The effect of religious commitment on suicide: A cross-national analysis." *Journal of Health and Social Behavior* 24:362–74.

Stack, S., & Rockett, I.R.H. (2018). "Are suicide note writers representative of all suicides? Analysis of the National Violent Death Reporting System." *Suicide and Life-Threatening Behavior* 48(1):12–20.

Stafford, K., Morrison, A., & Ma, A. (2023). "Medical racism in history causes health inequalities for Black Americans." *US News & World Report*, May 23. https://projects.apnews.com/features/2023/from-birth-to-death/medical-racism-in-history.html.

Stanistreet, D., Taylor, S., Jeffrey, V., & Gabbay, M. (2001). "Accident or suicide? Predictors of coroners' decisions in suicide and accident verdicts." *Medicine, Science and the Law* 41(2):111–15.

Stier Adler, E., & Clark, R.D. (2015). *An invitation to social research: How it's done* (5th ed.). Stamford, CT: Cengage Learning.

Stoecker, W.V., Smith, C.L., & Connors, E. (2023). "Part II Missouri's fentanyl poisonings rise to record levels." *Missouri Medicine* 120(1):10–14.

Stone, D.M., Holland, K.M., Bartholow, B., Logan, J.E., McIntosh, W.L., Trudeau, A., et al. (2017). "Deciphering suicide and other manners of death associated with drug intoxication: A Centers for Disease Control and Prevention consultation meeting summary." *American Journal of Public Health* 107(8):1233–39.

Stone, D.M., Holland, K.M., Schiff, L.B., & McIntosh, W.L. (2016). "Mixed methods analysis of sex differences in life stressors of middle-aged suicides." *American Journal of Preventive Medicine* 51(5 suppl. 3):S209–18.

Szalavitz, M. (2016). "How many drug overdoses are actually suicides?" *VICE*, February 29. https://www.vice.com/en/article/how-many-drug-overdoses-are-actually-suicides/.

Tait, G., Carpenter, B., & Jowett, S. (2018). "Coronial practice, indigeneity and suicide." *International Journal of Environmental Research and Public Health* 15(4):765.

Taleb, N.N. (2010). *The black swan: The impact of the highly improbable* (2nd ed.). New York: Random House.

Taylor, S. (1982). *Durkheim and the study of suicide: Contemporary social theory*. London: Palgrave.

Temple, J. (2016). *American pain: How a young felon and his ring of doctors unleashed America's deadliest drug epidemic*. Guilford, CT: Lyons Press.

Thomas, J. (2009). "Death certificates incomplete for suicide victims." *HealthDay News*, April 17. https://www.healthday.com/health-news/general-health/death-certificates-incomplete-for-suicide-victims-626114.html.

Throssell, R. (1989). *My father's son*. Melbourne: William Heinemann Australia.

Timmermans, S. (2005). "Suicide determination and the professional authority of medical examiners." *American Sociological Review* 70(2):311–33.

Tøllefsen, I.M., Hem, E., & Ekeberg, O. (2012). "The reliability of suicide statistics: A systematic review." *BMC Psychiatry* 12:9.

Too, L.S., Spittal, M.J., Bugeja, L., Reifels, L., & Butterworth, P. (2019). "The association between mental disorders and suicide: A systematic review and meta-analysis of record linkage studies." *Journal of Affective Disorders* 259:302–13.

Torrey, E.F. (2014). *American psychosis: How the federal government destroyed the mental illness treatment system*. New York: Oxford University Press.

Tsai, A.C., Kiang, M.V., Barnett, M.L., Beletsky, L., Keyes, K.M., McGinty, E.E., et al. (2019). "Stigma as a fundamental hindrance to the United States opioid overdose crisis response." *PLOS Medicine* 16(11):e1002969.

Tufte, E.R. (1997). *Visual explanations: Image and quantities, evidence and narrative*. Cheshire, CT: Graphics Press.

Tufte, E.R. (2006). *Beautiful evidence*. Cheshire, CT: Graphics Press.

Ubelaker, D.H. (ed.). (2015). *The global practice of forensic science*. Singapore: Wiley Blackwell.

UCLA Advanced Research Computing. (n.d.). *Introduction to generalized linear mixed models*. https://stats.oarc.ucla.edu/other/mult-pkg/introduction-to-generalized-linear-mixed-models/.

US Drug Enforcement Administration. (2023). "DEA reports widespread threat of fentanyl mixed with xylazine." *Public Safety Alert*, December 10. https://www.dea.gov/alert/dea-reports-widespread-threat-fentanyl-mixed-xylazine.

US Public Health Service. (2001). *National strategy for suicide prevention: Goals and objectives for action*. Washington, DC: Department of Health and Human Services.

Utsey, S.O., Hook, J.N., & Stanard, P. (2007). "A re-examination of cultural factors that mitigate risk and promote resilience in relation to African American suicide: A review of the literature and recommendations for future research." *Death Studies* 31(5):399–416.

Vanatta, P.R., & Petty, C.S. (1987). "Limitations of the forensic external examination in determining the cause and manner of death." *Human Pathology* 18(2):170–74.

Värnik, P., Sisask, M., Värnik, A., Arensman, E., Van Audenhove, C., van der Feltz-Cornelis, C.M., et al. (2012). "Validity of suicide statistics in Europe in relation to undetermined deaths: Developing the 2–20 benchmark." *Injury Prevention* 18(5):321–5.

Vasudevan, A.K., Hanumantha, & Eccleston, L. (2020). "Psychological autopsy: The psychological assessment of the dead individual's role in the death." *Medico-Legal Update* 20(3):13–18.

Visentin, S., Massaro, L., Viel, G., Cecchetto, G., & Montisci, M. (2019). "Suicide identification during on-site inspection: Proposal and application of an interpretative method for death scene investigation." *Forensic Science International* 297:148–55.

Waldhoer, T., Berzlanovich, A., Vutuc, C., & Haidinger, G. (2003). "Rates of postmortem examination in Austria: The effect of distance between location of death and site of examination." *Journal of Clinical Epidemiology* 56(9):891–95.

Wall, M.M., Huang, J., Oswald, J., & McCullen, D. (2005). "Factors associated with reporting multiple causes of death." *BMC Medical Research Methodology* 5:4–17.

Ward, H., Toledano, M.B., Shaddick, G., Davies, B., & Elliott, P. (2012). *Oxford handbook of epidemiology for clinicians*. Oxford: Oxford University Press.

Warner, M., Chen, L.H., & Makuc, D.M. (2009). "Increase in fatal poisonings involving opioid analgesics in the United States, 1999–2006." *NCHS Data Brief* 22:1–8.

Warner, M., Paulozzi, L.J., Nolte, K.B., Davis, G.G., & Nelson, L.S. (2013). "State variation in certifying manner of death and drugs involved in drug intoxication deaths." *Academic Forensic Pathology* 3(2):231–37.

Warshauer, M.E., & Monk, M. (1978). "Problems in suicide statistics for whites and blacks." *American Journal of Public Health* 68:383–88.

Watanabe, M., & Tanaka, H. (2022). "Increased suicide mortality in Japan during the COVID-19 pandemic in 2020." *Psychiatry Research* 309:114422.

Weinberger, L.E., Botello, T.E., & Gross, B.H. (2018). "Psychological autopsy: Consultative tool for suicide determination." In *Multidisciplinary medico-legal death investigation: Role of consultants*, L. Sathyavagiswaran, C.B. Rogers (eds.), 119–37. London: Academic Press.

Weinstock, L.R. (2021). *COVID-19 and the U.S. economy*. https://sgp.fas.org/crs/misc/R46606.pdf.

Wekstein, L. (1979). *Handbook of suicidology: Principles, problems, and practice*. New York: Brunner/Mazel.

West Virginia University. (2021). "Death by suicide? Drug overdoses muddy waters for investigators, amplify mental health crisis." *WVUToday*, February 8. https://wvutoday.wvu.edu/stories/2021/02/08/death-by-suicide-drug-overdoses-muddy-waters-for-investigators-amplify-national-mental-health-crisis.

West Virginia University. (2022). "WVU researcher examines interstate characteristics associated with self-injury mortality." *WVUToday*, February 9. https://wvutoday.wvu.edu/stories/2022/02/09/wvu-researcher-examines-interstate-characteristics-associated-with-self-injury-mortality.

Westhoff, B. (2019). *Fentanyl, Inc.: How rogue chemists are creating the deadliest wave of the opioid epidemic.* New York: Atlantic Monthly Press.

Whitaker, R. (2010). *Anatomy of an epidemic: Magic bullets, psychiatric drugs, and the astonishing rise of mental illness in America.* New York: Crown.

White, T. (2022). "Costs more than triple for outside docs to perform RI autopsies." *Live Now*, December 12. https://www.wpri.com/target-12/costs-more-than-triple-for-outside-docs-to-perform-ri-autopsies/.

Whitlock, A. (1971). "Migration and suicide." *Medical Journal of Australia* 2:840–48.

Whitt, H.P. (2006). "Where did the bodies go? The social construction of suicide data, New York City, 1976–1992." *Sociological Inquiry* 76(2):166–87.

Wilcox, H.C., Connor, K.R., & Caine, E.D. (2004). "Association of alcohol and drug use disorders and completed suicide: An empirical review of cohort studies." *Drug and Alcohol Dependence* 76(suppl.):S11–19.

Wilson, K.D. (1992). *Cause of death: A writer's guide to death, murder and forensic medicine.* Cincinnati: Writer's Digest Books.

Winker, M.A. (2008). "Measuring race and ethnicity: Why and how?" *JAMA* 292:1612–18.

World Health Organization. (2004). *International classification of diseases, tenth revision (ICD-10).* Geneva: World Health Organization.

World Health Organization. (2019). *Suicide and self-harm.* Geneva: World Health Organization.

World Health Organization. (n.d.). *WHO ICD-11 mortality tooling.*

Xiang, Y., Zhou, W., Xiang, H., & Smith, G.A. (2012). "ED visits for drug-related poisoning in the United States, 2007." *American Journal of Emergency Medicine* 30(2):293–301.

Yip, P., Pitt, D., Wang, Y., Wu, X., Watson, R., Huggins, R., et al. (2010). "Assessing the impact of suicide exclusion periods on life insurance." *Crisis* 31(4):217–23.

Ylijoki-Sørensen, S., Sajantila, A., Lalu, K., Bøggild, H., Boldsen, J.L., & Boel, L.W. (2014). "Coding ill-defined and unknown cause of death is 13 times more frequent in Denmark than in Finland." *Forensic Sciences International* 244:289–94.

Yuan, K., & Fayyad, A. (2018). "Should we tell fewer stories about suicide or better ones?" *Atlantic*, June 11. https://www.theatlantic.com/membership/archive/2018/06/should-we-tell-fewer-stories-about-suicide-or-better-ones/562577/.

Zhang, S. (2017). "The one-paragraph letter from 1980 that fueled the opioid crisis." *Atlantic*, June 2. https://www.theatlantic.com/health/archive/2017/06/nejm-letter-opioids/528840/.

Zilboorg, G. (1936). "Suicide among civilized and primitive races." *American Journal of Psychiatry* 92:1347–69.

Index

www.ingramcontent.com/pod-product-compliance
Ingram Content Group UK Ltd.
Pitfield, Milton Keynes, MK11 3LW, UK
UKHW041051201225
466270UK00003B/3/J

9 781421 453644